OCULAR IMMUNOLOGY

Second Edition

OCULAR IMMUNOLOGY

Gilbert Smolin, M.D.
Clinical Professor of Ophthalmology, University of California, San Francisco, School of Medicine; Research Ophthalmologist, Francis I. Proctor Foundation for Research in Ophthalmology, San Francisco

G. Richard O'Connor, M.D.
Professor of Ophthalmology, Emeritus, University of California, San Francisco, School of Medicine; Former Director, Francis I. Proctor Foundation for Research in Ophthalmology, San Francisco

Little, Brown and Company
Boston/Toronto

Copyright © 1986 by Gilbert Smolin and
G. Richard O'Connor

Second Edition

Previous edition copyright © 1981 by Lea & Febiger

All rights reserved. No part of this book may be reproduced in any form or by any electronic or mechanical means, including information storage and retrieval systems, without permission in writing from the publisher, except by a reviewer who may quote brief passages in a review.

Library of Congress Catalog Card No. 85-82482

ISBN 0-316-80188-7

Printed in the United States of America

MV

*To my loving and supportive parents,
family, and friends*

G. S.

CONTENTS

Preface *ix*

1. Introduction to Immunology *1*

2. Immunologic Testing Procedures *103*

3. Atopic Diseases Affecting the Eye *135*

4. Immunologic Reactions Limited to the External Eye *193*

5. Systemic Immunologic Diseases Affecting the External Eye *255*

6. Corneal Graft Reaction *273*

7. Immunologic Diseases Affecting the Uveal Tract and Retina *307*

Index *347*

PREFACE

In this second edition of *Ocular Immunology* we hope to present a broader yet more detailed view of the immunologic background for various inflammatory diseases of the eye. The eye is often thought of as a special target of immunologic disease processes. In reality, it may be no more the subject of immunologic attack than other organs of the body. But while other organs may remain "silent" under conditions of attack, the inflamed eye generally makes itself visibly, and sometimes painfully, obvious. The rather labile vessels of the conjunctiva, embedded as they are in a nearly transparent medium, may dilate rapidly, giving the eye a "bloodshot" appearance; and chemosis, the gross accumulation of edema fluid in the conjunctiva, may actually cause the conjunctiva to prolapse between the lids. The normally transparent media of the eye, when affected by inflammatory processes of immunologic origin, become partially opaque, rendering the transmission of images to the retina imperfect. Even when images are clearly transmitted and visual acuity remains good, products of inflammation in the form of vitreous floaters may cast disturbing shadows on the retina, making the patient aware that something is wrong.

The heterogeneous structure of the three-layered eyeball with its tough, collagenous sclera, its highly vascular uvea, and its exquisitely sensitive retina may account, to some degree, for the special qualifications of the eye as a target organ. Thus rheumatic diseases, primarily directed against collagen, find the sclera and the peripheral cornea ideal as target tissues. The choroid, with its fine network of vessels in the choriocapillaris, may act as a trap for immune complexes in much the same way as the renal glomerulus or the choroid plexus of the brain. Finally, the retina, basically an outpocketing of the primitive brain, appears to be subject to the same kinds of autoimmune insults as the brain itself, manifesting perivascular inflammatory reactions in the case of such diseases as multiple sclerosis and Behçet's disease.

In the interval between the publication of the first edition of *Ocular Immunology* in 1981 and the present, a great deal of new information has been accumulated. The number of journals dealing with the general subject of immunology has more than doubled. Technological advances such as the development of monoclonal antibodies, the use of automated cell sorters for the determination of subtypes of lymphocytes, and the perfection of sophisticated chromatographic techniques have revolutionized our ideas about the nature and sequence of immunologic events, particularly in the target tissues. The reader of the second edition will profit from these innovations. They have substantially changed the material of Chapter 1, a general introduction to the subject of immunology, that summarizes the important discoveries in immunology, making this new knowledge, as well as the vocabulary applicable to it, available to ophthalmologists who may not have had the time or the inclination to keep up with advances in this field.

Certain new diseases such as the acquired immune deficiency syndrome (AIDS) have been covered in the second edition; and others, such as sympathetic ophthalmia and lens-induced uveitis, have been described in much greater detail than in the first edition. In every case the authors have tried to incorporate pertinent new source material into the body of each chapter, retaining certain old references for historical purposes only. Such older references are generally "classical" articles.

For residents in training, *Ocular Immunology* may serve as a stimulus to enter one of the many investigative fields that are now open to ophthalmologists interested in solving immunologic disease problems. Such unsolved disease problems are still legion. The failure of corticosteroid therapy to eliminate these problems, on the one hand, and the multiple complications of indiscriminate therapy on the other, are reasons enough to push for further investigations in a field where the difficulties continue to baffle the physician, in general, and the ophthalmologist in particular.

We thank Nancy A. Thomas for typing the manuscript.

G. S.
G. R. O'C.

OCULAR IMMUNOLOGY

1 INTRODUCTION TO IMMUNOLOGY

At the heart of any discussion of immunology lie cell memory, cell specificity, and the recognition of nonself. These three mechanisms are used by the host to survive in a threatening world. The ability to mount specific immune responses to potentially harmful agents is not confined to human beings; such responses have been found in many of the lower vertebrates as well. Even invertebrates possess phagocytic cells and can probably mount some kind of still-undefined immune response.

A discussion of general immunologic principles is presented prior to the discussion of ocular immunology.

IMMUNOLOGIC PRINCIPLES

Phylogenic Considerations

In vertebrates, Good and co-workers [1–5] found an association between functional immune reactivity and the morphologic maturation of the lymphoid tissues. They found that the sea lamprey displays a weak immune response to antigenic stimuli, serum gamma globulin, allograft rejection, and delayed allergic reactions [3]; that its primitive thymus consists of a few lymphocytes in the gills; and that no plasma cells develop. In the guitarfish they found an independent thymus, a definitive spleen, and circulating lymphoid cells [1]. This animal, moreover, can mount a vigorous antibody response to several antigens, develop delayed hypersensitivity lesions, and show immunologic memory (Fig. 1-1).

Farther up the phylogenetic scale the paddlefish has a well-developed thymus containing lobules, lobes, thymocytes, and Hassall's corpuscles. The paddlefish also has peripheral blood lymphocytes and a more developed spleen. In amphibians, plasma cells were found in the lamina propria of the intestine, and evidence was adduced that they might be the source of immunoglobulin type A (IgA). In addition to a thymus, the chicken has an outpouching of the avian intestinal tract [4]. This outpouching is known as the bursa of Fabricius, and it can produce anti-

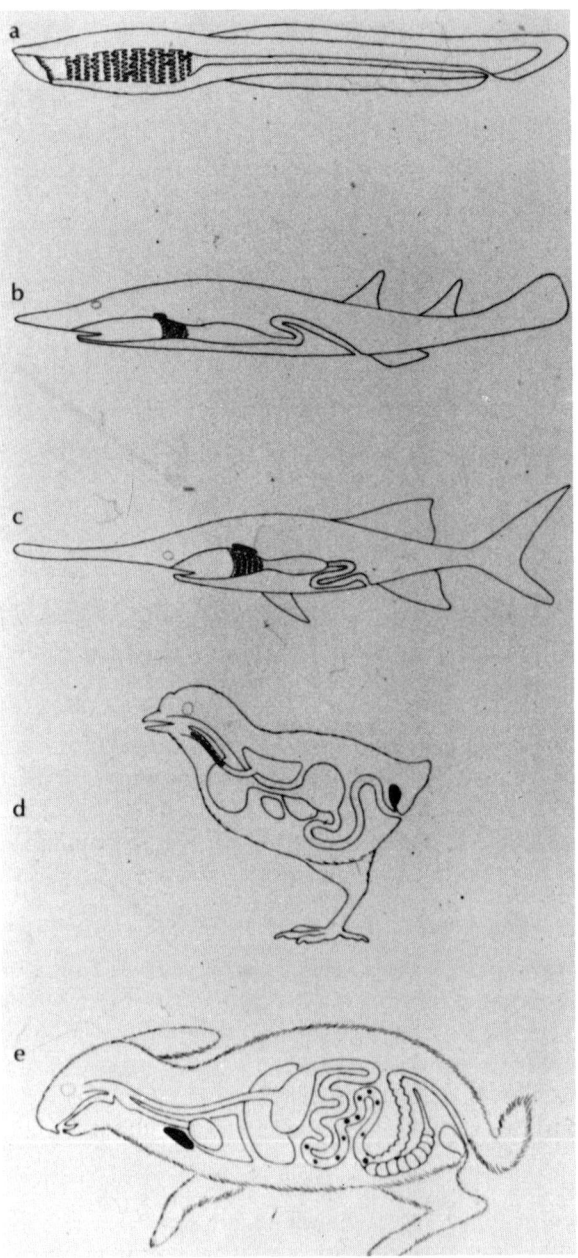

FIG. 1-1 Phylogenic considerations of the immune system: (a) Lamprey: a few lymphocytes in gills. (b,c) Guitarfish and paddlefish: independent thymus. (d) Chicken thymus and bursa of Fabricius for B cell production. (e) Rabbit Peyer's patches and thymus. (Modified from R. A. Good and D. W. Fisher (Eds.), *Immunobiology*. Stamford, Conn.: Sinauer Associates, 1971. Reproduced with permission.)

body. The chicken's thymus and bursa maintain two different cell populations, each with its own immunologic activity [5]. The thymus-dependent system is responsible for cell-mediated immunity (CMI), and the bursa-dependent system is responsible for plasma-cell-antibody immunity.

In the rabbit, Peyer's patches, which are histologically almost identical to the bursa, are present in the intestine. In fact, Peyer's patches and the tonsils are believed to be the mammalian counterparts of the bursa. The immune system of human beings consists of thymus-dependent lymphocytes, or T-lymphocytes, and thymus-independent lymphocytes (bursa-dependent), or B-lymphocytes. B-lymphocytes may be produced in the bone marrow.

The Immune Reaction

ANTIGENS. Both antigens and immunogens are substances that evoke immune responses when introduced into an organism. An antigen can combine only with an antibody and in that respect differs from an immunogen. The immune response may take one or more of the following forms: antibody production, cell-mediated immunity, or immunologic tolerance. The vast majority of antigens are proteins, but polysaccharides with molecular weights of 100,000 or more may also be antigenic. Lipids are never antigenic. The molecular weight of an antigenic protein may be as little as 1080 (dinitrophenylhepta-L-lysine is immunogenic in guinea pigs [6]) but is usually much greater.

The antigenicity of the protein tends to increase with increased molecular weight, probably owing to the greater number of variations in the composition and configuration of the component amino acids.

Because antibodies are stereospecific, the optical configuration of the antigen is important in determining its immunogenicity. The L-amino acid polymers seem to be more antigenic than the D isomers, perhaps owing to the slow and incomplete catabolism of the D-amino acid polymers [6]. Spatial folding of the proteins also plays a role in their antigenicity. Although an electrical charge on a macromolecule is not necessary for it to be immunogenic, the electrically charged side or end chains do play a role.

An antigen can be mixed with substances (adjuvants) that augment the immune response. Bacteria or their products can behave as adjuvants. Complete Freund's adjuvant (CFA) which consists of dead tubercle bacilli suspended in a water-in-oil emulsion, is one of the most frequently used adjuvants in experimental research. Adjuvants function by retaining antigen in the tissues and prolonging the period of immune stimulation [7]. The heightened antibody response after intravitreal injections of protein probably is due to the same mechanism of slow antigen release [8]. Adjuvants may also act as carriers by delivering potential antigens to antibody-forming cells. Because CFA seems to act partly by stimulating T-lymphocytes, it stimulates antibody production primarily in T-dependent classes.

Antigenicity ultimately depends on the host's ability to mount an immune response to the antigen regardless of its size, shape, charge, or other characteristics. The responsiveness of the host can vary from species to species, as noted in the discussion Phylogenic Considerations. It can also vary within species as a result of disease, drugs, aging, and other factors.

The body's own proteins do not normally elicit an immune response. In certain situations, however, this tolerance of self is lost, and the host's own tissue acts as an antigen (autoantigen). We discuss autoimmune diseases later in this section (page 70). Homologous or allogeneic antigens are proteins from another member of the same species, and heterologous or xenogeneic antigens are proteins from another species. Heterologous proteins tend to evoke a more intense immune response than homologous proteins.

Certain antigens are specific for a given organ in the same or different species and are called organ specific. Some of these are found in cornea and lens. Antigens common to members of a given species are called species specific, and antigens not common to a species but characteristic of a single individual are called individual specific. Heterophil antigens occur on the surfaces of tissue cells of many different animals, plants, and bacteria and show extensive interspecies cross relationships.

Some materials are not antigenic in themselves, but when linked covalently to carrier molecules (proteins), they function as antigenic groups (haptens) that direct the specificity of the immune response. Haptens are usually of low molecular weight and are not proteins (e.g., dinitrochlorobenzene [DNCB]).

Histocompatibility or human leukocyte antigens (HLA) in human beings are antigens carried on the surfaces of the nucleated cells of most tissues. Their differences constitute the major reason that tissues from unrelated donors cannot be freely exchanged without subsequent graft rejection. HLA antigens are determined by four subloci or alleles, one allele at each of two loci on each number 6 chromosome. The first histocompatibility locus has been called A, the second C, the third B, and the fourth D. HLA antigens whose identity is still debatable are called W (workshop) antigens.

The HLA antigens at these loci have been defined by serologic and cellular means. The HLA-A, B, and C loci code for antigens is present on almost all cells and is serologically defined (SD). These antigens are controlled by the class I genes. The D locus was originally defined by cellular techniques (proliferation in a primary mixed lymphocyte culture) and was designated LD. The D locus is controlled by the class II gene. Recently, serologically detected antigens associated with the D locus have been found in a limited number of tissues. The antigens associated with this locus are called immune associated (Ia) antigens. These antigens are present in ocular tissue (i.e., Langerhans' cells in corneal and conjunctival epithelium and macrophages).

Cellular defined antigens have been found associated with the A, B, and C loci. These loci are part of the major histocompatibility complex (MHC), which controls a variety of functions that play a critical role in numerous aspects of the immune response. The MHC was recognized as essential in transplantation when it was found that the capacity to reject transplanted cells or organs was determined by a single group of genes and their encoded cell surface antigens (HLA). Three broad classes of genes and molecules have been used to define the MHC. Class I products (controlled from loci A, B, and C) deal with immunosurveillance and the transplant antigen region. Class II genes and products (controlled at loci D) involve the immune response and regulation of T-cell, B-cell, and macrophage interaction. This region also deals with differentiation antigens. Class III products and genes control complement levels.

Class I products are glycoproteins, which are expressed on all nucleated cells and highly polymorphic (e.g., many different alleles determine structurally variant forms of the basic molecule). The class I products are the primary targets for cytotoxic T-lymphocytes that destroy organ grafts. Class I restricted cytotoxic T-lymphocytes are important in the lysis of virus-infected cells in which the cytotoxic T-lymphocytes recognize the viral antigen in association with class I antigens, such as influenza virus–infected cells. A dual recognition is also involved in the cytolysis of virus-induced tumor cells, cells with haptenic groups attached to them, and cytolysis of cells with minor transplantation antigens. Class I antigens are therefore involved in the effector phase of the cell-mediated cytolysis (target molecules).

Class II MHC products have a restricted distribution and exist primarily on lymphocytes. Cooperation between antigen-primed T cells and B cells require that the cells be syngeneic at this region. Interaction between T-cells and macrophages also requires recognition of antigen and D region products. Immune response genes probably reside in or near the HLA-D region in human beings. These genes have been shown to regulate the antibody response to specific antigens, delayed hypersensitivity responses, and T-cell proliferative responses. Evidence exists that they are very specific and regulate the response to a single antigen on a molecule. Thus far, these genes are autosomal dominant and MHC linked. IR gene regulation is functionally expressed on T cells, macrophages, and B cells. Monoclonal antibody studies have shown the presence of Ia antigens and HLA-A, B, and C antigens in tissues of 8-week old fetuses. These antigens reach their almost-complete tissue distribution after 32 weeks of intrauterine life [9].

Class III MHC products determine the structure and level of complement factors. Three complement factors have been identified that are regulated by this genetic locus: C2, C4, and Bf. (see page 40 for a discussion of these factors) These factors may play a role in the destruction of virus and bacteria as well as cells.

In human beings, certain diseases are associated with unusual frequencies to one or more of these HLA antigens, which may affect the host's susceptibility to the disease, resistance to it once it occurs, or both [10]. HLA antigens B8 and DRw3 are associated with adult celiac disease, dermatitis herpetiformis, chronic hepatitis, Hodgkin's disease, and myasthenia gravis. HLA-B27 is present in 90 percent of patients with ankylosing spondylitis. The complicating uveitis in these patients make this association especially meaningful for ophthalmologists. Other HLA antigens have been noted in association with conditions such as atopy, psoriasis, systemic lupus erythematosus, multiple sclerosis, and Sjögren's syndrome.

B-LYMPHOCYTES. B-lymphocytes, through their plasma-cell derivative, can form a soluble immunoglobulin (Ig) that will combine specifically with the provocative antigen. Each person is probably able to synthesize more than 10^5 different antibodies. Despite this remarkable diversity, certain structural and biologic features are common to all antibody molecules of a given class.

Antibodies act as though they had used the antigen as a template [11]. The combining region of the antibody fits closely to a part of the surface of the antigen (Fig. 1-2). Only substances that can fit into the combining region of the antibody can combine with it. The probable reason for the necessity of this closeness-of-fit of antigen and antibody is that the forces that hold them together are weak and work for only a short distance.

The participating forces are as follows:

1. The coulombic force (i.e., the electrostatic attraction between oppositely charged ionic groups on the two protein side chains, for example, an ionized amino group [NH_3^+] on one protein and an ionized carboxyl group [COO^-] on the other); permanent dipoles can also contribute to the energy of interaction
2. The hydrogen bonding between a proton donor on the antigen and an acceptor on the antibody, or the converse
3. The Van der Waals forces, which are due to the interaction between two atoms that are close, the atoms undergoing a mutual polarization with a resultant attractive force
4. The hydrophobic forces owing to the interaction of nonpolar surfaces

The lifespans of B-lymphocytes are measured in days, weeks, or months, so it is inappropriate to speak of an average lifespan [12]. The lifespans of the Ig molecules depend on the structure of the variable regions of these molecules [13]. Some Ig molecules are short-lived (days), whereas others are more stable and may possibly last for a year. The role of anti-idiotypic antibodies in the survival of the antibody molecule is discussed later in this chapter.

Tiselius and Kabat [14] first showed that precipitating antibodies in a strongly immunized rabbit were associated with gamma globulin. This fraction is known to include several serologically and functionally distinct classes of protein referred to as immunoglobulin. Despite some important differences, all immunoglobulins have a basically similar structure consisting of two identical heavy chains and two identical light chains (long and short chains of amino acids, respectively) covalently linked by interchain disulfide bonds.

Work with homogeneous myeloma proteins helped define the struc-

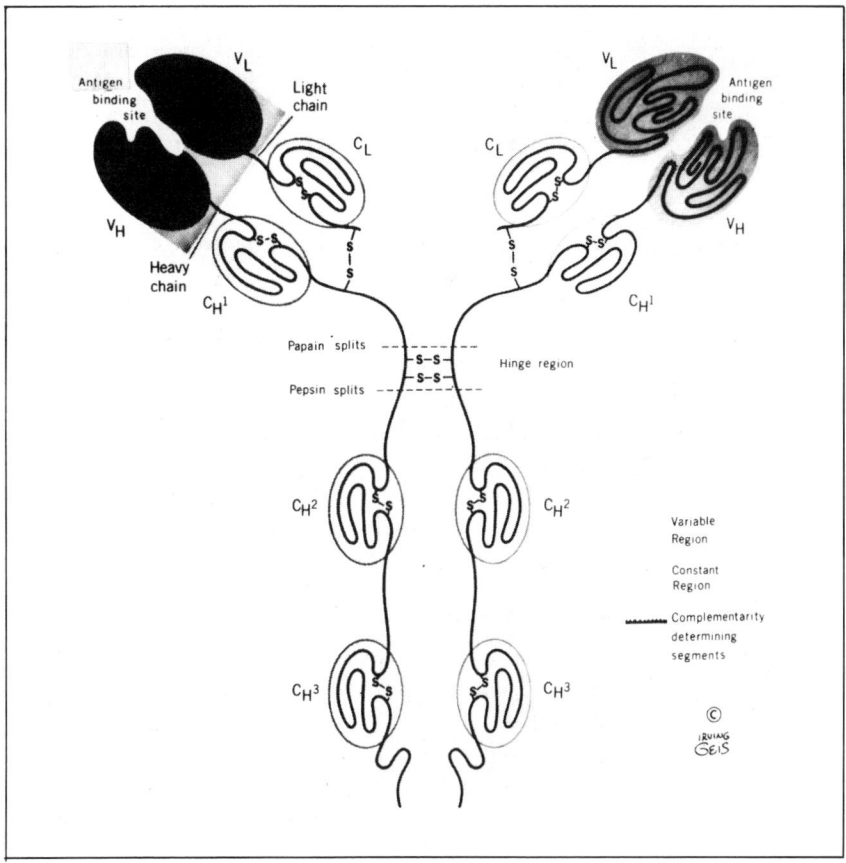

FIG. 1-2   Antibody structure demonstrating two Fab sections and the central Fc segment. The variable region of the end of Fab section can combine with antigen. V_L and V_H represent variable region of the light and heavy chain and C_L and C_H the constant region of the light and heavy chains respectively. (Drawing by Irving Geis. From R. A. Good and D. W. Fisher (Eds.), *Immunobiology*. Stamford, Conn.: Sinauer Associates, 1971. Reproduced with permission.)

ture further. When the amino acid sequence of one light chain from a given myeloma protein was compared with the sequence of another myeloma protein, an important relationship was noted: One-half of the light chain—the half with the terminal carboxyl group—seemed to have the same amino acid sequence from one light chain to another, whereas the other half—the half with the amino terminal end—had many different amino acid sequences from one end to the other. Such an arrangement illustrates the high degree of variability in this half of the light chain. Similar variations were found in the amino terminal half of the heavy chain.

In this variable region, certain areas exhibit hypervariability. These areas, three on the light chain and three on the heavy chain, lie relatively close to each other, probably forming the antigen-binding site. Their heterogeneity ensures diversity in the combining specificities through variations in the shape and nature of the surface they create.

Although antibody specificity of the Ig molecule seems to be determined by the heavy chain [15, 16], light chains must be present to combine with the heavy chains if the antibody molecule is to be active. One heavy chain and one light chain appear to be associated with each antigen-binding site [17], one pair of heavy chains and one pair of light chains accounting for the bivalent antigen-binding activity of the antibody molecules.

The Ig antibody can be split by papain into three fragments. Two are identical and are the areas that can combine with antigen ($F(ab)_2$ or fragment, antigen binding) [18]. The third fragment has no power to combine with antigen and is called Fc (fragment, crystallizable). Its ability to be crystallized attests to its uniformity. The Fc fragment is responsible for the capacity of the intact molecule to combine with complement, in some cases to pass the placental barrier, and to attach to skin, mast cells, macrophages, and staphylococcal antigen.

The antibody molecules can be thought of schematically as assuming a Y shape. On contact with antigen, the arms (Fab regions) of the Y open, using their attachment to the Fc region as a hinge (see Fig. 1-3). (Actually, the antibody molecule is globular.) This particular action may be responsible for activating the Fc region to perform some of its biologic functions.

Peripheral blood B cells have Fc receptors for both IgG and IgM and thus a single precursor cell may give rise to a clone producing antibodies of the IgM class and different IgG subclasses, all of which share combining sites [19, 20].

Ig molecules (IgG, IgM, IgA, IgD, and IgE) are incorporated into the cytoplasmic membranes of B-lymphocytes and behave as receptors for antigen, for antigen-antibody complexes, and for plant lectins. It appears that the T-cell receptor may also be an Ig molecule acquired by absorption rather than active synthesis.

Immunoglobulin G. The serum level of IgG is approximately 1000 mg/dl, which is about 80 percent of the total serum Ig level (Table 1-1). The IgG molecule has a molecular weight of about 150,000 [21]. The chain structure of IgG is the same as the chain structure of antibodies. The antigenic analysis of IgG myelomas showed four subclasses, now termed IgG_1, IgG_2, IgG_3, and IgG_4. IgG_1 is the predominant variant, and together with IgG_3 it possesses the ability to combine with complement, to bind to macrophages, and to cross the placenta. IgG_2, which is second in order of prevalence, has less complement- and macrophage-binding capacity and crosses the placenta with difficulty. IgG_4, the rarest variant, may function as a lymphocyte-dependent antibody and be concerned with killer cell (K-cell) function. K cells are lymphocytes that act nonspecifically on antibody-coated targets [22]; their origin is obscure.

During secondary response that follows a second exposure to the same antigen, IgG is the major immunoglobulin to be synthesized. Through its ability to cross the placenta, it provides a major line of defense against

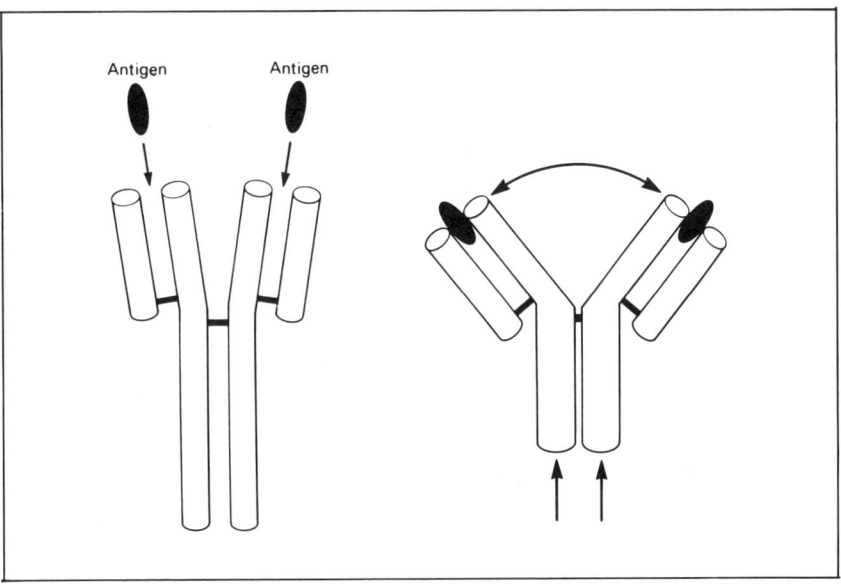

FIG. 1-3 Antibody combining with antigen. Antibody combining F(ab)$_2$ fragments are farther apart and constant or crystalizable (Fc) portion is shortened.

infection for the first few weeks of life, a line that can be reinforced by the transfer of IgG in colostrum across an infant's gut mucosa. Probably because of its relatively small size, IgG diffuses more readily than other immunoglobulins into the interstitial body fluids. There, as the predominant immunoglobulin, it carries the major burden of neutralizing bacterial toxins and of binding to microorganisms (especially streptococci, pneumococci, and staphylococci) to enhance their phagocytosis. The complexes of bacteria and IgG antibody can adhere to phagocytic cells, which have specialized surface receptors for sites on the Fc portion of IgG. B-lymphocytes also have surface receptors that can bind to the Fc regions of IgG. If red blood cells are coated with IgG, they can adhere to B-lymphocytes to form rosettes.

Immunoglobulin A. The serum level of IgA is approximately 170 mg/dl, or 15 percent of the total serum immunoglobulin. The molecule has a molecular weight of about 170,000 [23]. IgA tends to form dimers spontaneously through association with a cystine-rich polypeptide known as the "J chain." The antigen-combining power of IgA may be diluted by the formation of these dimers.

Two subclasses of IgA have been identified, IgA$_1$ and IgA$_2$. IgA$_2$ is unusual in that it lacks interchain disulfide bonds between heavy and light chains.

A special form of IgA is exocrine IgA—a combination of two IgA molecules with a secretory piece (also called "transport piece" or "T piece"), which is not an immunoglobulin (Fig. 1-4). The secretory piece is synthesized by local epithelial cells [24, 25], for example, lacrimal gland ep-

TABLE 1-1 Immunoglobulin Characteristics

Immunoglobulin	Half Life Days	Fixes Complement	Opsonic Activity	Crosses Placenta	Viral Neutral.	Sub Classes	Molecular Weight	Normal Serum Conc.	Primary Distrib.	Biologic Function
IgG	25–35	Yes	Yes	Yes	Yes	4	150,000	1,240 ± 220	Extracell. Fluids	Principal Serum Antibody
IgM	9–11	Yes	Yes	No	Yes	2	970,000	120 ± 35	Intravasc.	1st Antibody Response
IgA	6–8	No	No	No	No	2	170,000	390 ± 90	External Secretion	Secretory Antibody
Secr. IgA	6–8	No	No	No	Yes	1	400,000		External Secretion	Secretory Antibody
IgE	2	No	No	No	No	1	190,000	0.05	Reaginic Antibody	Anaphylactic Reactions
IgD	2–3	No	No	No	No	1	180,000	3 ± 2	Intravasc.	

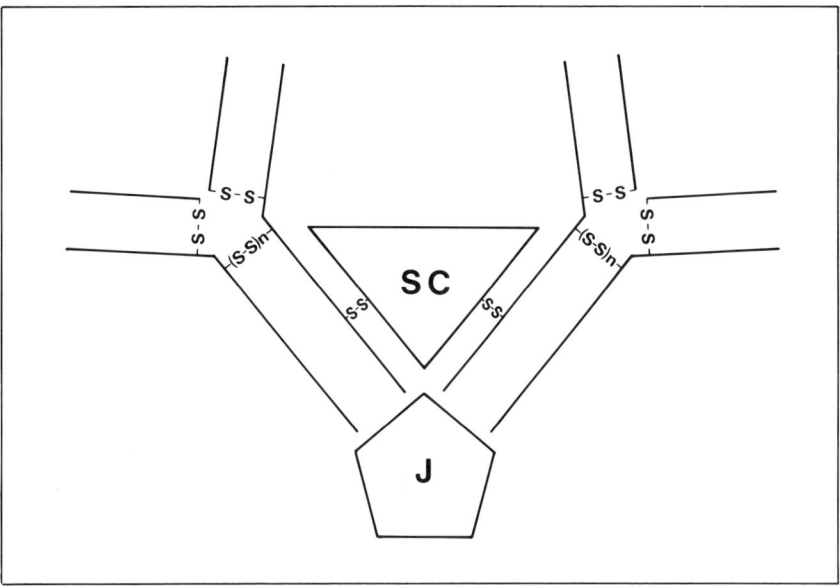

FIG. 1-4   Exocrine IgA has two IgA molecules with disulfide bonds (*S-S*) connected by a secretory piece (*SC*) and *J* chain.

ithelium [26], and has a single peptide chain with a molecular weight of 60,000 [27]. The exocrine IgA is stabilized against proteolysis, probably because of its secretory piece. This stabilization allows it to continue to act as an antibody in an environment rich in proteolytic enzymes. It appears in the seromucous secretions of the saliva, tears, nasal fluids, sweat, and colostrum, lung, and gastrointestinal tract. Exocrine IgA is probably the dominant antibody in the external secretions. The role of IgE in these secretions is being evaluated [28], and IgG is apparently abundant in some external secretions (e.g., bile, prostatic and vaginal fluid, and the fluid of the small intestines [29].

The principal role of the IgA antibodies is thus to serve as an "immunologic paint" on the body's external surfaces, and they may very well be the body's first line of defense against invading microorganisms [30, 31]. The evidence strongly suggests that for some infections of the external mucous membranes, local antibodies (possibly exocrine IgA) are more important in resistance to infection than circulating antibodies [32–34].

Specialized areas may be present in the lung, gastrointestinal tract and ocular tissues that serve as the main points of antigen entrance and IgA production. This mucous membrane–associated lymphoid tissue (MALT) may be present in the conjunctiva. After sensitization at these sites, the lymphocytes migrate to the draining lymph nodes and then "home" back to the original site of their production and possibly to the other MALT areas. Thus the ingestion of an antigen in a sensitized host

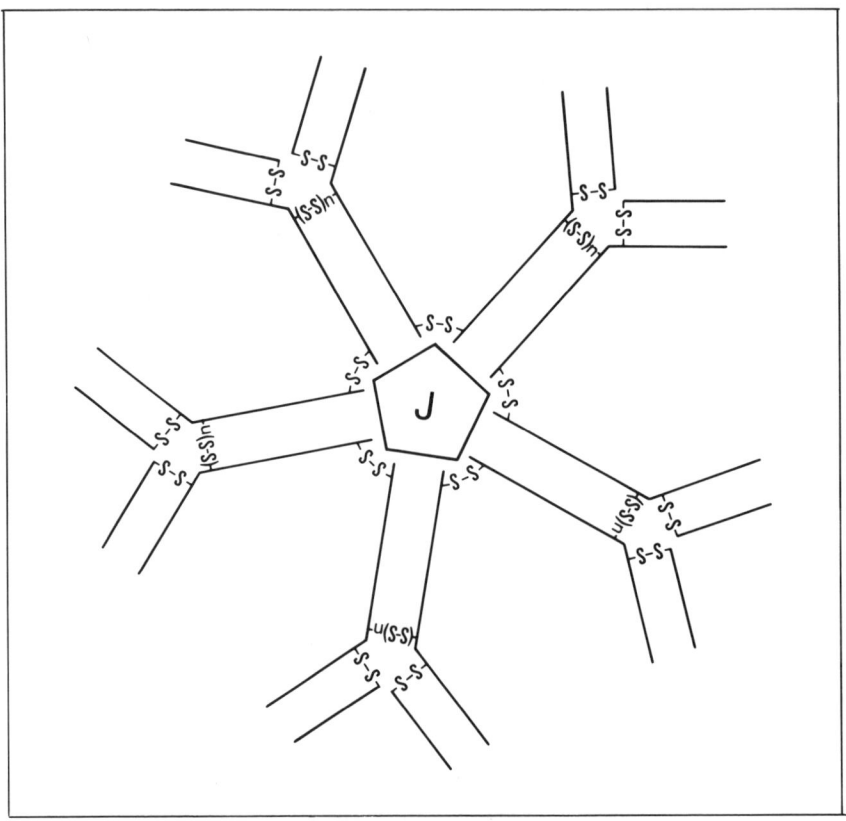

FIG. 1-5 Five basic antibody structures are joined together to form the IgM molecule.

can lead to the secretion of IgA antibodies to that antigen into the tear film from the lacrimal gland or conjunctiva.

There are also some interesting reports that IgA, lysozyme, and complement act synergistically in killing certain coliform organisms, and that aggregated IgA can bind polymorphonuclear leukocytes (PMNLs) and activate the complement system by the alternative pathway. IgA does not cross the placenta.

Immunoglobulin M. The serum level of IgM is approximately 100 mg/dl or 5 percent of the total Ig level. The IgM molecules, with a molecular weight of 970,000, are the largest of the immunoglobulins. Often referred to as macroglobulins because of their size, the IgM molecules are pentamers with a high valency or antigen-combining capacity (Fig. 1-5). Because of their high valency, they are extremely efficient agglutinating and cytolytic agents. IgM is also efficient in fixing complement [35] and is the first type of antibody to be formed after the initial encounter with antigen. Because it appears early in the response to infection and is confined mainly to the bloodstream, it probably plays a major role in combating bacteremia. It does not cross the placenta.

The isohemagglutinins (anti-A, anti-B), cold agglutinins, many natural antibodies to microorganisms, rheumatoid factor, antibodies against O antigens (or somantic antigens) of gram-negative bacteria, and the "WR" (Wassermann reaction) antibodies in syphilis are all characteristically IgM.

Immunoglobulin D. The serum level of IgD is approximately 3 mg/dl or 0.5 percent of the total Ig level, and its molecular weight is approximately 180,000. There are now reports of IgD antinuclear antibodies in systemic connective tissue disorders. The demonstration of IgD on the surface of a proportion of cord-blood lymphocytes suggests that it is an early receptor that later gives way to IgM and other immunoglobulins [36, 37–39]. IgD is a major immunoglobulin on B cells and does not cross the placenta.

Immunoglobulin E. The serum level of IgE is from 0.001 to 0.007 mg/dl, and its molecular weight is approximately 190,000. It does not fix complement and may cross the placenta. Anaphylactogenic skin-sensitizing antibody is carried by IgE [40], and IgE antibodies remain firmly fixed for a long time when injected into human skin where they are probably bound to mast cells. Contact with antigen leads to degranulation of the mast cells with release of vasoactive amines, for example, heparin and histamine. The physiologic role of IgE is not well understood, but it has been noticed that its serum level rises considerably in the presence of infection with certain parasites, particularly helminths. It has been suggested that contact between the parasite antigens and mast-cell–bound IgE antibody in the gut wall results in vasoactive-amine release and facilitates ejection of the invading parasites.

MONOCLONAL ANTIBODIES. Monoclonal antibodies were first described as a pathologic abnormality of excessive production of homogeneous antibody by myeloma cells. The production of myeloma antibody in vitro has now been controlled for the production of highly purified and specific antibodies to a variety of antigens. The technique involves fusing spleen cells and myeloma cells by means of exposure to polyethylene glycol. The replicating cell line must have two distinct properties: it must both lack Ig production or secretion and the enzyme hypoxanthine phosphoribosyl transferase. After fusion by polyethylene glycol, the hybrid cell has the combined genome of the parent cell lines. Selection of hybrids is accomplished by waiting for the natural death of the splenocytes while the myeloma cell line is killed by exposure to hypoxanthine, aminopterin, and thymidine. The surviving hybridoma cell lines are assayed for antibody production. Clones positive for antibody to a specific antigen are recloned and then used for mass production of antibody or subsequently frozen for future use.

The production of monoclonal antibody has been an important advance in immunology. Potentially, monoclonal antibody can be used in treating drug toxicity by administering monoclonal antibodies directed against a specific drug used for neutralization. Certain malignant disorders have been treated with monoclonal antibodies. The monoclonal antibody may be directed against a specific antigen on tumor cells or may be directed toward an idiotypic antigenic site on the patient's own tumor cell. Potentially, monoclonal antibodies could be used for more specific treatment of infectious diseases such as rabies and tetanus. Monoclonal antibodies may also be used to modulate the immune response with antibodies directed toward helper or suppressor T cells. Graft control has been accomplished effectively through the use of monoclonal antibodies directed toward T cells. Monoclonal antibody has also been used to remove graft-versus-host–producing cells from bone marrow prior to transplantation into patients. An important use of monoclonal antibodies has been in the development of diagnostic techniques for the identification of specific antigens on cells or in tissue as well as the identification of subsets of cells. Monoclonal antibodies have also been successfully used in a variety of radioimmunoassays.

ANTIBODY RESPONSE. The simplistic concept that there is an initial contact between antigen and a clone of B-lymphocytes, and that this contact results in the formation of specific antibody, is probably rarely borne out. (The roles of macrophages and T cells are discussed later in the chapter.) Four or 5 days elapse after contact with an antigen before antibody is detected in the serum. In this interval, the antigen is recognized and immune-cell sensitization occurs. A considerable amount of antibody synthesis must occur before circulating antibody becomes detectable.

When B-lymphocytes are sensitized, they develop prominent Golgi apparatus and a considerable increase in the amount of rough-surfaced endoplasmic reticulum. These transformed lymphocytes are called immunoblasts and eventually develop into plasma cells. In response to antigenic stimulus, the initial antibody is IgM. IgG antibody, once it is synthesized in adequate amounts, "shuts off" or slows down IgM synthesis [41].

Subsequent exposure to the same antigen causes an accelerated and much more prolific production of antibody. This secondary response is characterized by IgG formation from the outset, in contrast to the response that follows the initial exposure when IgM production predominates. This accelerated response probably is due to T-lymphocyte memory cells. These cells cooperate with or help B-lymphocytes form plasma cells, when then form immunoglobulin. A single plasma cell can produce more than one type of immunoglobulin at a given time (i.e., IgM, IgG, and IgD).

ANTIGEN-ANTIBODY COMPLEXES. Antigen-antibody or immune complexes can be triggered by a variety of endogenous as well as exogenous antigens. Antibody may react with structural antigens that form part of the intracellular or membrane structure. Antibody can also react with secreted antigens or with soluble antigens in the circulation to form immune complexes that are deposited in various organs. Circulating immune complexes may be deposited in the glomerulus, skin, synovium, vascular basement membrane, or eye.

The pathogenicity of immune complexes may be related to a variety of factors. The chronicity of immune complex formation is an important determinant of pathogenicity. Continued exposure to antigen may lead to chronic disease, such as chronic serum sickness. The antigenicity of the immune complex is a second important factor in determining pathogenicity. Strong antigens evoke an intense antibody response and result in rapid elimination of antigen from the circulation. In contrast, weak antigenicity results in protracted circulation of immune complexes. Immune complexes that localize in specific areas may produce notable tissue damage (i.e., uveitis). For example, DNA has affinity for basement membranes, providing a mechanism for localized immune complex disease.

Certain antigens may evoke an antibody response of only certain classes of antibodies. The class of antibody determines the ability to activate complement, the ability to bind to cellular Fc receptors, and the affinity of antibody for antigen.

The ratio of antigen to antibody is another important factor in determining the biologic activity of immune complexes. Immune complexes formed in large antigen excess do not fix complement and fail to initiate inflammatory reactions. Immune complexes formed in antibody excess are large, fix complement well, and have inflammatory potential. However, as they are rapidly phagocytosed and catabolized, they have limited pathologic potential. In contrast, immune complexes formed in slight antigen excess are soluble, disseminate as they circulate, fix complement well, are not rapidly phagocytosed, and have great inflammatory potential.

Immune complexes may produce pathologic changes in tissue by direct combination of antigen and antibody in that tissue. These complexes have the ability to activate complement, cause platelet aggregation, and activate the kinin system. An example of this process would be the Wessely ring in the cornea. Immune complexes that lodge in tissue or membranes may produce pathologic changes in a more localized manner. As an example, the peripheral infiltrates of the cornea in Wegener's granulomatosis is a result of localized deposition of immune complexes.

Immune complexes may also regulate the immune system. As immune complexes are formed, they are phagocytized by macrophages. The Fc fragments of immune complexes released from macrophages may selectively stimulate helper and suppressor T cells, amplifying or suppressing the immune response. Alternatively, the Fc portion of circulating immune complexes may directly stimulate helper or suppressor T cells. Immune complexes may interfere with immune mechanisms by adhering to the Fc receptors of effector cells, thereby blocking cytolytic effects.

There are a variety of receptors for immune complexes that can be divided into humoral or cellular receptors. As immune complexes form, the C1q component of complement (discussed in detail on page 41) binds to the Fc portion of the complex. Rheumatoid factor and IgG or IgM antibodies directed against IgG have a higher affinity for immune complexes IgG than for polyclonal IgG.

Receptors for immune complexes also exist on cells. The Raji is a lymphoblastoid cell with B-cell characteristics. It possesses low affinity Fc receptors for binding immunoglobulin but high affinity complement receptors. Circulating immune complexes interact with platelets and result in platelet aggregation. Macrophages will ingest immune complexes as well as aggregated IgG. Ingestion is based on the presence of Fc receptors on the cell surface membrane.

Although receptors for humoral and cellular components have important biologic functions, they have also served as a method for developing immune complex assays. The requirements for an ideal immune complex assay are numerous. The assay should be specific for immune complexes so the method does not detect the presence of antibody or complement not associated with immune complexes. The method should be sufficiently sensitive to detect low levels of immune complexes in the circulation. An ideal assay should also be able to differentiate between immune complexes formed in response to different antigens. The assay should detect immune complexes of all Ig classes. As not all immune complexes fix complement, the assay should be capable of detecting both complement-fixing and noncomplement-fixing immune complexes. Finally, the assay should be able to detect immune complexes of varying sizes. No one assay fulfills all of these criteria, but a variety of assays have been developed. The major assays in use are listed in Chapter 2.

T-LYMPHOCYTES. In the human being, monoclonal antibodies have been used to determine both functional T-cell subsets and maturational changes that occur in T-cell subsets. Monoclonal antibodies of the OK or Leu series have been extensively used.

All T-lymphocyte populations are derived from stem cells found in the bone marrow, liver, and fetal yolk sac and that pass through the thymus. During differentiation the early thymocytes bear the OKT10 and 9 antigens. As maturation proceeds to common thymocytes the OKT9 antigen is lost and the OKT8, 6, 5, 4 antigens appear; in the mature thymocytes the OKT6 is lost and the OKT3 and I antigens are expressed [42] (Fig. 1-6). Most T-lymphocytes have multiple antigens.

Several monoclonal antibodies recognize antigens on the majority of T cells and are termed "pan" T-cell reagents. These include OKT1, OKT3, OKT11, Leu 7, Leu 4, and Leu 5. The E rosette (sheep red blood cell) receptor is identified by OKT4, Leu 3a, and Leu 3b monoclonal antibodies, while T suppressor and cytotoxic cells are identified by OKT8, Leu 2a, and Leu 2b. Approximately 65 percent of peripheral blood lymphocytes are helper cells and 35 percent are suppressor cells (Table 1-2). OKT10 identifies early hematopoietic cells, prothymocytes, myeloblasts, promyelocytes, and activated T and B cells. Thus it is not a specific marker of T cells. Similarly, OKT9 identifies early hematopoietic

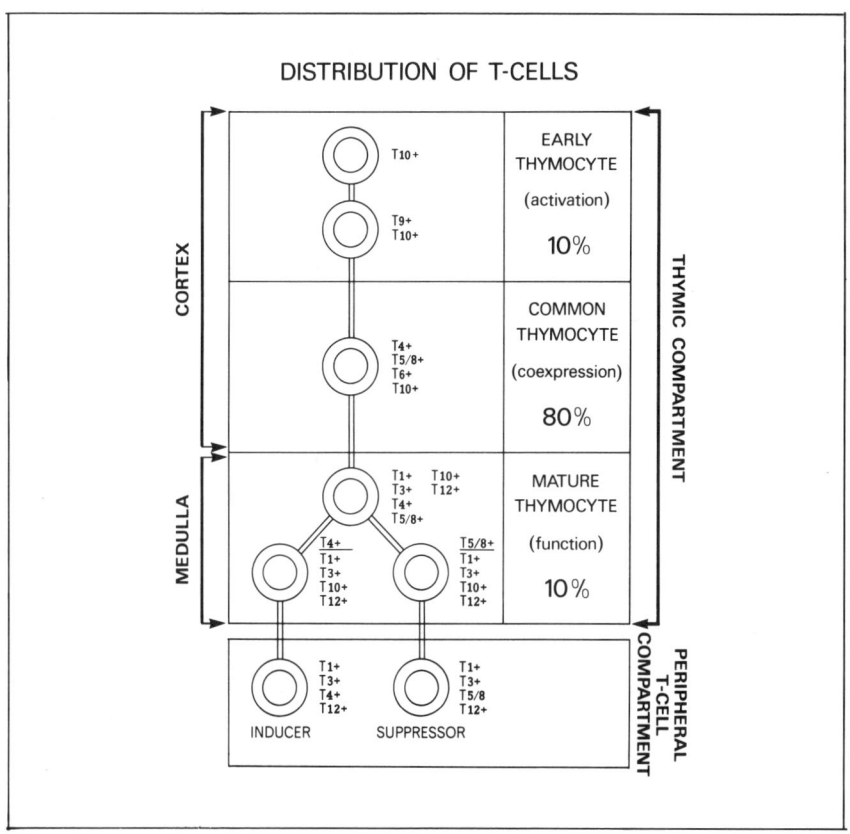

FIG. 1-6 Distribution of T cells.

cells, activated lymphocytes, and neoplastic cells. Activated T cells and B cells can be identified using OKIa1, whereas monocytes are identified by OKM1.

Using monoclonal antibodies, the functional activity of T-cell subsets has been defined. Helper-inducer activities are in the OKT4 (Leu 3) population. These cells respond to allogeneic cells, mitogens, and antigens. Suppressor-cytotoxic activities are in the OKT8 (Leu 3) population of cells, which also respond to allogeneic cells, mitogens, and antigens. OKT4 and OKT8 cells are within the OKT3 population. Thus OKT3 cells possess all of the aforementioned activities.

T-Cell Subsets. At least four major subsets of T cells can be identified on the basis of cell-surface differentiation markers, recognition repertoire, and functional capacities. The helper T cell (T_H) was the first to be identified unequivocally on the basis of its function; in fact, its recognition resulted in the concept of cell-to-cell interaction as a necessary part of the immune response. It is characterized by its ability to help B cells produce primarily IgG antibody and to help other T cells in their function. As previously noted, it bears the surface differentiation antigen T4 in human beings. It is restricted in its antigen-perception repertoire

TABLE 1-2 Surface Markers on Human Peripheral Blood T Cells

Marker	Method of Detection	T Cells Expressing Marker (%)	Proposed Function
Receptor for sheep erythrocytes (E)	Rosetting	100	Total T-cell function
Fc receptor for IgM	Rosetting with IgM antibody coated E	60–70	Helper; cytotoxic T-lymphocyte (Tc) precursors
Fc receptor for IgG	Rosetting with IgG antibody coated E	10–20	Suppressor; K and NK activity
Histamine receptor	Adherence to histamine column	10–20	Suppressor
OKT11	Immunofluorescence	100	Total T-cell function
OKT3	Immunofluorescence	85–95	Total T-cell function
OKT4	Immunofluorescence	50–60	Helper
OKT8	Immunofluorescence	20–30	Suppressor, precursors and effector
Anti-Leu 1	Immunofluorescence	95–100	Total T-cell function
Anti-Leu 2	Immunofluorescence	20–40	Suppressor; Tc precursors
Anti-Leu 3	Immunofluorescence	40–60	Helper

K = killer cell; NK = natural killer cell.

by the class II molecules of the MHC. Thus, the requirement for an interaction between T_H cells and B cells in most antibody responses readily explains why antibody responsiveness is markedly diminished in T-cell–deficient animals.

The cytotoxic T cell (T_c), or killer T cell, can kill target cells after making intimate contact with them. Among potential target cells are virus-infected cells and cells that differ from their host at one or other of the MHC gene products (allogeneic cells). The T_c cell is characterized by the surface antigenic marker T8 in human beings. It is restricted by class I MHC antigens.

There is a close association between binding and the killing activities of T_c cells. Damage occurs at the target cell membrane owing to direct damage or is a secondary event after intracellular damage occurs. Nonspecific killing of target cells by T_c cells can be enhanced by the presence of mitogenic lectins [43, 44] or if the cells are subjected to mild oxidation.

The suppressor cell (T_s) is a regulatory cell that can suppress the action of other lymphocytes, T or B. Some bear the surface marker T8 in human beings. They are said to release factors, some of which are antigen specific and others are not. These several subsets of T_s cells differ in their characteristic properties, target cells, and MHC restriction.

The cells involved in the inflammatory responses of delayed-type hypersensitivity are T cells (T_D). They act by releasing lymphokines at the site of antigen deposition, chemotactic for monocytes, and arresting their

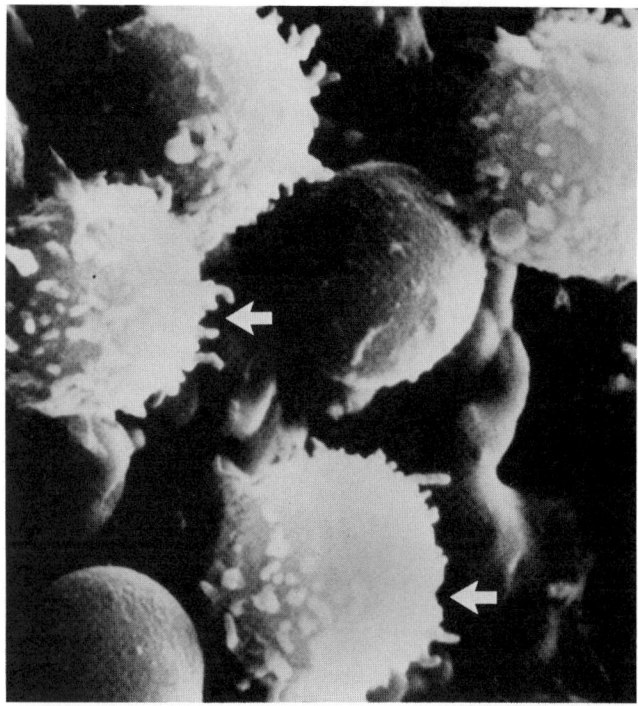

FIG. 1-7 Scanning electron micrograph of T and B cells shows tendency of B cells to have more turbulent surfaces (*arrows*) than T cells. Surface smoothness cannot be used to differentiate the two cell types because of cell variability.

further migration, thus leading to a local monocytic infiltration. Some T_D cells resemble T_H cells in their surface phenotype and MHC restriction specificity, and others resemble T_c cells. Presumably, it is the way in which antigen is presented that determines whether T_H or T_c cells are stimulated. One type, T_H cells, would recognize macrophage-processed antigen in association with class II MHC molecules; the other, would recognize cell surface antigen in association with class I MHC molecules [45].

T Cells versus B Cells. Morphologically, T-lymphocytes are difficult and sometimes impossible to differentiate from B-lymphocytes. When examined by the scanning electron microscope, the B-lymphocyte may have a more irregular, villous appearance than the T-lymphocyte [46], but recent observers have disputed this apparent difference (Fig. 1-7). In vitro, human T-lymphocytes can form spontaneous rosettes with uncoated sheep red blood cells [47]. B-lymphocytes, on the other hand, require the sheep red blood cells to be coated with IgG antibody. T and B cells can be separated by electrophoresis, by depletion of one by rosette formation, by affinity chromatography, and by fluorescent anti-Ig and anti–T-cell procedures.

Both types of lymphocytes react to a similar range of antigens, and the

TABLE 1-3 Surface Markers on Non-T Cells

Cell Type	Marker
Natural killer cells	OKM 1
	OKT 10
	Leu 7
B-lymphocytes	Leu 14
	B1
	OKB 2
	OKB 7
	BA- 1
	Cell Surface Immunoglobulin
Plasma cells	OKT 10
	Cytoplasmic Immunoglobulin
Monocytes-histiocytes	OKM 1
	OKM 5
	OKT 6 (Langerhans' cells)
	M 221

location of the antigen may determine the type of lymphocyte that predominates. For example, antigens in the circulating body fluids stimulate many more B-lymphocytes than T-lymphocytes, whereas fixed antigens in tissue allografts, solid neoplasms, and phagocytized bacteria stimulate many more T-lymphocytes than B-lymphocytes.

The percentages of circulating monocytes in the blood are as follows: T cells, 60 to 70 percent; B cells, 5 to 10 percent; macrophages, 15 to 20 percent, and null cells, 5 to 10 percent (Table 1-3).* Both types of lymphocytes have receptors for enkephalins and endorphins. The substances may act as humoral mediators between the central nervous and immune systems. These substances can influence antibody synthesis, lymphocyte proliferation, and natural killer (NK) cytotoxicity.

T-Cell Recognition of Antigen. A dual and single recognition hypothesis has been proposed to explain the ability of T cells to recognize specific antigen. Support for the dual recognition theory is found in T-cell–mediated cytolysis where recognition of both antigen and a histocompatibility antigen is required. In the single recognition hypothesis the immune response is directed toward a "neo" antigen, which is a result of macrophage processing or antigenic alteration induced by interaction between antigen and MHC products. The cooperative cell response occurs at two levels. Initially, macrophage processing of antigen presents antigen and a unique Ia determinant to the helper T cell. In responding, the T cell produces helper factors that may be antigen specific or antigen nonspecific. At the second level, the activated helper T cell in concert

---

* Null cells are a heterogenous group of mononuclear cells without T- or B-cell markers. They include natural killer (NK) and K cells.

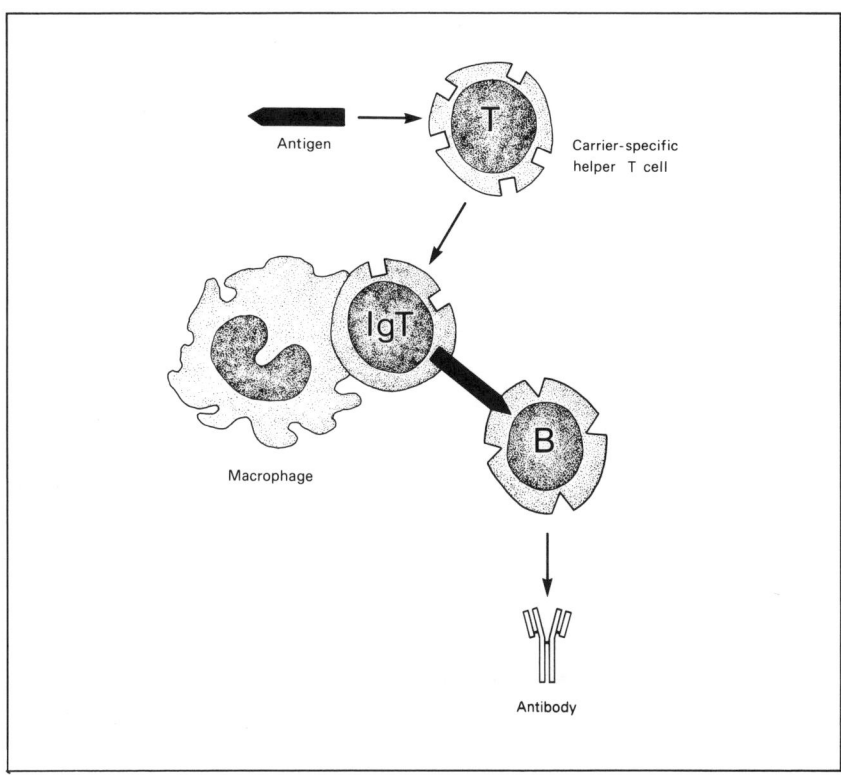

FIG. 1-8 Macrophage and helper T-cell stimulation of B cell to produce antibody.

with helper factors interacts with the B cell (Fig. 1-8). The antibody response is the result of T-cell recognition of specific antigen and Ia antigen and the action of helper cell factors. The control of the end product of the immune response, lymphokines (discussed later in this chapter) in relation to T cells, and antibody in relation to B cells is a result of interaction between helper and suppressor T cells and helper and suppressor cell factors. In addition, monocytes and macrophages may also exert both helper and suppressor control mechanisms [48].

T-Cell Activation by Antigen.. When T-lymphocytes come into contact with a processed antigen, they undergo lymphoblastic transformation and produce soluble factors called lymphokines [49]. A similar lymphoblastic transformation can be induced by a variety of plant mitogens (e.g., phytohemagglutinin [PHA] and concanavalin A [CON A]). These substances react with the T-cell surface nonspecifically, not as an antigen (Fig. 1-9).

LYMPHOKINES. Lymphokines are regulatory and effector substances produced primarily by T cells but may also be produced by B cells and monocytes and macrophages. The terms *monokines* and *cytokines* have been suggested as a broader definition or classification.

Some of the lymphokines produced affect macrophages (Table 1-4).

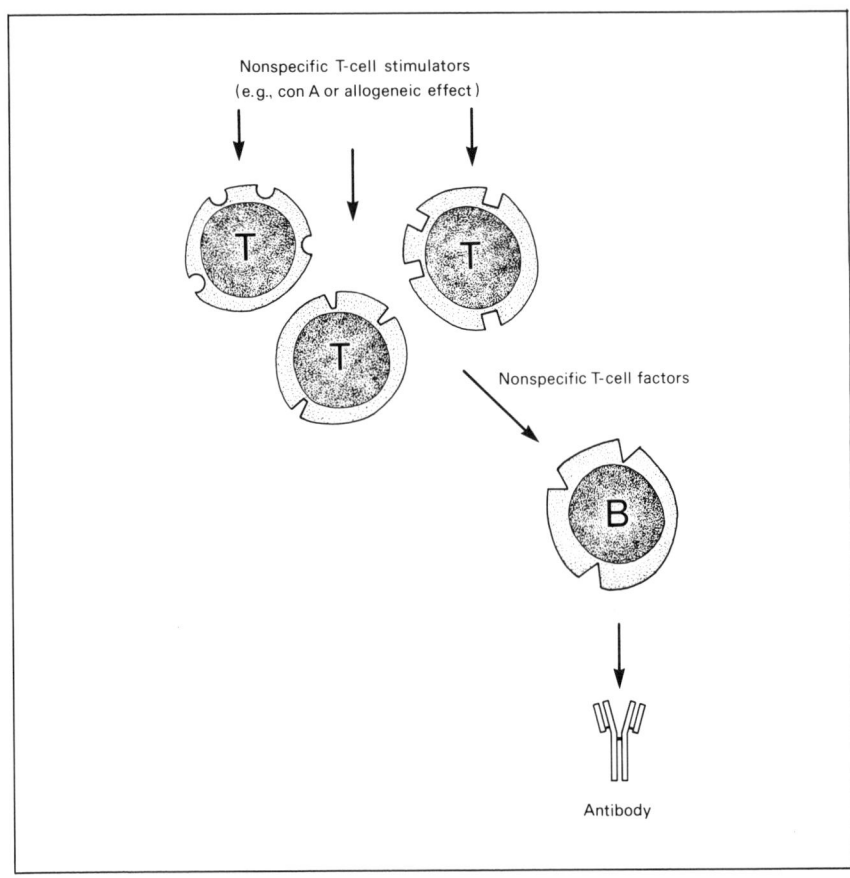

FIG. 1-9 Nonspecific T-cell stimulators induce lymphokine production, which can affect B-lymphocytes (con A = concanavalin A).

Migration-inhibition factor (MIF) prevents macrophages from leaving the scene of the interaction of the antigen (or mitogen) and the T-lymphocyte. This factor correlates with the CMI response. Only living lymphocytes produce MIF, and production can be blocked by inhibitors of protein synthesis (e.g., puromycin). The MIF produced by stimulating T-lymphocytes with a mitogen has similar properties. Active esterases on the surface of the macrophage alter the effect of the MIF on the cell and may regulate the response of the macrophages to the MIF. Macrophage-aggregation factor brings macrophages to this site of interaction, and macrophage-activating (or arming) factor (MAF) increases the biologic activity of the macrophage. MAF can alter macrophages in several ways by increasing the following: membrane stickiness, ruffled membrane activity, phagocytosis (selectively), the activity of adenyl cyclase (the plasma membrane enzyme), glucose oxidation, and the number of cytoplasmic granules. Some lymphokines can affect lymphocytes. Mitogenic factor enhances blastic transformation and the proliferation of sensitized T-

TABLE 1-4 Lymphokines

Mediators affecting macrophages
  Migration-inhibition factor (MIF)
  Macrophage-activating (arming) factor (MAF)
  Macrophage-aggregation factor
  Macrophage-spreading factor
  Chemotactic factor
  Antigen-dependent MIF

Mediators affecting neutrophilic leukocytes
  Chemotactic factor
  Leukocyte-inhibitory factor (LIF)
  Leukocyte-blastogenic factor

Mediators affecting basophils
  Chemotactic factor
  Migration-stimulation factor

Mediators affecting eosinophils: chemotactic factor

Mediators affecting lymphocytes
  Mitogenic factors (IL-2)
  Helper factors (B-cell growth factor, B-cell differentiating factor)
  Suppressor factors

Mediators affecting other cells
  Cytotoxic factors
  Growth-inhibitory factors
  Colony growth–stimulatory factors
  Osteoclast-activating factor
  P-stimulating factor

Skin-reaction factor

Transfer factor

Interferon

Immunoglobulin

lymphocytes; other enhancing and suppressing factors moderate B-cell activity.

Lymphotoxin (cytotoxin) is released by sensitized T-lymphocytes on contact with antigen and causes destruction of target cells. K cells also elaborate a lymphotoxin, which may be responsible for their ability to destroy tumor. The lymphotoxin may be released by the K cell directly into the proximate target cell or onto its surface membrane.

T cells also produce chemotactic and inhibitory factors for neutrophils, chemotactic factors for basophils (requiring the presence of antigen-antibody complexes), and chemotactic factors for eosinophils. There are a variety of colony-stimulating factors (CSF). CSF lymphokines are further designated by the target cell (e.g., granulocytes and macrophages are regulated by Gm-CSF). A potent lymphokine that affects linkages of hemopoietic cells (P stimulating factor; PSF) forms an important link between the immune and hemopoietic systems [50].

Another group of lymphokines are the interferons. These exist in three main forms. Interferon alpha was previously termed leukocyte or type 1 interferon. Production is induced by foreign or transformed cells as well as viruses. It is pH 2 stable. Interferon beta, or fibroblast interferon, is produced in response to viruses and nucleic acids. It is also pH 2 stable. Interferon gamma, or immune, type 2 interferon is produced in response to mitogens and antigens. It is pH 2 labile. Interferons have a number of biologic activities in addition to antiviral activity [51]. They may inhibit (1) differentiation of fibroblasts to fat cells, (2) bone marrow function, (3) formation of granulocyte progenitors, (4) differentiation of monocytes to macrophages, and (5) delayed-type hypersensitivity. Interferons may enhance (1) basophil secretion of histamine, (2) granulocyte-mediated antibody-dependent cellular cytotoxicity (ADCC), (3) macrophage vacuolation and phagocytosis, (4) macrophage cytotoxicity, (5) (or inhibit) antibody production, and (6) (or inhibit) T-cell proliferation [52–54]. Interferon induces blastogenesis and activates NK cells.

Considerable interest has been engendered by the use of interferon for the treatment of malignancy because interferon has been shown to inhibit the replication of neoplastic cells [55, 56].

A lymphokine designated IL-3 has attracted attention in recent years. It fosters the appearance of maturation markers on precursor T cells and the differentiation of some bone marrow precursors into histamine-containing basophil or mast cell-like cells [57]. Hematopoietic cell colonies in bone marrow cultures are also stimulated. IL-3 has a molecular weight of 41,000 [58, 59].

Other lymphokines are cytotoxic factors, growth-inhibitory factors, osteoclast-activating factor, skin reactive factor, and immunoglobulin. Lymphokines also have a variety of less specific actions on target cells and the organism (i.e., induction of hydrogen peroxide, production of fever and acute phase proteins) [57].

INTERLEUKINS.. Two distinct T-cell growth factors, or monokines, have been recently designated as interleukins. They are produced by mononuclear cells in response to a variety of stimuli.

Interleukin-1 (IL-1) is a macrophage or accessory cell-derived factor. It has been previously called lymphocyte-activating factor [60] and B-cell–activating factor. It is composed of a single peptide chain of molecular weight 12,000 to 16,000 [61]. The cells that are capable of producing IL-1 include macrophages (Kupffer's cells, adherent splenic and peritoneal cells), dendritic cells, Langerhans' cells, endothelial cells, transformed B-cell lines, melanoma cells, mesangial cells, astrocytes, neutrophils, keratinocytes, fibroblasts, and corneal and conjunctival cells [62]. Most of these cells (except fibroblasts, neutrophils, and corneal and conjunctival cells) express or can be induced to express Ia antigens. The majority of these cells (macrophages, dendritic, Langerhans', endothelial, and transformed B-cell lines) have accessory functions. These functions are discussed later (page 33). A number of agents are capable of stimulating macrophages to produce IL-1, including lipopolysaccharides, components of mycobacteria antigens, lectins, and activated lymphocytes. Exercise may also enhance IL-1 production [63]. Stimulation by activated lymphocytes is immune response gene restricted and requires Ia antigen identity.

There is no interspecies restriction of IL-1 activity. Although IL-1 is an antigen-nonspecific mediator, it functions as an essential activating signal in all T-cell–dependent, antigen-specific immune responses, the specificity of a given response being defined by the eliciting antigen [64, 65]. IL-1 and antigen presentation by an Ia identical macrophage are necessary signals for the activation of T cells [66]. (IL-1 can replace the macrophage requirement for the proliferative response of T cells to lectins.) Underlying the stimulatory effects of IL-1 is its participation in the production of interleukin-2 (IL-2), the T-cell–derived lymphokine that is ultimately responsible for the proliferation of T cells [67]. This link between IL-1 and 2 is essential because it involves the conversion of a primary macrophage-derived maturational signal into a secondary T-cell–derived proliferative signal that results in amplification of specific immune responses. The stimulation of IL-2 synthesis by IL-1 may be dependent on the presence of another activating signal, either a specific antigen or a polyclonal T-cell mitogen, such as concanavalin A.

IL-1 in concert with a specific antigen stimulates the clonal expansion of specific T helper and cytotoxic cells and B cells. This effect may be mediated by IL-2 (Fig. 1-10).

The mechanism of IL-1 action is not entirely understood. It may induce production IL-1 or IL-2 receptor expression (or both) after the initial signal for activation of the lymphocytes is received. IL-2 alone is sufficient to maintain T-lymphocytes in long-term culture. Human IL-2 is effective in doing this with lymphocytes from human beings and other species as well.

IL-1 also has many effects on nonlymphoid cells. It can markedly stimulate synovial cells to produce prostaglandins and collagenase [68]. Human dermal fibroblast proliferation is enhanced. Hepatocytes can be induced to produce acute phase reactants [69]. Fever induction is discussed in the section Macrophages (Adherent Cells). Serum amyloid A is elevated, possibly related to chronic inflammation.

IL-2 had been previously termed T-cell growth factor, K-cell helper factor, thymocyte-activating factor, T-cell mitogen factor, and T-cell replicating factor. Its molecular weight is 30,000. It is produced only if macrophages and IL-1 are present [70,71]. In addition to the actions previously noted, it can enhance natural K-cell activity without the presence of antigen and can boost development of T cytotoxic cells in concert with antigen [72].

T-Cell Activation by Mitogens. Mitogen action on lymphocytes is discussed earlier in the chapter, and the mechanism by which this occurs seems to be as follows: the initial phase of activation is characterized by

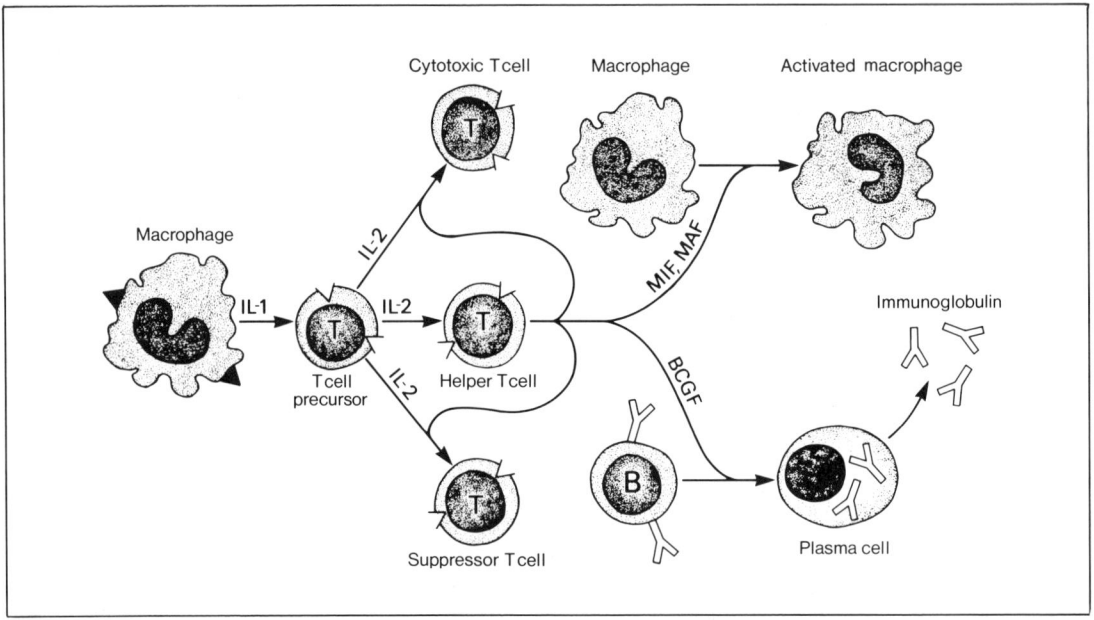

FIG. 1-10 Schema showing interleukin 1 and 2, migration inhibitory factor, macrophage activating factor, and B cell growth factor interactions affecting the macrophage, T and B cells.

nuclear activation with new RNA and protein synthesis and the appearance of IL-2 receptors; the second phase involves mitogen-dependent production of IL-1 by accessory cells, resulting in the production of IL-2 by T cells. The process involves a double signal—the first supplied by the mitogen, which moves the lymphocyte from a restricted G or G_0 phase of the cell cycle into a late G_1 phase and the second, supplied by IL-2, which moves the cell into the S phase and mitosis [13] (Fig. 1-11).

Mitogens induce calcium influx into lymphocytes and increases cyclic guanosine monophosphate (cGMP). The generation of cGMP derives from guanylate cyclase activation resulting from release of membrane arachidonic acid and its conversion to lipoxygenase products. The process enhances cellular activity [73].

IDIOTYPIC REGULATION. Before discussing idiotypic regulation of the immune response it is necessary to distinguish among isotypes, allotypes, and idiotypes. *Isotypes* are the antigenic differences that characterize the class and subclass of heavy (H) chains and the type and subtypes of light (L) chains. *Allotypes* are polymorphic allelic forms of the H and L chains. The antigenic determinants are usually localized to the C region of the Ig molecule. *Idiotypes* are antigenic determinants that distinguish one variable region of an Ig molecule from another and are located on the variable region of the H and L chains. A single individual has multiple

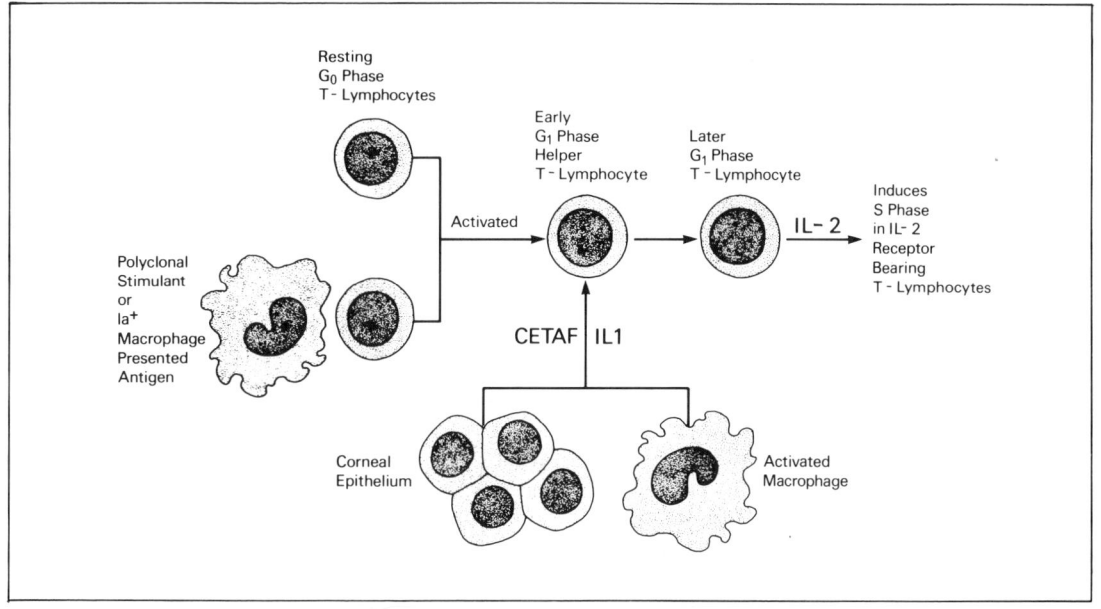

FIG. 1-11 Mitogen or macrophage present—antigen can stimulate lymphocyte to prophase from the G resting phase to the active S phase.

idiotypes. Idiotypes have been demonstrated on antibody molecules, receptors, and antigen-binding factors. An idiotype is made up of individual variations on the molecule termed *idiotopes*. As such, the same idiotope may occur on different idiotypes. In addition to idiotypic-positive antibody, it has been demonstrated that an antibody response may be directed against the specific idiotype of the first antibody. In turn, this second antibody may demonstrate a unique idiotype. Similarly, suppressor T cells or suppressor T-cell factors (T_s-1) may be generated in response to antigenic challenge. Both the cells and the factors have idiotypic representation. A secondary immune response may be generated by T_s-2 suppressor cells or suppressor cell factors (T_sF-2), which have anti-idiotype 1 activity. T_s-2 suppressor cells or suppressor cell factors in turn may have unique idiotypic features. Thus in terms of regulation of a T-cell response, antigen would stimulate suppressor T cells (T_s-1) to produce suppressor factors (T_sF-1). This factor would in turn stimulate a second population of T suppressor cells (T_s-2) followed by the production of a second T-cell suppressor factor (T_sF-2) and result in suppression of T-cell immunity. In the B-cell system antigen would stimulate a precursor clone of B cells with idiotype-1 to produce specific antibody (idiotype-1). The antibody would then stimulate anti-idiotypic B cells with anti-idiotypic-1 specificity. This would result in inhibition of further antibody production. Under certain circumstances, rather than inhibition, stimulation of the immune response has been observed. Idiotypic–anti-idiotypic responses are precise regulators of the immune response.

Dysfunction of T- and B-Lymphocytes

The diagnostic approach to the immune deficiency disorders begins with a history of recurrent, severe microbial infection. A family history is helpful in establishing a genetic basis. Once the diagnosis is suspected, in addition to the commonly available tests of T- and B-lymphocyte functions, monoclonal antibody tests directed at T-cell subsets are helpful. For example, in a recent study [74] several subtypes of disorders were found to occur in severe combined immunodeficiency, an autosomal recessive and x-linked disease. One type was associated with no lymphocytes with surface markers, another type with the failure to develop beyond early OKT9 and OKT10 stage of development, and a third type with a failure to differentiate beyond a late thymocyte stage (OKT3, 4, 5, 8, and 10).

The essential disorders caused by B-cell dysfunction are as follows:

1. Infantile X-linked agammaglobulinemia (Bruton's disease)
2. Transient hypogammaglobulinemia of infancy, a sporadically inherited disease
3. Selective immunoglobulinemia deficiency
4. X-linked immunodeficiency with hyper-IgM, an autosomal recessive inherited disease
5. Common variable hypogammaglobulinemia with low IgA, autosomal dominant, autosomal recessive, and sporadic inheritance pattern, and low IgG subclass with the same inheritance pattern
6. Secondary deficiency in nephrotic syndrome, chronic malnutrition, chronic lymphatic leukemia, myeloma, myotonic dystrophy, and selective immunosuppressive therapy

The essential disorders caused by T-cell dysfunctions are (1) congenital thymic-parathyroid aplasia (Di George's syndrome; sporadically inherited); (2) episodic lymphopenia with lymphocytotoxin; and (3) secondary deficiency owing to Hansen's disease (leprosy), Hodgkin's disease, chronic lymphocytic leukemia, several virus or parasitic infections, and cartilage-hair hypoplasia (autosomal recessive).

Combined B- and T-lymphocyte dysfunction occurs in (1) thymic aplasia with low IgA (ataxia telangiectasia; autosomal recessive); (2) immunodeficiency with normal or hyperimmunoglobulinemia; (3) X-linked T-cell dysfunction with low IgM (Wiskott-Aldrich syndrome); and (4) immunodeficiency secondary to severe chronic protein deprivation, radiation, the use of immunosuppressive drugs, and aging.

With aging there is a decrease in the total number of lymphocytes, both T and B cells. The response of T cells to phytohemagglutinin and concanavalin A and the mixed lymphocyte tumor cell culture reaction is also diminished. The percentage of T helper cells increases as does synthesis of IgG and plasma levels of IgG and IgA [75, 76].

In addition to B- and T-cell dysfunction, stem-cell dysfunction can also occur in patients with (1) severe combined immunodeficiency (Swiss type; autosomal recessive X-linked), (2) immunodeficiency with one or more normal immunoglobulins (Nezelof's syndrome; sporadically inherited, autosomal recessive), and (3) immunodeficiency with hematopoietic hypoplasia [77].

T-lymphocyte or B-lymphocyte deficiencies (or deficiencies of both) may be caused by enzyme defects. Recently, adenosine deaminase deficiency has been discovered in some patients with these disorders. The mechanisms involved in causing suppression of the immune system are still to be evolved.

Some malignancies are associated with certain lymphocyte types. Waldenström's macroglobulinemia, chronic lymphatic leukemia and Burkitt's lymphoma are B-cell tumors. Some lymphosarcomas are associated with B and null cells. Lymphoblastic leukemia in children, mycosis fungoides, and Sezary's disease are associated with T cells infiltrates.

Patients with Sjögren's syndrome may have polyclonal B-cell infiltrates.

Immunologic Tolerance

Potential antigens reach the lymphoid cells curing their developing, immunologically immature phase in the perinatal period and suppress in some way any future response to that antigen when the animal reaches immunologic maturity. By this means, unresponsiveness to one's own bodily components (self) can be established. Any foreign cells introduced into the body during this period can trick the animal into treating this foreign nonself material as self. The animal then has immunologic tolerance to this nonself material.

Immunologic tolerance can be induced in the adult as well. There are two levels of antigen dosage—very high and very low—at which tolerance (referred to as "high zone" or "low zone" tolerance) can be achieved within a few hours. In the absence of persistent antigen, it can last from 4 to 7 months. Weigle [78, 79] has pinpointed the T cell as the target of tolerance at low-antigen levels. Several possible explanations of this phenomenon have been suggested: (1) There may be a special type of T cell that suppresses potentially reactive lymphocytes, (2) T cells that are responding to the antigen may be eliminated; or (3) immune complexes may block the receptor sites of the T cells.

Both B- and T-lymphocytes can be made unresponsive at high-antigen doses. The period of induction is relatively long, and in the absence of persistent antigen, tolerance is short-lived. The greater difficulty in making B cells tolerant may be related to the higher concentration of surface receptors. B-cell tolerance can be attributed to the depletion of specific B-lymphocytes after their interaction with antigen or the suppression of B-lymphocytes by the T cells of tolerant animals.

Tolerance can be more readily established if immunosuppressive drugs such as cyclophosphamide are given. Cyclophosphamide has a cytotoxic effect on antigenically stimulated dividing B cells that would otherwise be difficult to make unresponsive. Soluble antigens are more tolerogenic than aggregated or particulate antigens.

IL-2 administration during the induction of tolerance to a specific hapten/skin sensitizer dinitrofluorobenzene can reproducibly intervene and partially reverse the tolerance induction.

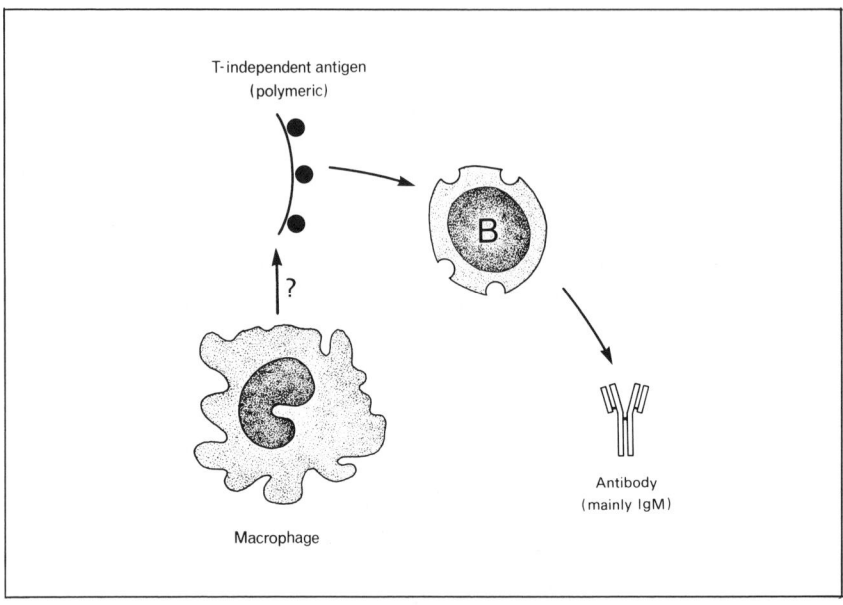

FIG. 1-12   B cells triggered without help.

Immunologic Enhancement

Enhancement is the achievement of increased survival of foreign (nonself) antigens. Enhancing antibodies, administered or produced under appropriate conditions, combine with the surface antigens of the target cells, which are then no longer accessible to the receptors on the sensitized aggressor lymphocytes. This combination avoids the activation of complement or of nonspecific K cells. The suppression of CMI may also be an important factor in immunologic enhancement.

T- and B-Lymphocyte Interaction

B-cell maturation, from stem cells to antibody secreting cells, is a stepwise process in which changes in the distribution of cytoplasmic and membrane immunoglobulin occur. Pre-B cells contain cytoplasmic IgM and, as maturation proceeds, the immature B cells express surface IgM and subsequently IgG and IgD. B-cell activation and maturation occur as a result of specific stimulation of B cells and expansion of factors produced by T helper cells. B cells may be activated by antigen, anti-idiotype, mitogens, or anti-Ig.

Rarely antigens seem able to go directly to B-lymphocytes and trigger them for antibody production (Fig. 1-12). They do not require the collaboration of T cells, and for the latter reason are called *T-independent antigens*. These antigens are such substances as pneumococcal polysaccharide, dextran, and (polyvinylpyrrolidine). All are polymers, and there are some unusual behavior patterns in the antibody responses to them: They are almost exclusively IgM, little or no "memory" is produced, and tolerance is readily induced.

How can T-independent antigens be explained? Some observers believe that B cells require two signals for efficient triggering: the specific

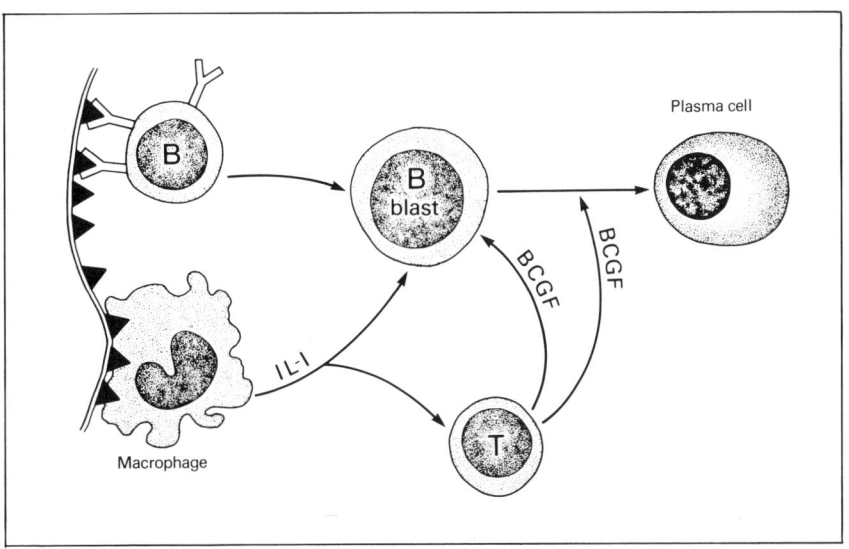

FIG. 1-13 Macrophages, T cells, and antigen can stimulate B cells (B cell growth factor).

signal (the antigenic determinant that the B cell is programmed to recognize), and a nonspecific signal that helps trigger the B cell or causes its differentiation and proliferation. Because adjuvants seem to be potent auxiliaries in antibody production, the nonspecific signal has been called adjuvanticity. Because T-lymphocytes regularly produce these helper or nonspecific signals, how do the T-independent antigens work? It seems possible that they serve also as general B-cell mitogens, that they carry their own adjuvanticity, and that they thus trigger both signals without T-cell help. Macrophages may play an important role in this situation.

But most antigens are not like these T-independent ones. Most antigens are not polymers; in contrast, they induce both IgG and IgA as well as IgM antibody responses, memory is produced, tolerance is not easily produced, and the antibody responses to them are thymus-dependent.

Helper T cells recognize antigen in the context of Ia determinants on macrophages [80] and as a result of this recognition soluble factors are produced that act on B cells. Antigen specific, Ia-restricted interactions with macrophages lead to the production of these antigen-nonspecific factors. These factors act only on activated B cells or blasts. The B cells become activated after recognizing antigen. Specifically, once activated B cells express a receptor for B cell growth factor (BCGF), this factor and IL-1 are required to drive the B cells into the S phase (replication) [70] (Fig. 1-13). There is little information about the receptor for the IL-1 or BCGF on the B cells. Under the influence of BCGF, proliferation of B cells occurs with the expression of a receptor for B cell differentiation factor (BCDF), also produced by helper T cells. This factor induces polyclonal maturation of B cells to Ig secretion without replication [70, 80].

Helper T cells grown in the absence of macrophages (accessory cells)

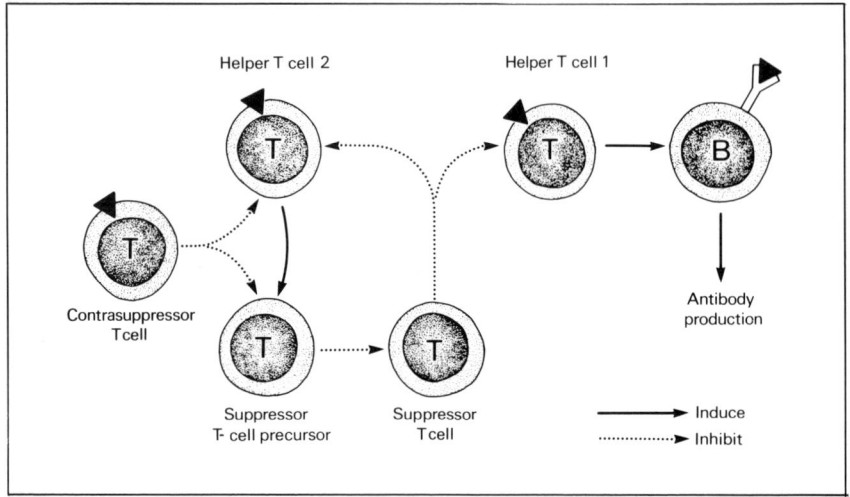

FIG. 1-14 The complex interaction of suppressor and helper T cells is depicted. The contrasuppressor T cell when stimulated by antigen can inhibit helper T cell and suppressor T cell precursor activity. Suppressor T cells can inhibit helper T cell activity.

and antigens but in the presence of IL-2 can be induced by certain mitogens to produce BCGF and BCDF [80].

This interaction of helper T cells, antigen, and macrophages mimics mitogens in their stimulatory capacity to activate B cell blasts in a polyclonal fashion [80].

The effect on nonspecific T-cell stimuli can also be seen in other situations: Mixtures of allogeneic cells can stimulate each other to produce nonspecific T-cell products, and these products can substitute for T cells in triggering B-cell responses to T-dependent antigens.

It has been recognized that suppressor T cells act as negative regulators of B-cell maturation, inhibiting the process. These cells have been implicated in virtually all of the known immunologic regulatory mechanisms [81, 82] (i.e., maintenance of tolerance, antigenic competition, control of antibody responses to thymus-dependent and thymus-independent antigens, and control of IgE-antibody responses). We now know that many immunodeficiency and autoimmune diseases are associated with disorders of this negative regulatory or suppressor-cell system [83, 84], and suppressor cells have been implicated in the immunologic enhancement of tumor growth [85].

Suppressor T cells can generally be differentiated from helper T cells because of their high density, radiation resistance, steroid resistance, and Fc receptor for IgG, whereas helper T cells are low density, are radiation and steroid sensitive, and have an Fc receptor for IgM (Fig. 1-14).

Suppressor T cells need IL-2 and cofactors for growth and differentiation [86].

A population of suppressor B cells has been recently described [87]. These cells inhibit primary and secondary humoral immune responses and inhibit contact and delayed-type hypersensitivity to a variety of extrinsic antigens.

Natural Killer Cells

NK activity has been described in human beings and other species. NK activity does not require MHC products to be present on target cell membranes and previous sensitization to produce cytotoxicity against target cells [88]. This contrasts with the cytotoxic T cells and K cells. The K cell is a lymphocyte without T- or B-cell surface markers (null cell), which can be differentiated from NK cells by a monoclonal IgM antibody (HNK-1) [89].

NK cells have characteristics distinct from other lymphoid cells. NK cells are closely associated with the large granular lymphocytes. They are neither phagocytic nor plastic adherent (nonmacrophage), and they lack surface immunoglobulin and receptors for the third component of complement (non-T or non-B). They do contain receptors for the Fc portion of IgG, a property that enables them to bind to antibody-coated target cells and mediate ADCC. (A number of other cells have cytotoxic capacities toward antibody-coated target cells, including macrophages, PMNLs, platelets, fetal liver cells, and K cells; Fig. 1-15.) Functionally, this mechanism would be expected to be important when the targets, for example, solid tumors, transplants, and large parasites, are too large for ingestion by phagocytosis.

NK cell activity is greater in males and in the young and can be decreased in certain disease states (i.e., lupus erythematosus) [90]. Isolation of NK cells for study and therapy may be accomplished by lectin binding and fluorescence-activated cell sorting (FACS) [91].

The soluble factors that can regulate NK cell activity include the interferons (alpha, beta, and gamma) [92], the interleukins (IL-1, 2, and 3) [93], thymic serum factor, prostaglandin E_2 and other cyclic adenosine monophosphate (cAMP) elevators [94], hormones (diethylstilbestrol, estradiol, hydrocortisone), immune complexes, antibodies, endotoxins, certain proteolytic enzymes, phospholipase A, and phorbol ester [95]. Thymocytes, macrophages, and granulocytes may also regulate NK cell activity. Natural cytotoxic cells are another type of effector cell in mice that may be related to the NK cells [96].

Macrophages (Adherent Cells)

Ia antigen-bearing (Ia^+) nonlymphocyte cells that trigger immune responses are called accessory cells or antigen-presenting cells almost interchangeably. Accessory cells not only mediate lymphocyte response to foreign antigens or mitogens but also directly stimulate T-cell proliferation to cause a mixed leukocyte reaction. Ia^+ macrophages are accessory cells, because accessory-cell activity usually resides in the adherent cell population and macrophages are the classical adherent cell. Recently, however, studies on Ia^+ nonmacrophage cells have indicated that dendritic cells and epidermal Langerhans' cells [97] serve as accessory cells

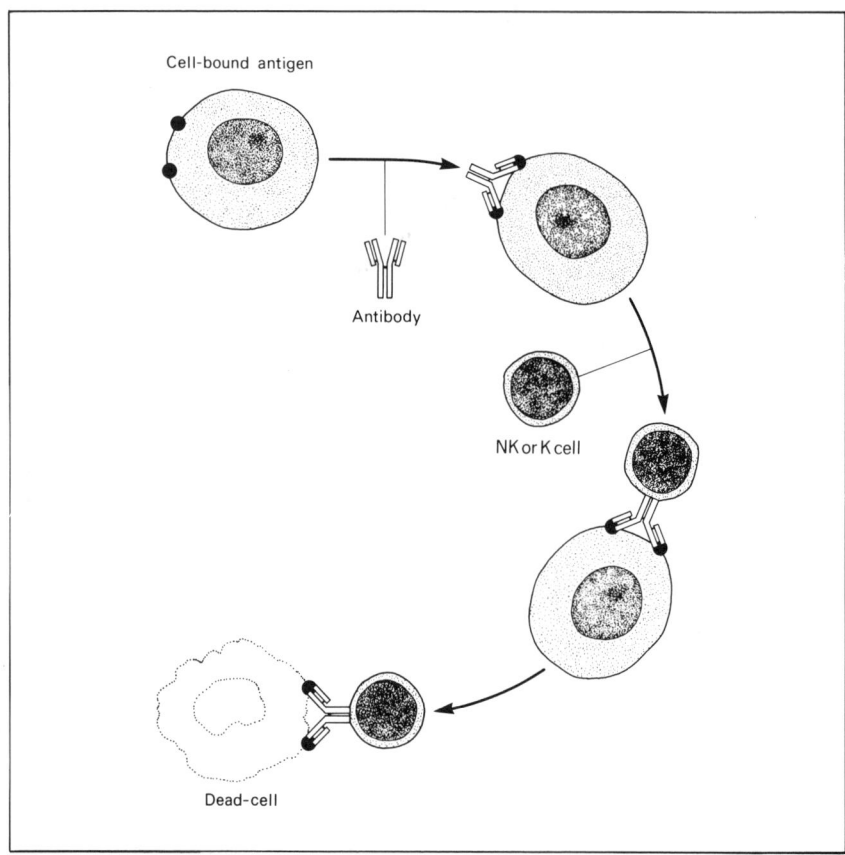

FIG. 1-15 The Fab segment of the antibody molecule can combine with cellular antigen leaving the FC portion exposed. Killer or natural killer cells can adhere to this exposed segment of the molecule activating the antibody to cause cell death. (Modified from an illustration by Gerald Weissmann, M.D., that appeared in R. A. Good and D. W. Fisher (Eds.), *Immunobiology*, Stamford, Conn.: Sinauer Associates, 1971. Reproduced with permission.)

as well [98]. Langerhans' cells can express Fc IgG and C_3 receptors as well as Ia^+ [99], whereas dendritic cells do not [100].

Macrophages are essential for the development of cellular and humoral immunocompetence. First, the induction of T-lymphocyte proliferation requires the physical association of these cells with macrophages-bearing antigens as previously noted. Second, the macrophage is a principal site of control by the immune-response gene [101]. Third, macrophages have receptors that augment the killing and phagocytosis of infectious agents, and fourth, macrophages secrete a wide range of biologically active molecules that influence development of the afferent limb of the immune response.

Macrophage membranes possess receptors for the Fc portion of certain classes of antibodies. An antibody that fixes in this way to macrophage membranes is called a cytophilic antibody and may play a major role in immune reactions, for example, hemolytic anemia and infections.

Subpopulations of macrophages express Fc receptors for IgE. The relatively low binding affinity of monomeric IgE to this receptor suggests that the function of this receptor on the macrophage may be to interact predominantly with performed IgE immune aggregates such as soluble immune complexes or IgE-coated parasites [102].

Mackaness and colleagues [103] substantiated several theories of the role of lymphocytes and macrophages in immune responses to infection. T-lymphocytes are the vectors and macrophages are the effectors of CMI. Macrophages have no memory for a previously encountered antigen but may acquire memory by interacting with lymphocytes and their products (lymphokines). Macrophages are necessary for the production of some lymphokines (e.g., macrophage-activating factor and monocyte chemotactic factor). Clones of T-lymphocytes have receptors for antigen on their surfaces, and some of these receptors may be transferred to the macrophage.

Macrophages have characteristics that fit them particularly well for the functions noted previously. For example, they have well-developed phagocytic activity, an ability to adhere to charge surfaces, motility, lysosomal enzymes, membrane receptors for the Fc portion of certain complement components (C3) and the Ig molecule, and they respond to chemotactic stimuli. Many of these characteristics are more prominent when the macrophage is activated [104, 105]. In animal studies, macrophage activation is associated with increases in cell size, in the ability to spread on glass and adhere to a charged surface, in phagocytic activity, in microbiocidal and digestive capacities, in glucose oxidation, and in the release of some of the lysosomal enzymes.

Activated macrophages secrete complement proteins (C1, C2, C3, C4, and factor B), colony-stimulating factor, macrophage growth factor, angiogenesis factor, hydrogen peroxide, interferon, plasminogen activator, collagenase, elastase, lysozyme, bacteriocidins, endogenous pyrogen (IL-1; a stimulatory factor for leukocyte production), hyaluronidase, leukotrienes, prostaglandin E (PGE), and other products [106]. As a result, fibrin meshworks, collagen and elastin fibers, and probably ground substance can be lysed as the macrophage proceeds toward its target. PGE may inhibit T-cell proliferation, rosette formation, cytotoxicity, and the release of lymphokines from activated T cells, acting in this way as a negative feedback mechanism (Fig. 1-16). PGE may also inhibit the responses of NK cells and even macrophages. Clonal proliferation of macrophage stem cells may be inhibited as well as the expression of Ia-like antigen on their surface. Interestingly, PGE may enhance some T-cell populations, such as suppressor cells [107]. Preliminary work in patients with Hodgkin's disease reveals that macrophage prostaglandins may play a major role in suppressing the CMI. Macrophage suppressor activity may be important in suppressing inflammation in patients with chronic diseases.

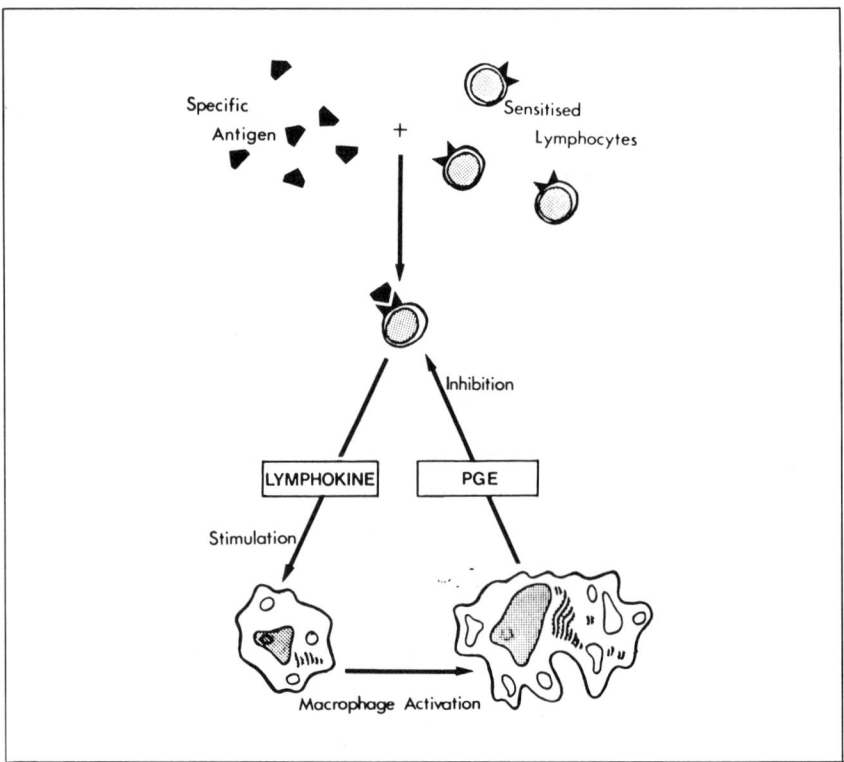

FIG. 1-16 Activated macrophages can release prostaglandins, which inhibit lymphokine production by sensitized lymphocytes.

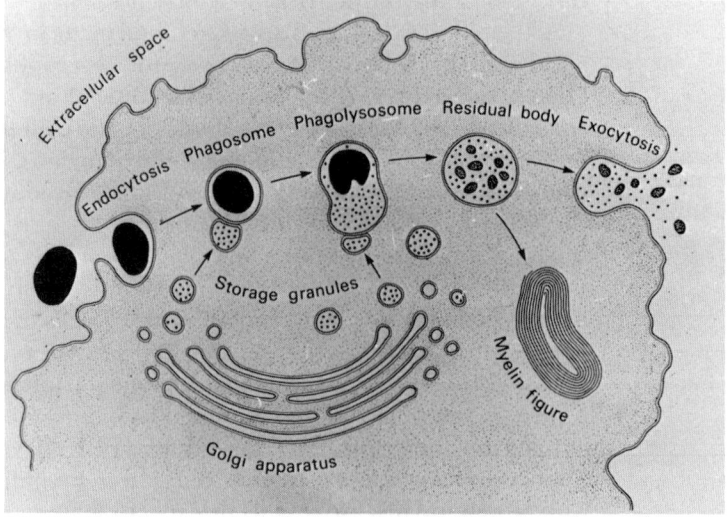

FIG. 1-17 Phagosome activity. (Modified from an illustration by Gerald Weissmann, M.D., that appeared in R. A. Good and D. W. Fisher (Eds.), *Immunobiology*, Stamford, Conn.: Sinauer Associates, 1971. Reproduced with permission.)

Phagocyte
Function

Both macrophages and PMNLs function as phagocytic cells.

The rapid attraction of large numbers of phagocytes to target sites is undoubtedly crucial to the host defense against microorganisms. Phagocyte function can be divided into six interdependent steps: (1) random movement, (2) chemotaxis, (3) attachment to material, (4) ingestion, (5) activation of the phagocyte, and (6) destruction of the foreign material.

1. *Random movement.* Random movement is the nondirectional movement of cells [108] and is measured by their migration through a capillary tube or porous filter. Random movement and chemotaxis are separate events, the former one is normal while the latter is abnormal, for example, in Chédiak-Higashi syndrome [109].

2. *Chemotaxis.* There are two steps in chemotaxis: activation of the phagocytic cell membrane by the chemotactic agent and cell movement [110, 111]. Measurement of chemotaxis is usually performed in a Boyden-type chamber. This chamber consists of two compartments separated by a single membrane with small pores; the upper compartment contains the cells, the lower the chemotactic substance.

Defective chemotaxis is noted in the following disease entities: lazy leukocyte syndrome [112], Chédiak-Higashi syndrome [113], familial chemotactic defect [114], Wiskott-Aldrich syndrome [115], malignant melanoma [116], hyperimmunoglobulinemia E syndromes, chronic mucocutaneous candidiasis [117], Job-Buckley syndrome [118], atopic dermatitis [119], chronic granulomatous disease, staphylococcal abscesses [120], diabetes [121], acrodermatitis enteropathica, Down's syndrome, mannosidase deficiency, sepsis, malnutrition, lupus erythematosus, and rheumatoid arthritis.

3. *Attachment to material.* The phagocyte must next seek out and attach itself to the foreign material. The adherence of microorganisms to phagocytic surfaces is called *enhanced phagocytosis*. The attached phagocytes can then transport particles from the extracellular space to within the phagocytes and their vacuoles (phagosomes). Defective adherence can occur in myotonic dystrophy or be drug-induced by salicylates, ethanol, or steroids.

4. *Ingestion.* Investigation of the process of ingestion has uncovered many facts about this complex series of events. Of special interest are the importance of cell-membrane receptors for IgG and C3 in the process of opsonization, the role of microtubules and the contractile proteins (actin and myosin) within the cell, and the importance of the divalent cations— manganese, cobalt, magnesium, and calcium—in the phagocytic process [122] (Fig. 1-17).

5. *Activation of the phagocyte.* Activation of the phagocyte's intracellular metabolism is required for the destruction of foreign material. The metabolic events are a dramatic increase of glucose utilization through the hexose monophosphate shunt, an uptake of oxygen, and the production and release of superoxide and hydrogen peroxide [123]. This "respiratory burst" can be detected within seconds of contact between cells and phagocytic particles.

6. *Destruction of the foreign material.* The destruction of foreign material by neutrophilic polymorphonuclear leukocytes is caused by oxygen-dependent and oxygen-independent factors [124]. The oxygen-dependent factors are myeloperoxidase-mediated or myeloperoxidase-independent (mediated by peroxidase, hydroxyl radicals, singlet oxygen, or superoxide); the oxygen-independent factors are acid hydrolases, neutral proteases, lysozyme, lactoferrin, and cationic lysosomal proteins [125]. The myeloperoxidase system, which uses hydrogen peroxide and superoxide, remains the most important microbicidal activity studied to date.

A variety of stimuli can cause granule exocytosis by normal human PMNLs which results in the destruction of the foreign material. Phagocytosis, interaction with an opsonized nonphagocytosable surface, bacterial toxins, hydroxyeicosatetraenoic acid (HETE), and lectins (concanavalin A) are some examples.

Defects in microbicidal activity occur in Chédiak-Higashi syndrome, chronic granulomatous disease, myeloperoxidase deficiency, diabetes, malnutrition, and sepsis.

Antibiotics may affect neutrophil function. Phagocytosis can be depressed by systemic administration of tetracycline, amphotericin B, or polymyxin B; oxidative metabolism can be depressed by sulfonamides, tetracycline, amphotericin B, and polymyxin B; and microbicidal activity can be hindered by sulfonamides and aminoglycosides. Chemotaxis can be enhanced by the systemic administration of nafcillin, bacitracin, lincomycin, clindamycin, and chloramphenicol. Clindamycin, chloramphenicol, rifampin, tetracycline, and amphotericin B can also depress chemotaxis of PMNLs.

Although phagocytes can perform all their functions without the help of complement or antibody, both of these substances improve their performance.

Interestingly, PMNLs can delay corneal epithelial wound healing in vitro [126].

Inflammation

There are neurogenic and nonneurogenic causes of vasomotor activity. The capillaries, precapillaries, and smaller arterioles are affected by chemical materials, and the large vessels proximal to the terminal arterioles are affected by the nervous system. Of the complicated, nonneurogenic causes, the most important are (1) vasoactive amines, including histamine, leukotrienes, chemotactic factors, and serotonin; (2) serum proteases and polypeptides known as *kinins;* and (3) PGE and PGF. In specific types of inflammation, some mediators play more prominent roles than others.

KININ, FIBRINOLYTIC, AND CLOTTING SYSTEMS. The kinins are a family of vasoactive polypeptides that can elicit pain, increase vascular permeability and produce edema, contract intestinal smooth muscle, and alter vascular tone. The interrelationships of the kinin-generating system, the fibrinolytic system, the clotting system, and the complement

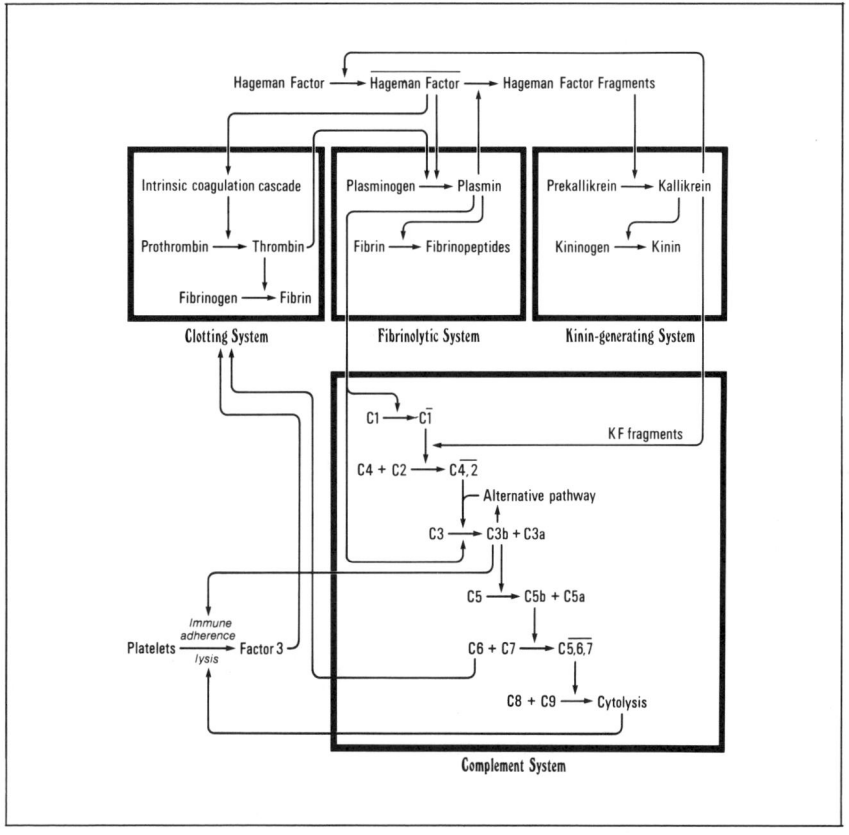

FIG. 1-18 Interactions among complement, clotting, fibrinolytic, and kinin-generating systems.

system are complex. Although the details of their interactions are not fully understood, the following facts are ample evidence that the four systems do indeed interact (Fig. 1-18).

As noted in Figure 1-18, Hageman factor (clotting factor XII) plays an important role in the clotting, kinin, and fibrinolytic systems. Activation of Hageman factor initiates both the intrinsic coagulation sequence (e.g., the thrombotic occlusion of small vessels) and the plasmin system. Plasmin, in addition to cleaving polymerized fibrin into vasoactive fibrinopeptides, cleaves activated Hageman factor. The cleaved fragments activate the kinin system, which increases vascular permeability, the chemotaxis of PMNLs, and the production of a fragment (KF) that makes C1 more efficient in the production of C4,2.

Plasmin also initiates the complement system by activating C1, and it can directly generate anaphylatoxin from C3. C1 esterase inhibitor inhibits plasmin, kinin generation, thrombin, and activated Hageman factor.

Finally, the clotting system can be activated by the immune adherence of platelets to C3b, and by the subsequent release of clot-promoting platelet factor (factor 3). C6 apparently also promotes clotting.

The plasma components of inflammation are coagulation, fibrinolysis, kinin-generation, and complement [127]. During acute phase response proteinase inhibitors (α_1-antitrypsin and α_1-antichymotrypsin), complement proteins (C1s, C2, C3, C4, C5, C56, C9, and B), coagulation proteins (fibrinogen, prothrombin, factor VIII, and plasminogen), transport proteins, and other substances (C-reactive protein, amyloid A, ceruloplasmin, fibronectin, and α_1-acid glycoprotein) are increased. The coagulation system can cause thrombosis, generate kinin, activate complement, release platelets, and induce chemotaxis [128, 129]. The fibrinolytic system can cause thromobolysis, generate kinin, induce chemotaxis, activate complement, and increase proteolytic activity [130]. The kinin system can cause edema and vasodilation, chemotaxis, and proteolytic activity [131]. The complement system can cause cytolysis, chemotaxis, immune adherence, lysosomal release, histamine release, lymphocyte stimulation, thrombolysis, and proteolytic activity [132].

COMPLEMENT SYSTEM. During the study of the lytic properties of antisera early in the history of immunology, it was discovered that both a specific antibody and complementary nonspecific factors found in fresh serum were required for cell lysis. These factors were called the *complement system* or simply C.

The classic complement system consists of nine separate components, C1 through C9. When activated, these components interact sequentially with one another in a so-called cascade similar to the coagulation sequence. The individual components were numbered in the order of their discovery, which is not precisely the same as the order of their activation: C4 is out of sequence; because it is second in the sequence of activated components, the order of activation is C1, C4, C2, C3, C5, C6, C7, C8, and C9.

Classical Pathway of Complement Activation. In general, the activation of the components of the complement system requires the enzymatic cleavage of each component into two fragments. The larger of the two joins the preceding activated component, which generates new enzymatic activity that can cleave the next component. The smaller fragments in the earlier steps frequently have inflammatory properties of their own. For example, C4 and C2 fragments have kininlike activity, C3b enhances phagocytosis, C3A and C5A produce an anaphylatoxin and cause chemotaxis, and C567 also causes chemotaxis (Fig. 1-19).

Antibody plays three roles in immune cytolysis by complement: (1) It selects the target for the complement task; (2) it serves as a site of attachment for the first component of complement; and (3) it triggers the conversion of inactive C1 to enzymatically active C1. Immunoglobulins vary in their ability to bind C1: IgG and IgM antibodies bind C1; IgA apparently does not. C1 has three subunits: C1q, C1r, and C1s. The interaction of C1q with antibody results in the conversion of C1r from a proenzyme

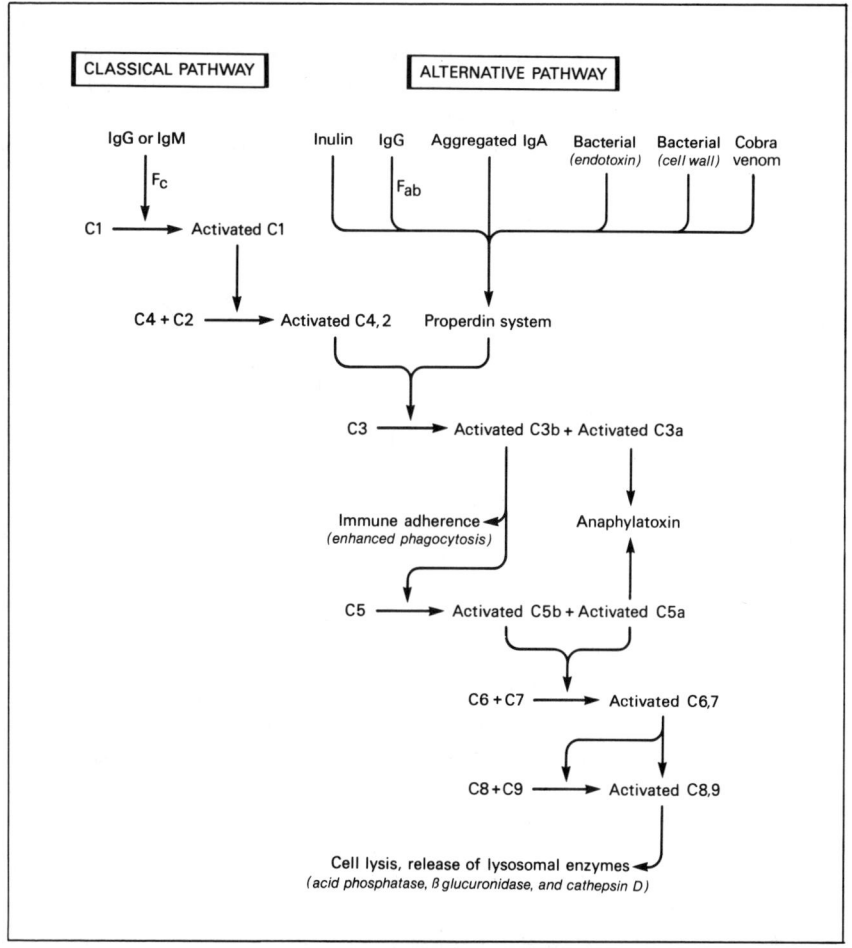

FIG. 1-19 The classical and alternative (properdin) pathways of the complement cascade are depicted.

to an active enzyme, which then converts the C1s enzyme from the precursor to the active form [133].

The binding of C4 to the cell surface is dependent on the action of $\overline{C1}$. (A bar over the numeral or numerals indicates activated complement components exhibiting enzymatic activity [134].) The formation of C1,4,2, from C1,4, and C2 takes place in two stages: Reversible binding of C2 in unaltered form is followed by enzymatic cleavage of C2 by $\overline{C1}$ [135].

The C1,4,2 complex is extremely labile [136]. Activated C4 and C2 form a bimolecular complex C4,2 (also called C3 convertase). This complex, through its C2 subunit [137], activates C2. This amplification step is important because one bimolecule of C4,2 can produce several hundred active C2 molecules [134]. The enzymatic activity of C4,2 on

Ce also produces a low molecular weight fragment (C3a), which is called anaphylatoxin because it can produce symptoms of anaphylaxis.

Another anaphylatoxin (C5a) is produced when C5 is activated by the peptidase-activated C3b. The activated C5 in turn interacts with C6 and C7 to form a trimolecular complex, C567 [138], which binds to the cell membrane and participates in cell lysis by serving as the focal point for the lytic action of C8 and C9. C567 may be bound to the cells with membrane-associated antibody and early C components, or it may exist in fluid form and can then react with unsensitized cells [139]. C567 is also chemotactic for PMNLs and thus participates in the inflammatory reaction. Once C567 becomes membrane-bound, C8 joins the complex, and six binding sites for C9 then develop on C8. The resulting complex produces functional holes in the cell membrane [140]. The binding of C5 to the cell's membrane produces a doubling of the membrane's thickness and a structural alteration that resembles holes. Studies carried out at the time of this step, however, have not uncovered any evidence of functional holes in the membranes. Functional holes appear only with the assembly of C8, but the addition of C9 greatly increases the velocity of the lytic reaction [141].

Alternate Pathway of Complement Activation. The alternate pathway, which is also called the properdin system, can be activated by a variety of substances, for example, aggregated immunoglobulins IgG 1,2,3, and 4; IgA; and IgE. The initiation site is the Fab area of the Ig molecule—in contrast to the initiation site in the classical pathway, which is the Fc area. The alternate pathway can also be initiated by bacterial endotoxins, bacterial cell walls, and polysaccharides (inulin). Properdin convertase, and then properdin, are activated sequentially. The active properdin then activates a factor D. The activated factor D in turn activates a factor B, which with C3b can activate C3. Activated factor D is also called "glycine-rich beta glycoproteinase"; and activated factor B is also called "glycine-rich gamma glycoprotein". The end result is thus an enzyme, distinct from C4,2, that activates C3 and the remainder of the complement sequence, bypassing C1, C4, and C2 of the classical pathway.

Regulation. Once activated, the complement sequence does not continue to cascade endlessly. Regulation is afforded by the following mechanisms:

1. The natural instability of C2, C3, C4, and C5, which are only transitorily activated by their respective activating enzymes [142]
2. The inhibitors of the hemolytically active forms of C1 [143], C3 [144], and C6 [145] that are normally present in the serum
3. *Immunoconglutinins,* which are autostimulated antibodies to autologous complement, are directed specifically against antigenic groups of bound-complement molecules [146], and have been described for C3 and C4
4. The local concentration of certain enzymes to which some of the complement components are sensitive (e.g., C3 is inactivated by trypsin [147]

Biologic Activity of Complement. Cytolysis can occur in three ways:

1. The classic mechanism of membrane damage by complement, referred to as immune cytolysis, requires antimembrane antibody and all the components of complement
2. Cytolysis independent of antibody occurs with the attachment of C567 to the cell surface [148]
3. Cytolysis results from interaction between complement and unsensitized mononuclear leukocytes [149]

The anaphylatoxins are derived from C3a and C5a. They can contract smooth muscle, can change capillary permeability, and are inhibited by antihistamines.

Kininlike activity has been mentioned as a product of C2 [150].

Chemotactic activity has been noted in the C3a fragment, the C5a fragment, and the macromolecule complex C567 [151]. A fragment of guinea pig C3 also stimulates lymphocytes to produce a chemotactic lymphokine [152].

Antigen-antibody complexes, plus C3b, can cause immune adherence of platelets and the subsequent release of their vasoactive amines. Complement-dependent mechanisms of histamine release, which are thought not to involve the anaphylatoxins, have been reported. Release of the vasoactive amines by the platelets may be one of the mechanisms.

Phagocytosis can be enhanced by C3b.

Complement may more directly affect the immune reaction by assisting in the processing, presentation, and trapping of antigen. Activation and differentiation of the B-lymphocyte (second signal) may be affected by complement as is the cyclical antibody response, the switch of IgM to IgG, and the generation of B memory cells [152, 153]. The specific antibody production to sheep red blood cells and polyclonal antibody production can be either enhanced or suppressed by the actions of C5a or C3a respectively [154].

T-cell proliferation and differentiation can be effected by complement (e.g., the induction of T suppressor cells and T helper cells). T-cell–mediated cytotoxicity may be enhanced or suppressed by C5a or C3a respectively. Monocytes are activated, and the production of IL-1 and prostaglandins are enhanced [152, 155]. Mitogen blastogenesis may also be enhanced.

Complement Defects. Serum from patients with hereditary angioneurotic edema lacks the inhibitor of C1 esterase [156]. The deficiency is inherited as an autosomal dominant trait.

C1r deficiency has been associated with dermatitis, necrotizing vasculitis, increased susceptibility to pyogenic infections, and renal disease that involves pseudolupus vasculitis of the kidneys [157, 158].

C2 deficiency is associated with a variety of syndromes resembling lupus erythematosus and other diseases that cause vasculitis of collagenous tissue. There is a delay in the generation of chemotactants and frequently an increased incidence of bacterial infections [159].

Three separate mechanisms resulting in C3 depletion have been described.

1. There is a failure of the synthesis of C3, and the addition of C3 to the serum of affected patients in vitro corrects the defect [160].
2. In a second form of C3 depletion, a deficiency of the C3b inactivator results in continuous activation of the properdin system and in the consumption of C3 [161]. This situation in turn results in faulty generation of the chemotactic substance C3a and the opsonin C3b. The addition of C3 to the serum of affected patients does not correct the defect because the added C3 is rapidly consumed.
3. In the third type of C3 deficiency, a proteolytic enzyme (a C3ase) is present. Addition of C3 to the serum of a patient with this defect also fails to correct the defect [162]. The homozygous C3 deficiency is associated with recurrent bacterial infections and with defective chemotaxis and phagocytosis.

Infants with C5 deficiency fail to thrive and have diarrhea and severe dermatitis (Leiner's disease) [163]. They are also susceptible to pyogenic infections. In the members of two families with this problem, C5 was present in their sera but was not functioning (i.e., did not generate C5a chemotactic factor); replacement of C5 by fresh plasma alleviated the symptoms of the disease [164].

In animals, a C6 deficiency has been reported in rabbits [165] and a C567 deficiency in mice [166]. Recently a C8 deficiency was reported in human beings as well as C789 deficiency in some patients with generalized gonorrhea.

CELLULAR FACTORS. The cellular components of inflammation are platelets, PMNLs, macrophages, and lymphocytes [167]. The platelets can cause adhesion (infarction) and can release lysosomal enzymes, adenosine phosphate, catecholamines, prostaglandins, cationic proteins, and procoagulants [168]. The PMNLs are phagocytic and can release proteolytic enzymes, synthesize prostaglandins and pyrogens, and activate complement [169, 170]. The macrophages are also phagocytic and can release proteolytic enzymes and modulate lymphocyte function (see earlier discussion). Lymphocyte activity is discussed in detail earlier in the chapter.

Arachidonic acid metabolites were first linked with inflammation in studies showing that the mechanical irritation of rabbit eyes released a mediator, called irin, into the anterior chamber of the eye. Irin has been now identified as PGE_2 and $PGF_{2\alpha}$. A list of arachidonic metabolites is shown in Figure 1-20. Although these metabolites help "drive" inflammatory reactions of all types, they are more important in some types of inflammation than in others [171]. For example, prostaglandins play a major role in the sunburn reaction, and the early stages of this reaction can be completely reversed by the topical application of the cyclooxygen-

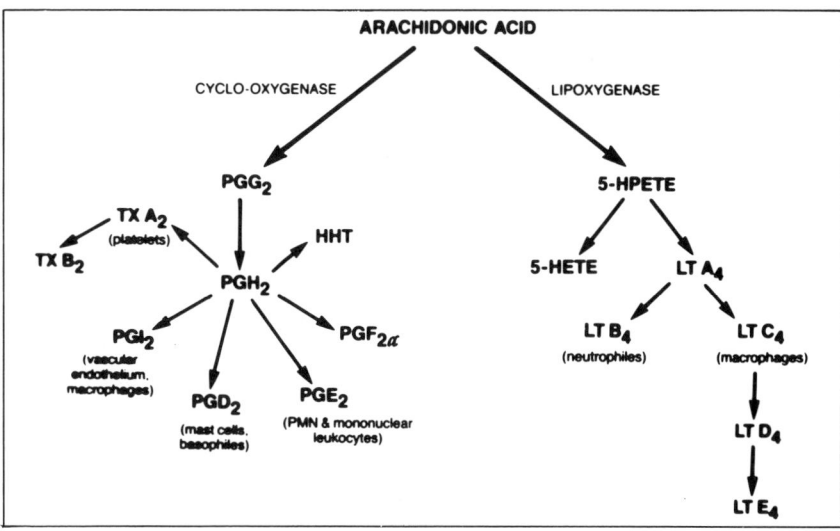

FIG. 1-20 Arachidonic acid can be broken down by the cyclooxygenase and lipoxygenase pathways into various pharmacologically active metabolites. (PG = prostaglandin; TX = thromboxane; HPETE = hydroxyperoxyeicosatetraenoic acid; HETE = hydroxyeicosatetraenoic acid; LT = leukotriene.)

ase inhibitor indomethacin [172]. The later stages are promoted by mediators released by the infiltrating PMNLs.

Prostaglandins also play an important role in allergic diseases, suppression of T-cell activity (lymphokine production, etc.) [173], and enhancing antibody production by inhibiting T suppressor cell actions [174].

All cell types seem to be able to generate prostaglandins, which they disgorge at the slightest provocation. Prostaglandins cause either vasoconstriction or vasodilatation, depending on the type of prostaglandin, vascular bed, or animal species. (Vasodilatation is the more frequent event.) Two features of the vascular effects of prostaglandins however, are not shared by other putative mediators of inflammation. The first is their sustained action and the second their ability to counteract the vasoconstriction caused by such substances as norepinephrine. Prostaglandins can cause hyperalgesia, and certain of them (e.g., PGE_1) may be leukotactic. The newly arrived leukocytes may then release more prostaglandins, further aggravating the vasodilatation, hyperalgesia, and fever, and in chronic inflammatory states, prostaglandins (e.g., PGE_1) may increase granuloma formation as well.

ANTI-INFLAMMATORY AGENTS. The anti-inflammatory agents presently available are nonsteroidal, steroidal, or cytotoxic, and their effect on the immune system may be specific or nonspecific.

Essentially all of the currently available nonsteroidal anti-inflammatory agents (NSAIAs) block the microsome cyclooxygenase enzyme system that modifies arachidonic acid to produce prostaglandins and thromboxanes. Thus by not affecting the lipoxygenase pathway, these agents have limited effectiveness. Newer NSAIAs are being developed that, in fact, may block both pathways. Most of the NSAIAs on the market are derivatives of salicylic acid, pyrozolin, indoleacetic acid, pyrrolic acid, propionic acid, anthranilic acid, and oxicam. These include aspirin and diflunisal (Dolobid); phenylbutazone (Butazolidin); indomethacin (Indocin) and sulindac (Clinoril); ibuprofen (Motrin, Rufen), fenoprofen (Nalfon), naproxen (Naprosyn), ketoprofen, and benoxaprofen; mefenamic acid (Ponstel); and piroxicam (Feldene) respectively. It has been shown that the administration of arachidonic acid analogs such as fish oils will also diminish prostaglandin and leukotriene release and may be helpful in altering the effects of these latter agents [175]. The enhancing inflammatory effects of the prostaglandins include sustained vasodilation, fever, granuloma formation, increased vascular permeability, and hyperalgesia. In addition, prostaglandins can counteract vasoconstriction caused by substances such as norepinephrin or angiotensin. The leukotrienes and HETEs can cause leukocyte chemotaxis and increased vascular permeability.

The NSAIAs have been effective in a variety of ocular disorders [176]. These agents can ameliorate or prevent elevation of the intraocular pressure (IOP) after arachidonic acid administration, aqueous flare and cells and miosis after trauma, elevation of the IOP after alkali burns of the cornea, reduced IOP after trauma, inflammation after paracentesis, elevation of IOP in herpetic uveitis, cystoid macula edema, and neovascularization of the cornea [177–179]. The side effects include renal damage [180], fixed drug eruptions, photosensitivity, toxic epidermal necrolysis, serum sickness, urticaria [181], and enhancement of ocular herpetic infection [182].

Corticosteroids are transported to the target tissue through the bloodstream or tissue fluids (e.g., tears). They enter the target cell and each molecule is then bound to a specific intracytoplasmic receptor. The corticosteroid-receptor complex is translocated to the nucleus where it is bound to the target cell genome. The target cell then responds by increased or decreased synthesis of specific messenger RNA. The messenger RNA is shifted to the cytoplasm where protein synthesis takes place with subsequent expression of the corticosteroid effect on the target cell. Action of the corticosteroid through these receptors accounts for a wide range of diverse effects on the target cells, including alteration of cellular enzymes, cell surface structures, and secretion of extracellular products [183].

The receptor has a differential binding affinity for various steroid compounds resulting in different relative potencies of the steroids. The least potent group includes cortisone and hydrocortisone; the intermediate group includes prednisone, prednisolone, methyl prednisolone, and triamcinolone; and the most potent glucocorticoid group includes betamethasone and dexamethasone. The steroid-induced response may persist for a considerable period of time (hours to days) after the agent is no longer present in the target cell, depending on the half-life of the products regulated by the steroid. This persistence may partially account for the need for infrequent steroid administration to control some ocular inflammatory processes. This low dosage may allow a separation of beneficial steroid effects from harmful ones where different dose-response relationships exist.

The relative potency of the steroids to elicit a response is in general agreement with the receptor-binding activities of the steroid.

Steroidal anti-inflammatory agents can block both the cyclooxygenase and lipoxygenase pathways by causing the cells to produce a protein called lipomodulin that inhibits phospholipase A_2 production, which in turn inhibits the release of arachidonic acid [177]. Steroids increase the levels of adenyl cyclase, increase the levels of cAMP in human leukocytes, enhance the cAMP response produced by PGE, and potentiate the effect of β-adrenergic catecholamines [184–186]. All these actions diminish the release of the vasoactive amines (e.g., heparin, platelet-activating factor, histamine, eosinophil chemotactic factor, and others) from the mast cells and basophils. The histamine content of the tissues is reduced [187], and eosinopenia and basophilopenia can occur. Steroids also constrict the blood vessels [188], and this action diminishes vascular permeability and postinflammatory neovascularization [189]. This reduction can affect favorably both the afferent and efferent limbs of the rejection phenomenon. Steroids can reduce complement levels and perhaps antagonize the kallikrein-kinin system [183]. Neutrophil chemotaxis [190] is diminished and stabilization of the lysosomal enzymes [191] is enhanced, and these processes in turn reduce the amount of necrosis and subsequent neovascularization. There is also a drop in the number of both the blood monocytes and the monocytes at the inflammatory sites [192].

Steroids also affect the immune system directly. They can cause transient lymphopenia, which reaches its maximum effect in 4 to 6 hours and lasts for 24 to 72 hours [193]. The T-lymphocytes are more sensitive to the steroids than are the B-lymphocytes [194]. Steroids can diminish the number of NK cells present in the serum. The lymphopenia can be due to the lysis or more likely to the redistribution of the lymphocytes to other body compartments, particularly the bone marrow. Lymphocyte proliferation, function, and circulation are also inhibited [195, 196], and the proliferative response to mitogenic stimulation by phytohemagglutinin and to antigenic stimuli [197, 198] can be depressed in vitro as is the mixed lymphocyte reaction. Decreased IL-2 production mainly is due to macrophage inhibition rather than to T-cell suppression [199]. IL-1 activity may also be reduced. Steroids can reduce the metabolism of the macrophage, impede its release from the bone marrow and its circulation, and interfere with antigen retention on the macrophage surface [200]. The bactericidal and fungicidal activity is diminished as is endocytosis and reticuloendothelial clearance. Lysosomal membrane stability occurs. Inhibition of macrophage spreading on glass has been reported. IL-1 production is decreased.

In addition, steroids can reduce the movement of antigen-antibody complexes across basement membranes.

The complications of systemic corticosteroid therapy are multiple. These include pseudotumor cerebri and psychiatric disorders; glaucoma and cataracts; thinning of the skin; osteoporosis and aseptic necrosis of bone; myopathies; peptic ulceration, pancreatitis, and intestinal perforation; fluid imbalance, hypertension, sodium retention, and hypokalemia; inhibition of wound healing; hypersensitivity reactions and suppression of host defenses (especially toward viral infections and tuberculosis); growth failure, hyperglycemia, hyperlipidemia, alteration of fat distribution (cushinoid appearance), fatty infiltration of the liver, and secondary amenorrhea [183].

Among various other anti-inflammatory agents are gold salts, penicillamine, the anticoagulants (heparin and coumarin), and the profibrinolytic agents (phenformin and ethylestrenol).

Cyclosporine and the cytotoxic agents are discussed later in the section Immunosuppression.

Hypersensitivity Responses

There are five types of hypersensitivity response.

TYPE 1: ANAPHYLACTIC RESPONSE. When anaphylactic hypersensitivity response (type 1) occurs, the participating antibodies are primarily IgE (IgG is rarely involved). On contact with the antigen (allergen), the IgE triggers a reaction in the mast cells and basophils, which causes the release of several important pharmacologic mediators (Fig. 1-21).

The hallmark of atopic disease is the rapidity of the onset of symptoms once a sensitized person is brought into contact with the allergen to which he or she is responding. When the allergen is airborne (inhalant allergy) the reaction is primarily in the respiratory tract and eyes; when the allergen is ingested (food allergy), the reaction is in the gastrointestinal tract and sometimes in the skin; and when the allergen is applied to the skin, the reaction occurs there.

Nearly 10 percent of the population suffers in one degree or another from this type of allergy. Sensitivity is normally assessed by the response to intradermal challenge with antigen. The release of histamine and the other mediators rapidly produces a wheal and flare, maximal within 30 minutes and then subsiding.

HLA Antigen Associations. There are conflicting views as to whether any specific HLA antigen predominates in atopic individuals. Levine and colleagues [201] clearly documented an association between HLA antigens and human allergic disease. But although they found certain HLA types associated with certain allergic disease, in the families they studied no preferential association existed between one particular HLA type and the immune response gene that determines ragweed hayfever. Marsh and associates [202], on the other hand, found an association between HLA-B7 and the IgE response to ragweed antigen; and in other studies, HLA-A1, 3, and 9 and HLA-B5, 8, and 12 have also been reported to be associated specifically with atopic disease in human beings.

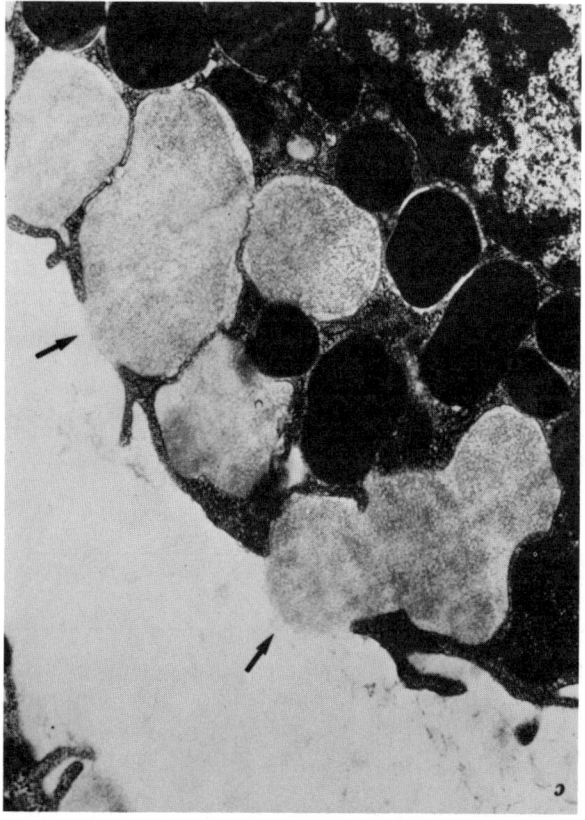

FIG. 1-21 Release of vasoactive amines from mast cell or basophil. Arrows point to areas where substances are being released from the cell.

Mechanisms. Basophils and mast cells play an integral part in type 1 hypersensitivity reaction. Basophils can be distinguished from mast cells by their small diameter (10–14 μm vs 12–30 μm), the multilobular nature of the basophilic nucleus, the margination of chromatin in the nucleus, and the large pink granules (1–1.2 μm) in the cytoplasm; in contrast, mast cells are elongated, have one nucleus (usually oval), often a nucleolus, and smaller (0.1–0.4 μm) more numerous granules that tend to stain dark purple [203]. Basophils, which are circulating cells (0.5–1% of the circulating PMNLs), arise in the bone marrow from the same stem cells as the other PMNLs. The origins and fate of the mast cells are still obscure.

The responses of these cells may also differ. Basophils will respond to PGD_2 to release histamine whereas mast cells usually do not. Basophils release small quantities of arachidonic acid metabolites whereas mast cells release substantial quantities [204].

Interestingly, mast cells from different sites differ in pharmacologic mediator content and release.

It is evident that the mast cells and basophils (and occasionally eosin-

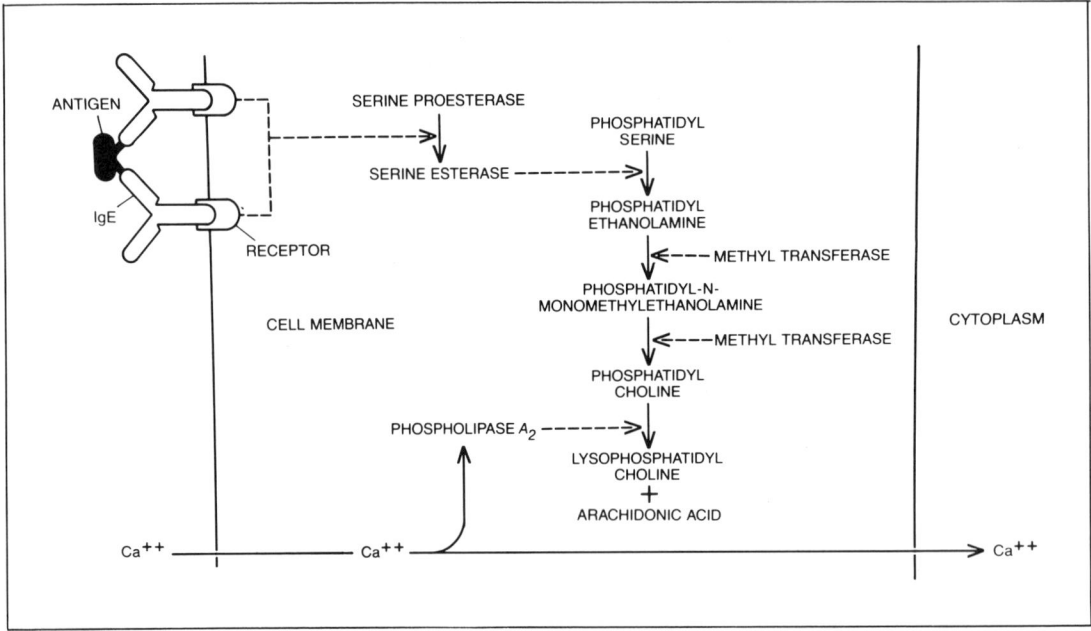

FIG. 1-22 Mast cell or basophil membrane can be altered by the adherence of immunoglobulin E and antigen resulting in calcium influx into the cell.

ophils [205]) can become coated with a particular type of antibody (homocytotrophic) whose Fc region can bind specifically to sites on the cells' surfaces. The most effective antibody belongs to the IgE class, but IgG can perform the same function.

The expression of IgE on either IgM-bearing virgin B cells or IgM-IgD double bearing B cells does not require the participation of T cells or antigen and occurs in fetal or early neonatal life [206]. This population of cells is relatively large. Once the IgE is expressed on the cell surface, these B cells are committed for IgE formation after differentiation. This formation requires helper T cells and is regulated by suppressor T cells [207].

Mucosal (conjunctival) mast cells have intracytoplasmic IgE as well as surface IgE in contrast to connective tissue mast cells, which only have surface IgE. The IgE may be locally produced in the mucosal tissue [208].

The number of receptors for IgE on the target cells ranges from 1000 to 400,000 (average 100,000) [204]. Mast-cell receptor density is higher than that of the basophils. It is apparently essential that there be two adjacent antibodies on the same mast cell that will form a bridge on contact with bivalent antigen. This arrangement induces changes in the Fc region of the immunoglobulin and configurational alterations of the cell surface that can activate a molecule that is a precursor of a protein-digesting enzyme, serine esterase; when the precursor, serine proesterase,

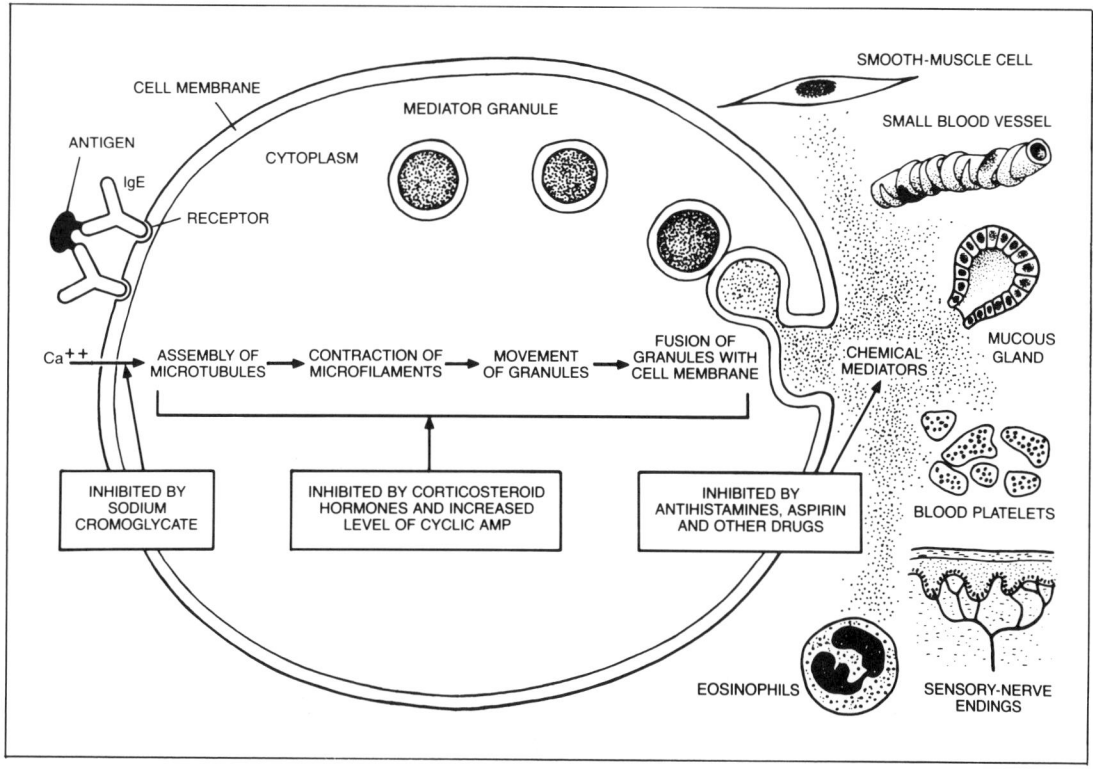

FIG. 1-23 Calcium entrance into the mast cell or basophil allows for the release of the pharmacologic mediators of allergy.

is activated, it is converted into the enzyme. Serine esterase initiates a chain of reactions that results in the generation of lecithin (phosphatidylcholine). This sequence of events modifies the mast cells' outer membrane, which becomes permeable to calcium ions. Calcium enters the cell and activates the enzyme phospholipase A_2, which causes metabolism of lecithin to lysolecithin (lysophosphatidylcholine) and arachidonic acid [209] (Fig. 1-22). The role of the metabolites of arachidonic acid in inflammation is discussed earlier in the chapter.

The entry of the calcium ions also activates enzymes that release energy and cause the intracellular granules to move to the mast-cell membrane, fuse with it, and disgorge their contents (i.e., pharmacologic mediators of allergy; Fig. 1-23). These biochemical changes, including increased membrane permeability to calcium and alteration of cAMP, can occur within 5 to 15 seconds [209].

Aside from the direct action of IgE, it is also probable that complement is nonspecifically activated, and that by means of C3a and C5a products, it contributes to mast-cell degranulation [210]. In addition, endotoxin (working through the complement system) [211] and both concanavalin A [212] and phytohemagglutinin [213] (working through a direct cell-surface reaction), can cause mediator release.

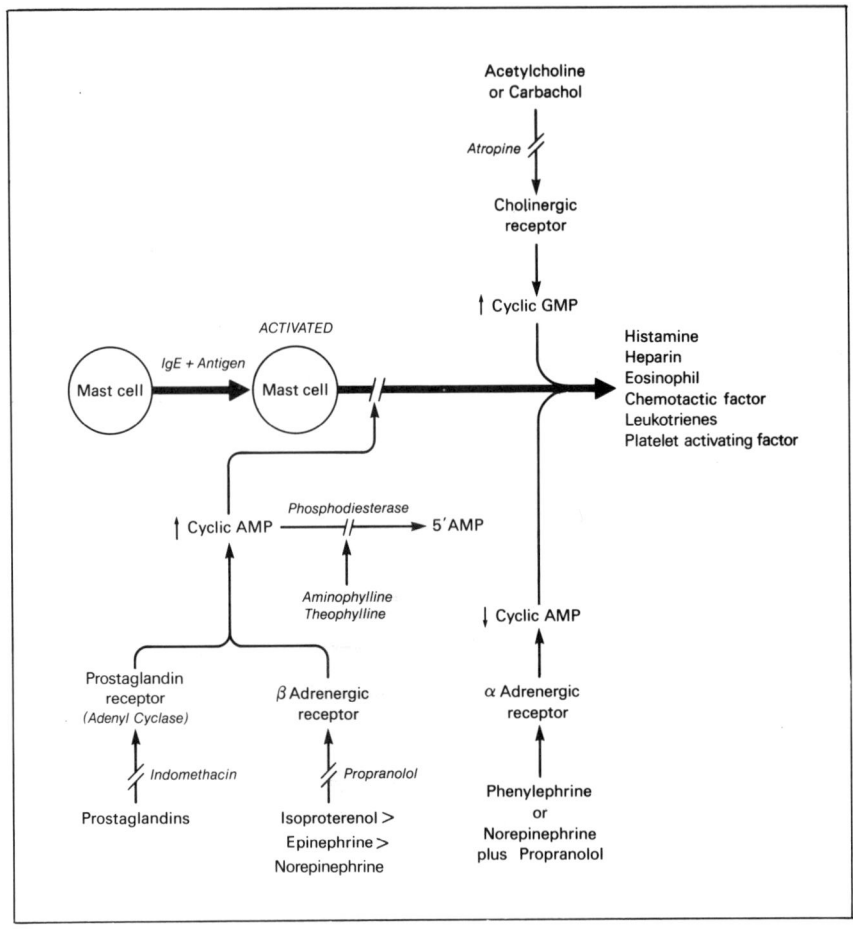

FIG. 1-24 Effect of various factors on cyclic adenosine monophosphate in the mast cell or basophil, and ultimate effect on release of the pharmacologic mediators of allergy. (AMP = adenosine monophosphate; GMP = guanosine monophosphate.)

Cyclic Adenosine Monophosphate. Mediator release from mast cells and basophils is directly influenced by the levels of cAMP (elevated levels inhibit release) and by the levels of cGMP (elevated levels enhance release; Fig. 1-24).

PGE_1 and PGE_2 act through membrane-bound adenyl cyclase to increase the levels of cAMP (and thus inhibit mediator release). Stimulation of the β_2-adrenergic receptor also increases the levels of cAMP. As a result, isoproterenol, epinephrine, or norepinephrine (with decreasing effect) can elevate the cAMP level in the mast cell and basophil. Stimulation of the α- (or α_2) adrenergic receptor can reduce the level of cAMP. Phenylephrine or norepinephrine, plus propranolol (a β blocker), can bring this about [213]. Phosphodiesterase breaks down cAMP to 5'AMP. Inhibitors of this action, such as caffeine, aminophylline, papaverine, and theophylline, can elevate the levels of cAMP. The cholinergic receptor, which can be stimulated by acetylcholine or carbachol, leads to elevated levels of cGMP and mediator release. Substances such as ascorbate, IL-1, serotonin, thymic hormones, and plant lectin mitogens can increase cGMP levels. Atropine can block the stimulation of the cholinergic receptor and thus inhibit mediator release.

By elevating the level of cAMP or reducing the level of cGMP, the symptoms of allergy from the pharmacologic mediators can be alleviated. Cromolyn sodium, which is useful in the treatment of allergies, may work by preventing calcium influx or by inhibiting the phosphodiesterase breakdown of cAMP. Prostaglandins are a normal constituent of ocular tissue [214] and may play a role in ocular allergy [215, 176].

Pharmacologic Mediators of Anaphylaxis. The currently recognized chemical mediators of allergic reactions are preformed molecules and mediators being formed and activated during the release reaction. The release of these substances (degranulation) is a noncytotoxic process that involves sequential exocytosis of granules and granular material into the extracellular spaces. Glycolysis and calcium are necessary for this release, which is accompanied by a drop in the cellular level of cAMP.

The substances that are preformed and rapidly eluted under physiologic conditions in human beings include histamine, eosinophil chemotactic factors of anaphylaxis, chemotactic factors for neutrophils, T-lymphocytes and B-lymphocytes, superoxide anions, lysosomal hydrolases (arylsulfatase A, glucuronidase, hexosaminidase), kininogenase, and tryptase. The secondary or newly generated mediators include leukotrienes (C, D, and E), HETE, hydroxypentaeicosatetraenoic acid (HPETE), prostaglandin, thromboxane, prostaglandin-generating factor, and platelet-activating factor. The preformed, granule-associated mediators include heparin, chymotrypsin and trypsin, arylsulfatase B, and chondroitin sulfate [216–218].

Basophils can also release prekallikrein activator, kallikrein, and Hageman factor activator.

Some of these pharmacologic mediators account for the signs and symptoms of allergy (Table 1-5). Mucous secretion is enhanced by $PGF_{2\alpha}$, PGE_1, PGI_2, PGD_2, PGA_2, HETE, leukotrienes C and D, histamine, and prostaglandin factor of anaphylaxis. Acetylcholine and α-adrenergic agonists can also enhance mucous secretion. Vascular permeability is increased by PGE_2; leukotrienes C, D, and E; histamine (H_1 receptor); and bradykinin. Vasodilation is enhanced by PGE_2; leukotrienes C, D, and E; and histamine (H_1 and H_2; H_1 and H_2 receptors are present on the ocular surface in human beings [219]). Platelet aggregation is caused by thromboxane. Smooth muscle contraction is enhanced by PGG_2, H_2, $PGF_{2\alpha}$, and PGD_2; thromboxane A_2; leukotrienes C, D, and E; histamine (H_1); and bradykinin. Eosinophils and neutrophils are attracted to the area of mediator release by HETE, PGI_2, leukotriene B_4, histamine, eosinophil, and neutrophil chemotactic factors of anaphylaxis. Elevation of cGMP and enhanced mediator release can be caused by PGG_2, and PGF_2 [220–222]. Leukotriene B_4 can stimulate suppressor T cells. In general, the

TABLE 1-5   Physiologic Effects of Arachidonic Acid Metabolities

---

Smooth muscle contraction: PGG_2, PGH_2, TXA_2, $PGF_{2\alpha}$, PGD_2, LTC, LTD, LTE
Smooth muscle relaxation: PGE_2, PGI_2
Increases in cAMP: PGI_2, PGD_2, PGE_2
Increases in cGMP: PGG_2, $PGF_{2\alpha}$
Chemotactic attraction of eosinophils and neutrophils: HETEs, PGI_2, LTB_4
Platelet aggregation: TXA_2
Inhibition of platelet aggregation: PGI_2
Increased mucous secretion: $PGF_{2\alpha}$, PGE_1, PGI_2, PGD_2, PGA_2, HETEs, LTC, LTD
Decreased mucous secretion: PGE_2
Augmentation of mediator release: $PGF_{2\alpha}$, HPETE
Inhibition of mediator release: PGE_2, PGD_2 (rat)
Increased vascular permeability: PGE_2, LTC, LTD, LTE
Vasodilation (hypotension): PGE_2, LTC, LTD, LTE
Inhibition of T-cell secretion of lymphokines: PGE_2
Inhibition of lymphocyte transformation and lymphocyte-mediated cytotoxicity: PGE_2

PG = prostaglandin; TXA_2 = thromboxane A_2; LTC = leukotriene C; LTD = leukotriene D; LTE = leukotriene E; cAMP = cyclic adenosine monophosphate; cGMP = cyclic guanosine monophosphate; HETEs = hydroxyeicosatetraenoic acid; LTB_4 = leukotriene B_4; HPETE = hydroxyperoxyeicosatetraenoic acid.

leukotrienes are notably more potent (1000 times?) than histamine and are nonresponsive to the histamine stimulator 48/80.

The phospholipids in the cell membrane can be converted to lysoglycerylphosphorylcholine, which produces platelet-activating factor.

Platelet-activating factor is produced by neutrophils, eosinophils, macrophages, and platelets as well as basophils and mast cells. In addition to its effect on platelets, this factor can attract and activate PMNLs, stimulate monocytes and cause smooth muscle contraction and increased vascular permeability [223].

Feedback Inhibition. Histamine, which stimulates muscle contractions in target tissues through its interaction with specific H_1 receptors, also interacts with histamine H_2 receptors on the surface of reacting target cells. Interaction with H_2 receptors leads to an increase in intracellular cAMP and thus to the inhibition of mediator release.

PGI_2, PGD_2, and PGE_2 can also elevate cAMP and inhibit mediator release. PGE_2 can also cause decreased mucous secretion and smooth muscle relaxation. Platelet aggregation can be inhibited by PGI_2. Heparin can bind histamine and also inhibit complement activation. Chondroitin sulfate can also bind complement [216].

Later eosinophils move into the target area, become immobilized, and continue to accumulate. Lymphokines, complement fragments, leukotriene B_4, HETE, histamine, eosinophil chemotactic factor of anaphylaxis, and platelet-activating factor can cause chemotaxis of the eosinophils to the target area. The eosinophils can phagocytize immune complexes, especially allergen IgE complexes, and serve as an inhibitor of the allergic response. Eosinophils contain major basic protein, Charcot-Leyden crystals, peroxidase, cationic proteins, neurotoxin, histaminase, phospholipase B and D, arylsulfatase B, and numerous other enzymes [224]. An eosinophil-derived inhibitor (EDI) can prevent histamine release [225]. Interacting with PGE receptors present on mast cells or basophils, EDI activates adenyl cyclase, and this increases cAMP and inhibits mediator release.

The major basic protein can bind heparin and may inactivate leukotrienes C, D, and E. Eosinophil peroxidase inactivates leukotrienes C, D, and E. Some of the cationic proteins can bind heparin. The histaminase can destroy histamine, and phospholipase D can inactivate platelet-activating factor.

There may be a third set of immunoregulatory mediators released from lymphocytes. Lymphocytes can produce lymphokines that mobilize both eosinophils and basophils. Helper and suppressor T cells may play an equally important role in this response. Histamine may also affect T-cell function; there is evidence that it can inhibit the production of MIF, prevent lymphocyte transformation, and E rosette formation [226–228]. B cells may release these mediators, again causing the inhibitory feedback.

Immunoglobulin A and Allergy. An association exists between IgA deficiency and allergy. Infants who become allergic by 1 year of age have lower levels of serum IgA at 3 months of age than infants who do not develop allergy. The mechanism by which the absence of secretory IgA at mucosal surfaces contributes to or prevents allergic sensitization is not clear. Reduced IgA may reduce opsonization and phagocytosis, thereby permitting excessive absorption of potential allergens that can provoke IgE formation [229]. In addition, maternal IgG may suppress infant IgE [230].

Helper and Suppressor T cells. T cells exercise a dual control on the production of IgE.

1. They affect the initiation of IgE production. (Neonatally thymectomized animals fail to produce IgE.) The helper T cells that participate in the synthesis of IgE antibodies to a given antigen are not identical to the helper T cells that participate in the synthesis of IgG antibodies to the same antigen.
2. Suppressor T cells are apparently the major factor regulating the production of IgE [231, 232]. The concept of elevated IgE levels secondary to a reduction in the regulatory function of T cells is supported by the observations of elevated serum IgE levels in anergic patients with Wiskott-Aldrich syndrome [233], in patients with Di George's syndrome, and in patients with recurrent infections and impaired cellular immunity [234]. In each of these disorders, the elevated IgE levels are associated with defects in T-cell function in patients who can still syn-

thesize Ig molecules, including IgE. Although allergic diathesis has many other possible explanations, it is quite possible that allergic persons are deficient in suppressor T cells that influence IgE responses.

Further circumstantial evidence includes the deficiency of suppressor T cells in the hyper IgE syndromes [235], the increase of antigen-specific suppressor T cells after desensitization treatment [236], and the poor suppressor T-cell response to histamine in atopic persons compared with normal persons [237].

This concept involving suppressor cells may be responsible for the rationale of employing transfer factor and levamisole to treat atopic disease. Beneficial therapeutic effects have been attained with the use of these agents.

TREATMENT. The treatment of anaphylactic hypersensitivity reaction is discussed in Chapter 3. It consists of the pharmacologic control of the intracellular level of cAMP and of interference with calcium influx. The effects of pharmacologic mediators (e.g., histamine and leukotrienes) can be neutralized by competitive inhibition by certain drugs (e.g., antihistamines), and corticosteroids can elevate the intracellular levels of cAMP, suppress inflammation, and suppress immune responsiveness.

Attempts to desensitize patients immunologically by treating them repeatedly with allergens has proved to be worthwhile in a notable proportion of patients. The purpose of the inoculations is to boost the synthesis of blocking IgG antibody the function of which is to divert the allergen from contact with the mast-cell–bound IgE. But because T-cell cooperation is important in IgE synthesis, the beneficial effects of allergen injections may also be mediated through an induction of tolerance in the appropriate T-lymphocytes.

TYPE II: CYTOTOXIC RESPONSE. Cytotoxic hypersensitivity response (type II) is the response that participates in the immune protection of the host from pyogenic bacteria. The antigen is on the surface of the cell (e.g., bacterium, transplanted cell, and tumor cell). The combination of this antigen with antibody (usually IgG_1, IgG_3, or IgM) causes the death of the affected cell by promoting its contact with phagocytes. This contact is accomplished by (1) a reduction in surface charge, (2) opsonic adherence directly through the Fc portion of the antibody, or (3) immune adherence through bound C3b (Fig. 1-25). Cell death may also occur as a result of activation of the complement system up to C8 and C9 (see Fig. 1-19). These two fragments cause cell damage by digesting cytoplasmic membranes and precipitating osmotic lysis. The release of C3 and C5 fragments attracts neutrophilic polymorphonuclear leukocytes, which in turn cause tissue damage by the release of lysosomal hydrolases. The bacterial polysaccharides are frequently absorbed on the surfaces of tissue cells where they can activate complement through an alternative pathway.

Another cytotoxic mechanism is available [238]: Target cells coated

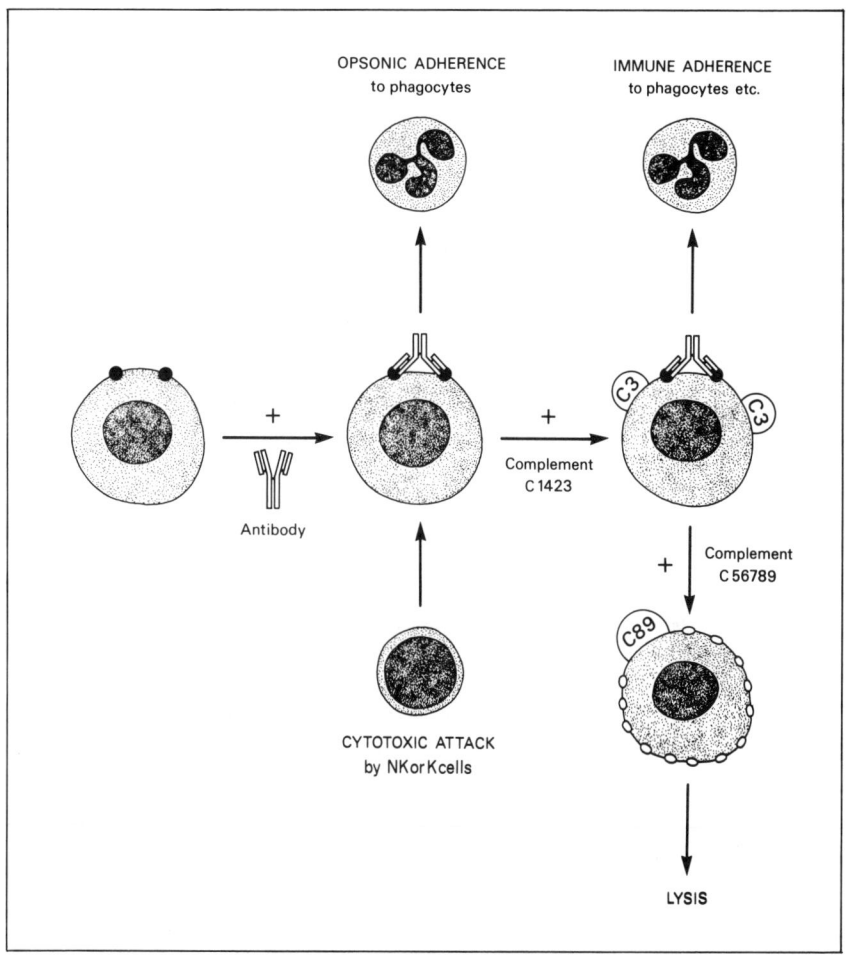

FIG. 1-25 Type II (cytotoxic) hypersensitivity. (NK = natural killer; K = killer.) (Modified from I. Roitt, *Essential Immunology*, London: Blackwell, 1971.)

with IgG antibody can be killed "nonspecifically" through an extracellular, nonphagocytic mechanism in which nonsensitized K cells bind to the target by their receptors for the IgG Fc fraction (ADCC). Phagocytic macrophages may act in this way. K-cell activity occurs in other cells that are neither T-lymphocytes nor Ig-bearing B-lymphocytes. Some observers [239] have even classified K-cell activity as type VI hypersensitivity [239].

Some of the many other cytotoxic hypersensitivity reactions are transfusion reactions, rhesus incompatibility, organ transplantation (in part), autoimmune reactions, and possibly systemic lupus erythematosus, acute nephritis, and acute endocarditis.

Certain drug reactions are also examples of this type of hypersensitivity response. Many drugs adhere to red cells and function as haptens.

The red cell-hapten complex induces an immune response, and there are cytotoxic reactions to the red cells or to the red cell–drug complex [240]. By another mechanism, some drugs such as quinidine bind loosely to red cells. Antibody-quinidine complexes can dissociate from red cell surfaces and then pass in complex form from one red cell to another. The destruction of red cells occurs as a "bystander" reaction. Components of complement may be detected on the affected cells in the absence of detectable antibody. Other drugs such as methyldopa alter red cells so that they become autoimmunogenic. The antibody produced reacts with the patient's own red cells in the absence of bound drug. Normal red cells may also be destroyed during a hemolytic drug reaction because they bind activated complement components (i.e., components released from cells that have been antigenically altered and have reacted with antibody and complement) [241].

Other drug reactions may be expressions of other types of hypersensitivity response. Some drugs couple to body tissue and become full antigens (not haptens), which then sensitize the person. If IgE antibodies are formed, anaphylactic reactions occur. Other drugs couple to serum proteins, and complex-mediated reactions occur. In reactions to topically applied ointments, the cell-mediated immune response may play a major role.

Circulating cytotoxic antibodies can be demonstrated in vivo by the passive transfer of antibody-containing serum into a normal recipient. In vitro, adding the patient's serum to the target cells in a test tube, or adding the patient's serum to normal cells in the presence of antigen, produces agglutination or lysis if complement is present. Sometimes the antibody fails to produce agglutination unless a second antibody is added. Such nonagglutinating antibodies are called "incomplete" and may be detected by the Coombs' test [242].

TYPE III: IMMUNE-COMPLEX RESPONSE. In immune-complex hypersensitivity (type III) response, the injured cells of tissues are innocent bystanders and do not possess the antigenic determinants that can combine with the antibody initiating the injury. The antibody reacts with its antigen, and the resulting immune complex directly or indirectly injures tissues that are in the vicinity. The distribution of tissue injury is determined by the sites of formation or deposition of the immune complexes. The damage that occurs is complement mediated (Fig. 1-26).

The mechanism of immune complex–induced injury is complicated. The size of the immune complex is important: Large immune complexes are readily phagocytized by the reticuloendothelial system and do not have a chance to localize in tissues; small immune complexes, although persisting in the circulation, are too small to localize in tissues. The size and solubility of the immune complex are determined by the ratio of antigen to antibody; for example, antibody excess produces large, insoluble complexes.

Immune complexes must also persist in the circulation to localize in tissues, and apparently the permeability of the blood vessels must be in-

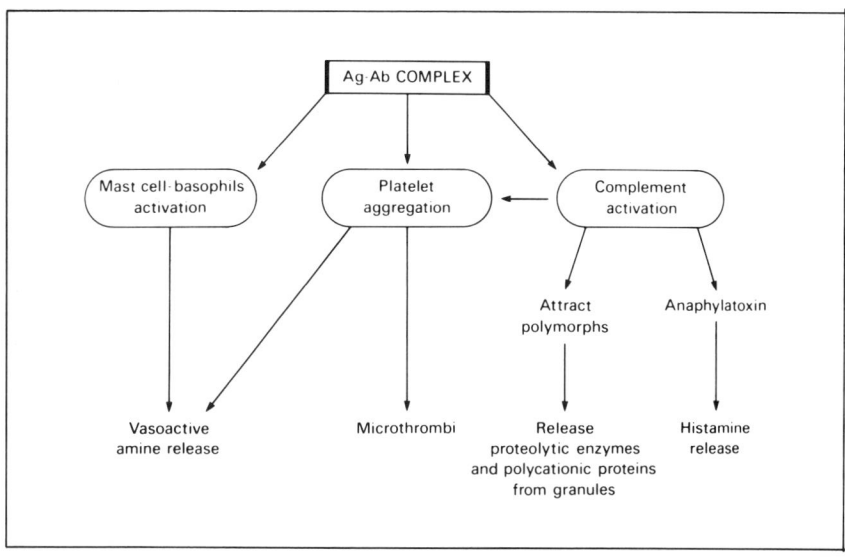

FIG. 1-26 Type III (immune-complex–mediated) hypersensitivity. (Ag-Ab = antigen-antibody.) (From I. Roitt, *Essential Immunology*, London: Blackwell, 1971.)

creased before circulating complexes can localize in extravascular areas. Vascular permeability may be increased by the release of vasoactive amines. In accordance with one mechanism, mast-cell–bound or basophil-bound IgE reacts with the introduced antigen to release the vasoactive amines. This process increases vascular permeability and allows the introduced antigen-IgG complex to pass into the tissue [243]. Platelets (a source of vasoactive amines) and complement anaphylatoxins both increase vascular permeability. Previous damage (nonimmunologic) to the blood vessels can increase their permeability and pave the way for the subsequent deposition of antigen-antibody complex in the surrounding tissues (Auer reaction).

Several hours after the deposition of the immune complexes in the vessel walls of tissues, complement is activated and polymorphonuclear leukocytes are attracted. Much of the resultant tissue damage is due to the release of proteolytic enzymes from these leukocytes, but large complexes may also cause damage by raising blood viscosity [244]. The antigen-antibody complexes can activate Hageman factor, and the interrelationship between the clotting, fibrinolytic, kinin-generating, and complement systems plays an important role in the resultant tissue changes. (This interrelationship is discussed in detail in the section Inflammation.)

Antigen Excess (Serum Sickness). The introduction of relatively large doses of soluble antigen, commonly in the form of heterologous serum protein, can produce immune complexes with IgG or IgM antibodies in the blood. These soluble complexes, combined with complement, can cause lesions in the walls of the blood vessels and in the perivascular spaces. Serum sickness after the injection of a foreign protein arises approximately 1 week after the injection. The clinical picture consists of fever, swollen lymph nodes, a generalized urticarial rash, and painful joints associated with a low serum-complement level and transient albuminuria.

Serum sickness is a generalized disease characterized by complement-fixing immune complexes in blood vessel walls [245]. Although the localization of the immune complexes is complement independent, the vasculitis that occurs (a disruption of the basement membrane or internal elastic lamina, and necrosis of the media owing to the infiltration of PMNLs) is complement dependent. (Serum-complement levels may fall while the disease is actually occurring [246].)

The same mechanism operates in *nephrotoxic nephritis*, which is self-perpetuating. Complement is fixed to these immune complexes in the kidney, and leukocytes are then attached. Tissue damage follows. Serum-complement levels are also likely to be reduced in this condition [247].

If nonglomerular antigen-antibody complexes are trapped and localized in the kidney, experimental serum sickness (a similar type of nephritis) occurs. In this process, however, PMNL infiltration is not a prominent feature.

Acute poststreptococcal glomerulonephritis probably is due to immune complex deposition and is similar in its pathology to the nephritis of serum sickness. Gamma globulin and complement are bound to the kidney tissue, and the serum levels of complement may be depressed [248].

In some patients with chronic glomerulonephritis, gamma globulin and C3 are deposited on the glomerular basement membrane, and the C3 serum levels are reduced [249].

Systemic lupus erythematosus is probably caused by circulating complement-fixing immune complexes that become trapped and localized in blood vessels in the various organs and in the glomeruli. The pattern of the deposition of gamma globulin and complement in these blood vessels is similar to the pattern in serum sickness [250], and the serum-complement levels are often depressed. The antigen-antibody complexes found in the kidney include DNA-anti-DNA [251]. Complement has also been found bound to the skin in areas of lupus rash.

In *rheumatoid arthritis,* complement activation occurs within the joint space and could explain the inflammatory symptoms. The serum-complement levels are elevated or normal, but the levels of complement in an actively inflamed joint are often markedly depressed [252].

In the autoimmune hemolytic anemias, complement has also often been incriminated [253].

Antibody Excess (Arthus Reaction). Maurice Arthus discovered that the injection of soluble antigen intradermally into rabbits hyperimmunized with high levels of precipitating antibody produced an erythematous and edematous reaction that reached a peak in several hours. The injected antigen precipitated with the antibody (often within the venule), binding complement and causing an intense infiltration with PMNLs.

Anaphylatoxin generation and platelet aggregation cause vasoactive amine release. This reaction can be blocked by the depletion of either complement or the neutrophilic PMNLs. For example, in lepromatous leprosy, large numbers of degenerating leprosy bacilli combine with circulating antibody to form the nodules [254].

Intrapulmonary Arthus-type reactions to inhaled antigen appear to be responsible for farmer's lung, pigeon-fancier's disease, and similar conditions. In patients with farmer's lung severe respiratory difficulties occur within hours of exposure to the dust from moldy hay. The patients are found to be sensitized to thermophilic actinomycetes present in the dust from the hay, and immune complexes are formed. Extracts from the organisms give precipitin reactions with the patient's serum, and after intradermal injections of the extracts, Arthus reactions occur.

The role of complement has been elucidated in several experimental situations. In the Arthus reaction complement is an essential participant. In this immune vasculitis, the role of complement is to attract PMNLs chemotactically to the site of the immune complexes in the walls of the blood vessels [255].

TYPE IV: CELL-MEDIATED IMMUNE RESPONSE. Type IV, or cell-mediated immune (CMI), response is due entirely to the activity of T-lymphocytes, and its onset is delayed clinically. It cannot be transferred from sensitive to nonsensitive persons with serum antibody; lymphoid cells or soluble transfer factor are required [256].

Because T-lymphocyte sensitization usually occurs in response to fixed rather than to soluble antigens, it is predictable that it will be encountered in reactions to many bacteria, viruses, fungi, tissue allografts, neoplasms, and simple chemicals bound to the cell.

There seems to be two types of this delayed hypersensitivity response: (1) the classical, tuberculin type, and (2) the cutaneous, basophil type (previously called the Jones-Mote reaction). In the classical, tuberculin type basophils and mast cells are scarce, and in the cutaneous, basophil type basophils and mast cells are abundant. In both types of reaction mast cells are activated by antigen-specific T-cell factors with resulting inflammatory changes [257].

The reaction is probably initiated by combining an antigen (associated with or processed by a macrophage) with the receptors on the surface of an appropriate T cell, which is present as a memory cell after previous exposure to the antigen. The cell membrane becomes activated, and the signal is transmitted to the interior of the cell, which is transformed into a large blast cell and undergoes mitosis. A number of lymphokines are then released and further mediate the response. (Some of these factors can also be released by B cells.) The effects of these lymphokines are documented in the literature [258–267].

Tissue damage can be caused by these lymphokines as well as by the C8 component of complement bound to the target-cell membrane. Histologically, the classic CMI responses are characterized by perivascular cuffing with lymphocytes, particularly early in the course of the reaction, and by a granulomatous response later. Usually a core of macrophages (many of them engorged with ingested antigenic material and called *epitheloid cells*) is surrounded by the lymphocytes. The chemotactic mediators account for the presence of PMNLs, eosinophils, and basophils.

T cells can also cause mast cells to release their vasoactive amines, in this way making it easier for the T cells to pass from the bloodstream into the tissue (presumably the site of the immune response).

Impaired Cell-Mediated Immune Responses. A variety of conditions are associated with defects in the CMI response. These are discussed earlier under Dysfunction of T- and B-Lymphocytes. People in technologically advanced countries live longer because of high-quality health care, and there is wide use of immunosuppressive therapy, especially in connection with transplantation operations. These two factors account for a large number of people with impaired delayed hypersensitivity responsiveness [268], and offset to a considerable extent the advantages of the technologic advancement.

Numerous assays are available to test the CMI response [269].

Contact Dermatitis. The skin is a major interface between human beings and their environment. Contact dermatitis serves as a clinical model of the adverse effects of environmental agents. The sensitizing substances are haptens; that is, they must combine with a carrier protein to sensitize [270]. They are of low molecular weight, can penetrate the skin (i.e., are lipid soluble), and can form strong covalent bonds with proteins (e.g., of the skin) [271].

Some of the commonest sensitizers are the following (listed in decreasing order of frequency): nickel sulfate, topical anesthetics, potassium dichromate, peruvian balsam, thimerosal (sometimes an ingredient of ophthalmic solutions), paraphenylenediamine, ethylenediamine hydrochloride, thiram, neomycin sulfate, and ammoniated mercury [272, 273]. The conjugates formed in the skin reach the regional lymph nodes by way of the lymphatic system [274]. In the epidermis Langerhans' cells enlarge and actively process the antigen. Subsequently keratinocytes take over as the major Ia positive cells in the epidermis [275]. The accessory cells present the antigen to the T cell and then the T cell is processed by the macrophage, undergoes blast transformation, and forms clones of committed T cells. Within 12 to 24 hours, lymphocytes and monocytes accumulate in the area of the skin where the sensitizer was applied.

It has been suggested that basophils play an important role in contact dermatitis. They appear late, however, and make up only a small percentage (5% or less) of the inflammatory cells [276].

Sensitivity may persist for as short a time as 1 year in patients who are only slightly sensitive to an uncommon sensitizer, but in patients sensitive to more commonly encountered sensitizers, it may last for many years. Multiple sensitivities are common, perhaps because of a genetic predisposition.

Identification and removal of the offending antigen are the most important components of any treatment regimen. Even after the offending antigen has been removed, the dermatitis may persist for 2 or 3 weeks,

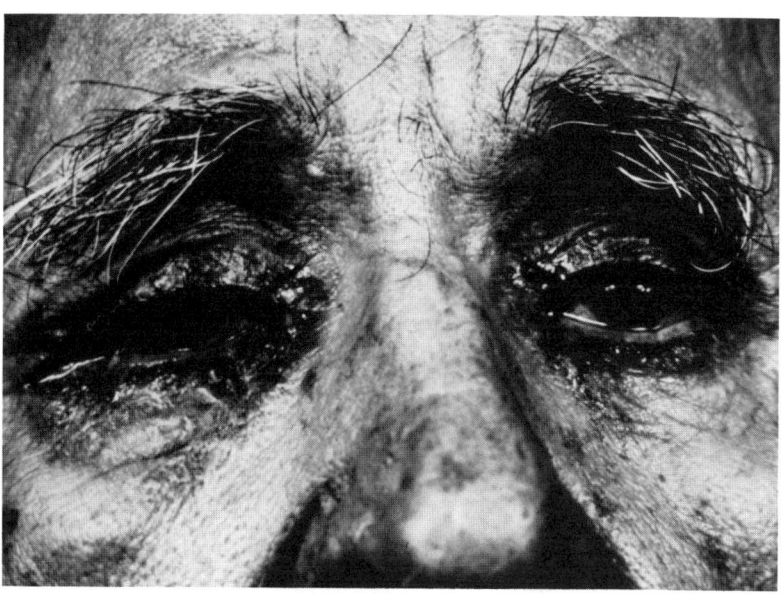

FIG. 1-27 Contact dermatitis around both eyes of a patient using an ophthalmic ointment.

and the use of anti-inflammatory agents such as corticosteroids may be necessary to relieve the symptoms (Fig. 1-27).

There remains the important roles played by the CMI response in transplantation reactions (to which we devote Chapter 6) and in both infections and tumors, which are discussed in the following sections.

Infections. For infectious disease to occur, microorganisms must penetrate the host's barriers. Once they are breached, the organisms can be disseminated by the bloodstream, by the lymphatic system, or by tissue migration (of the organisms themselves or of the phagocytic cells containing them) [277].

Virulence is the term usually applied to an organism's ability to produce disease. The infecting organisms can exert their virulence in a number of ways: Some produce exotoxins, some possess antiphagocytic factors, some possess endotoxins as part of their cell walls, some produce fibrinolysins, some (in the presence of antibiotics) may be converted to L-phase variants (viable bacteria minus cell walls) only to reemerge as fully virulent organisms when the antibiotics are withdrawn, and some can undergo antigenic changes in their coats in vivo. Certain viruses can induce a virus-specific suppressor T cell that is reactive against cell-mediated immune responses.

The host's three main lines of defense against microorganisms are (1) the barriers provided by intact skin and mucous membranes, (2) nonspecific immune defenses, and (3) specific immune defenses. Constitutional factors (probably related to the HLA antigens) may also make one person susceptible to certain infections and another resistant.

1. *Skin, conjunctival, and mucous membrane barriers.* Most bacteria do not survive long on the skin because of the direct inhibitory effect of the lactic acid and fatty acids in sweat and sebaceous secretions and the effect of the low pH that these substances generate. The ciliated epithelium in the respiratory tree prevents the bulk of inhaled organisms from reaching the alveoli, and the expulsion forces of sneezing and coughing protect the host mechanically. Mucous secretions inhibit the penetration of cells by viruses by competing for the viral enzyme, neuraminidase.
2. *Nonspecific immune defenses.* The role of secretory IgA alone or with complement is discussed earlier in the chapter. "Natural antibodies" (largely IgM) are present in the sera of normal persons and almost certainly appear in response to repeated contact with the many bacterial antigens present normally in the gut. Lysozyme is an antibacterial substance that somewhat inhibits bacterial activity in the eye. Most gram-positive organisms are affected, but *Staphylococcus aureus* is an exception. Cells may produce interferon in response to viral infection, and the interferon blocks translation of viral messenger RNA. The roles of phagocytosis and of the acute and chronic inflammatory responses to infection are discussed earlier under Phagocyte Function.
3. *Specific immune defenses.* Humoral immunity and CMI responses may be operative either together or singly against any particular pathogen. Humoral antibody plays a major role in resistance against a number of microorganisms and their toxins. Among them are bacteria such as group A streptococci, pneumococci, and *Hemophilus influenzae;* viruses such as influenza virus and poliovirus; and the toxins produced by *Corynebacterium diphtheriae* and *Clostridium tetani.*

Opsonizing antibody and C3b are necessary for the adherence of bacteria to PMNLs. Some gram-negative bacteria that have a lipoprotein outer wall can initiate the complement cascade by the alternate pathway. Antibodies can also neutralize extracellular viral particles.

The CMI response appears to be important in the host's defense against the following organisms:

Bacteria—mycobacteria, *Salmonella* sp., *Listeria monocytogenes, Francisella tularensis, Brucella* sp., and *Treponema pallidum*
Viruses—herpes simplex, herpes zoster, cytomegalovirus, rubeola, and vaccinia
Fungi—*Candida* sp., *Aspergillus* sp., *Coccidioides* sp., *Histoplasma capsulatum*
Protozoa—*Toxoplasma gondii, Plasmodium* sp., and some helminths

Contact between T-lymphocytes and antigen occurs either at the site of infection or in lymph nodes draining the area invaded by the organism. The antigens most likely to induce sensitization of the T cells are proteins found on the membranes of living cells (e.g., viral antigens).

Specifically sensitized T-lymphocytes may function in several ways to protect the host. They may produce lymphokines (as previously discussed), they may lyse infected host cells directly, or they may enhance antibody production by B-lymphocytes. When previously sensitized T cells are able to lyse virus-infected cells, antibody to the virus may in certain circumstances block the cytotoxicity, presumably by shielding the antigen from recognition by the cytotoxic T cell [278].

In viral infections the host can destroy infected and noninfected cells so that the virus is forced to become extracellular. Although the extracellular virus can then be destroyed by circulating antibody, the viral antigen incorporated into the cell membrane is destroyed by sensitized T-lymphocytes. In some experimental animals, the viral antigen acts as a foreign antigen, apparently because the virus changes the normal antigen on the membranes of infected cells (i.e., the H-2 histocompatibility antigen) so that it is recognized as foreign by host lymphocytes and is subsequently lysed [279, 280].

Cytotoxicity may be beneficial or detrimental, depending on the tissue attacked. In lymphocytic choriomeningitis (LCM), T cells are sensitized by LCM-infected cells and are then directly cytotoxic for these cells. This cytotoxicity is actually detrimental to the infected host because it is directed against vital tissues—the ependyma, meninges, and choroid plexus. The virus itself apparently does not harm the infected tissue directly but induces cytotoxicity to virus-infected host cells by immunologic mechanisms. The rationale for the use of immunosuppressive agents (corticosteroids) in corneal stromal herpes simplex is based partially on this concept; that is, that the cytotoxicity to vital tissue is due in large part to immunologic mechanisms. It must be remembered, however, that herpes simplex virus itself is cytotoxic; that the immunosuppression enhances viral (as well as other microbial) growth and spread (in part by suppressing ADCC); that the unaltered course of the disease is limited (especially in uncompromised hosts); that healing may be delayed; and that the healed tissue may ultimately result in an eye with surprisingly good visual acuity.

Nonimmune mononuclear cells (probably macrophages) lyse herpesvirus-infected cells in the presence of serum containing high titers of antibody against herpesvirus [281]. In this situation, antibody may increase the cell-to-cell contact between macrophage and virus-infected cell.

Immune interferon is produced by lymphocytes in response to viral infections [282]. It may bind to host ribosomes, and by preventing translation of viral RNA, it can prevent viral multiplication and spread. Interferon may also affect the absorption and penetration of the virus into the cell. Local interferon levels correlate with clinical recovery in human beings infected with herpes zoster varicellosus [283].

There is evidence that NK cells play a role in viral disease. Certain mice lines with low levels of NK cells are more susceptible to herpetic disease than mice with normal levels of NK cells. When herpes simplex recurs in human beings, the level of NK cells seems to be lowered. It is suspected that these NK cells play a major role in the immune surveillance process, which prevents recurrences of herpetic disease. Interferon and interferon inducers may augment the activity of NK cells. The CMI response also plays an important role in fungal [284] and protozoan infections [285].

Infection and CMI Depression. Known to depress delayed hypersensitivity skin reactions are the following: viral infections—mumps, chickenpox, measles, infectious mononucleosis, and influenza; bacterial infections—tuberculosis, brucellosis, leprosy, streptococcal infections, syphilis, bacterial pneumonia, and typhoid fever; fungal infections—histoplasmosis, coccidioidomycosis, and blastomycosis; and parasitic infections—toxoplasmosis [286]. In addition to depressing delayed hypersensitivity skin reactions, these infections may depress in vitro lymphocyte transformation and the chemotaxis of monocytes [287].

Two events that accompany infection may be responsible for the development of immunosuppression.

1. The number of circulating T-lymphocytes is notably reduced.
2. Certain viruses are predisposed to infect transforming lymphocytes. The virus may interfere with the DNA synthesis of the transforming lymphocyte and may in this way suppress lymphocyte transformation and proliferation [288].

Tumors. The CMI also plays an important role in tumor control. The immune system polices the body's cells, keeping watch for altered cells, which may become neoplastic. The immunologic surveillance mechanism works because cancer cells possess different surface antigens. Tumor cells carry a wide variety of cell surface antigens and only some of these are either tumor-associated antigens or tumor-specific antigens. Furthermore, only a portion of these may function as tumor-specific transplantation antigens (TSTA), which mediate host resistance against tumor growth [289]. Altered cytoplasmic antigens play an insignificant role in this process [290].

TUMOR-SPECIFIC TRANSPLANTATION ANTIGENS. The varieties of TSTA are as follows:

1. *Viral TSTA.* Cells infected with oncogenic viruses have new transplantation antigens on their surfaces that are characteristic of the infecting virus. The sequence of events may be as follows: (a) each virus selects specific cellular targets according to the presence or absence of viral receptors; (b) the virus acts partly as a mitogen on the target cell; (c) proliferation rather than lyses occurs in these cells; (d) various cofactors (ultraviolet light, exposure to carcinogens, etc.) may be present; (e) the host immune defect allows for cell proliferation; and (f) conversion of polyclonality to monoclonality occurs [291]. Viruses capable

of transforming cells from a normal to oncogenic phenotype include herpes simplex, type 2, Rous-associated, Y73 avian, UR2 avian, Moloney murine, Harvey murine, Kirsten murine, McDonough feline, simian, UR2, 3G11 murine sarcomas, and others causing myeloblastosis, myelocytomatosis, reticuloendotheliosis, erythroblastosis, and leukemia. Importantly, all tumors induced by viruses contain the same new tumor-specific antigens [292]. Tumors induced by other viruses have other antigens, although they too may have some in common with tumors induced by closely related viruses. Immunization with one tumor confers resistance to subsequent challenge with any other syngeneic tumor induced by the same virus.

2. *Chemical TSTA.* The action of chemical carcinogens is apparently largely a random interaction with the native cell DNA. As a result, these tumors are all antigenic but show a high degree of individual specificity. (Even two tumors induced in the same animal by the same carcinogen appear to differ antigenically [293].) Some chemical carcinogens are benzpyrene, methylchloanthrene, and dimethylaminoazobenzene.

3. *Embryonic TSTA.* Tumors derived from the same cell type often have a common "differentiation" antigen also present on embryonic cells. These are called *oncofetal antigens*. Examples are the α_2-fetoprotein in hepatic carcinoma [294] and the carcinoembryonic antigen in cancer of the intestine [295].

4. *Cell-division TSTA.* Antigens on the cell surface may change during cell division. The oncofetal antigens are sometimes "division" antigens.

IMMUNE RESPONSE TO TUMORS. Apparently immunologic processes are operative in cancer in human beings. For example, (1) cytotoxic antibodies, which have been found in the sera of a proportion of patients with malignant melanoma, apparently act to prevent metastasis of the tumor; (2) the presence of lymphoid reactions in the draining lymph nodes, the infiltration of lymphocytes into a resected primary tumor site, and the peripheral-blood-lymphocyte counts correlate with the prognosis in treated cancer patients [296, 297] (3) tumors can cause specific inhibition of the migration of autologous leukocytes in vitro (MIF tests); and (4) lymphoid cells from patients with neuroblastomas are sometimes cytotoxic for cells of other neuroblastomas in vitro.

There are numerous examples of the formation of specific circulating antibodies in response to malignant tumors [298, 299]. The antibodies are not necessarily damaging to the tumor. An antibody-cytotoxic death of a tumor is in fact rarely seen except in tumors of lymphoid origin. It seems that K cells and T-lymphocytes are needed for an attack on a solid tumor. Cell-mediated cytotoxicity seems to be the primary effector mechanism against antigenic tumors [300, 301], but the complex interrelationships of many of the lymphokines and tumor cells are still to be defined.

Interferon enhances natural and antibody-dependent, lymphocyte-mediated cytotoxicity against tumor cells [302] and exerts a direct inhibitory effect on the multiplication of tumor cells. It also increases the expression of tumor surface antigens [303].

Immune interferon is measurably more active than leukocyte or fibroblast interferon as an inhibitor of tumor growth. A combination of immune interferon and either of the others, however, is better than either type alone both in vitro [304] and in vivo [305].

Interferon is active in non-Hodgkin's lymphoma, multiple myeloma, breast cancer, osteogenic sarcoma and to a lesser extent in melanoma, Hodgkin's disease, and acute and chronic leukemia [306]. Both recombinant and natural interferons have been employed in these clinical studies.

Aside from T cells and their products, a variety of other cell types may play an important antitumor role. These include macrophages, NK cells, natural cytotoxic cells, and granulocytes.

Macrophages accumulate in considerable numbers in tumors and have natural and rapidly activatable ability to lyse or inhibit the growth in vitro of a wide variety of transformed cells. Adoptive transfer of activated macrophages in vitro or in vivo inhibits metastatic spread of certain tumor lines. Agents that depress macrophage function can enhance tumor growth, and nonspecific stimulation of macrophages is associated with decreased tumor growth or incidence [96].

NK cells, like macrophages, accumulate at the site of tumor growth and have natural and activatable ability to lyse tumor cells. NK cells may play an important role in resistance to metastases. Enhanced tumor growth is seen in patients with depressed NK cell activity [96].

The role of prostaglandin in tumor growth is unclear, but tumor cells can stimulate monocytes to produce large amounts of PGE [307]. As previously noted, PG may inhibit lymphokine production, and this action may be one mechanism responsible for the "escape" of tumor cells from immune surveillance [172].

Tumors succeed for the following reasons:

1. *Tumor antigenicity.* Although most tumors are antigenic, their antigens are relatively weak compared with the transplantation antigens. In the microscopic tumor trying to survive, selection pressures may occur so that the more antigenic cell lines are recognized by the immunologic surveillance mechanism and are destroyed. The less antigenic tumors, on the other hand, may survive.
2. *Host immune responsiveness.* Malignancies occur far more often in the immunodepressed than in the immunocompetent; for example, (a) in children with immunologic deficiency diseases [308] (who have an abnormally high incidence of leukemia, lymphoma, and reticulum-cell sarcoma); (b) in patients suppressed by drugs in attempts to prolong transplantation survival [309]; and (c) in the elderly, whose CMI responsiveness is diminished. Malignant neoplasms seen with increased frequency in immune-deficient patients include B-cell lymphoma, leukemia, squamous cell carcinoma, Kaposi's sarcoma, cervical carci-

noma, and hepatocellular carcinoma [291]. Lapses in a person's immunologic competence occur as a result of situations such as infections, operations, general anesthesia, and severe stress, and these periods of relative immunodepression, despite their brevity, may allow tumors to become established.

3. *Tumor effect on host's immune responsiveness.* Tumors themselves may depress CMI responsiveness nonspecifically, especially when they are far advanced [310]. IL-2 production and NK cell activity are both diminished in patients with cancer [311].
4. *Blocking Factors.* Under certain conditions, humoral factors thwart the CMI response so that an allogeneic graft (which is a tumorlike foreign antigen) can grow when it otherwise would not. The belief that these blocking factors were pure antibodies became untenable when it was found that they disappeared shortly after the tumor regressed or was surgically removed. In fact, the blocking factors are probably composed of antigen-antibody complexes, which may be aimed at the lymphocytes as well as at the tumor cells. The complexes can combine with specific receptors on sensitized T-lymphocytes, thus altering the T cells' ability to destroy the tumor [312]. They can probably also adsorb to the surface of the tumor cell and block the cytotoxic lymphocyte, preventing it from gaining access to the antigenic sites on the cell surface [313]. Which of these mechanisms plays the major role in blocking is still debatable.
5. *Tolerance.* With weak antigens, tolerance can be achieved by exposure to large amounts of antigen for short periods of time or to small amounts for long periods. The latter process may produce tolerance to tumors. A small tumor may escape immune destruction and survive for a long time, feeding small amounts of antigen into the system until specific tolerance is attained. If the immune response is delayed or inadequate, the tumor may "sneak through" and grow appreciably. When it has reached a certain size (by whatever mechanism), the host's CMI response may then not be able to handle it because of its mass.

THERAPY. Patients with tumors are treated in the following ways:

1. *Prophylaxis.* The ideal way to handle tumors would be to prevent them by vaccination. Oncogenic viruses are currently the most important targets for vaccination attempts.
2. *Surgical treatment.* Once the tumor is established, removing it entirely is curative. If complete removal is not possible, the tumor load should be reduced because (1) blocking factors can be reduced, (2) if the size of the tumor is reduced sufficiently, the tumor-CMI relationship may be altered favorably, and (3) tumor factors that suppress the CMI response can be reduced.
3. *Medical treatment.* Tumor antigenicity may be increased by coupling the tumor to a carrier and thus increasing the likelihood of its destruction.

Procedures leading to reduced serum-blocking activity may be therapeutically beneficial. Surgical removal of the antigen (tumor), as previously noted, or removing the antigen by plasmapheresis, may be effective. Either the inoculation of unblocking antibodies, or the stimulation of the formation of such antibodies, might be helpful. Because antibodies are needed for the formation of the blocking complexes, it is possible, at least in certain systems, that the inhibition of antibody formation (e.g., by the administration of drugs that diminish antibody formation) would be therapeutically beneficial [314].

If it is correct that the antigen-antibody blocking complexes have an excess of antigen, the addition of large amounts of antibody should lead to the formation of complexes with an excess of antibody that would no longer block [315].

Serum from a patient with a spontaneously regressing skin melanoma had a beneficial effect on other patients with melanoma [316]. The mechanism responsible for this effect—whether related to antibody excess, to unblocking antibodies, or to some other factors—is not clearly understood.

Many researchers are attempting to isolate and produce monoclonal antibodies to cancer cell antigen to destroy the tumor. It may be possible to attach anticancer drugs (i.e., Ricin), to these antibodies to increase their tumor-killing properties. Monoclonal anti-idiotype antibodies can be employed to treat B-cell lymphomas because the idiotypic area of each lymphoma clone may be considered a tumor-specific marker [317].

Increasing the patient's CMI responsiveness or reticuloendothelial system, or both, by thymosin [318], *C. parvum* [319], bacillus Calmette-Guerin (BCG) [320], or *Bordetella pertussis* [321] may inhibit tumor growth, prevent the induction of tumors by chemicals and viruses, and increase tumor rejection.

Immunotherapy for accessible tumors by means of delayed hypersensitivity reactions has been effective in skin cancers. DNCB oxazolone, purified protein derivative of tuberculin (PPD), and fluorouracil have been found successful in this way [322].

TYPE V: STIMULATORY RESPONSE. Type V stimulatory response may occur when cells receive instruction by an agent such as a hormone through surface receptors that specifically bind the agent. This combination may lead to allosteric changes in the configuration of the receptor or of adjacent molecules that become activated and send a signal to the cell's interior. For example, thyroid-stimulating hormone binds to the thyroid-cell receptors, causing an activation of adenyl cyclase in the cell.

Autoimmunity. Ehrlich [323] first suggested that there must be a way to prevent the body from producing antibodies against its constituent tissue antigens. When there is a breakdown in the control of this mechanism, autoantibodies (i.e., antibodies capable of reacting with "self" components) are produced. Many believe that autoantibodies are present in normal individuals, aiding in the disposal of cellular breakdown products but being kept under control so as not to cause disease [324]. The term *autoimmune disease* applies to disease clearly shown to be caused by autoantibodies. Some autoantibodies may be present after tissue damage without having caused the damage, however, and are apparently harmless (e.g., heart antibodies after myocardial infarction).

Suppressor T cells are thought to play a major role in preventing (or controlling) autoantibody production by the autoantigen-binding lymphocytes that are present in normal, healthy persons. The production of autoantibodies and autoimmune disease may be the result of (1) a breakdown of immune tolerance to self tissue, (2) a decline of suppressor T-cell activity (e.g., in the aged [325] or in thymectomized animals [326]), (3) a disturbance in the balance between helper and suppressor T cells [327], (4) a defect in the macrophage population, (5) genetic abnormalities, or (6) a combination of these factors. Hormonal factors may contribute to the pathogenesis of autoimmune diseases [328]. Abnormal estrogen metabolism is present in patients with lupus erythematosus, and androgens can suppress autoimmune models in mice [328].

Immune tolerance can be broken down by altering the established self antigens. Neoplasms can alter body tissue and form new antigens that can elicit immune responses. Chemical and physical agents can alter the configuration of protein molecules so that previously hidden antigenic determinants on the cell membranes can elicit an immune response to the cell. Intracellular viral protein can also elicit an immune response to the cell in which they reside.

Other factors that can cause autoimmunity are as follows:

1. Haptens can combine with host proteins to render them autoantigenic.
2. Exogenous cross-reacting proteins can produce autoimmune disease [329].
3. Antigen to which the host has not previously been exposed can produce an autoimmune response. Cloistered tissue (e.g., lens protein) can be suddenly exposed to the body's immune system, as after trauma or operation, and an autoimmune reaction may follow.
4. Ontogenic tissue that develops late and is not present during uterine life can act as a foreign protein and elicit an antibody response.
5. In addition to these tissue-related antigenic factors, it is possible that abnormal mutant clones of lymphocytes can form and attack self.
6. Virus infections may affect autoimmunity. Viruses may make some component of the infected cells foreign to the host, viruses may act on the immunoregulatory system (especially suppressor T cells), viruses may induce "molecular mimicry" (antibodies raised against viruses may cross-react with normal tissue antigens), viruses could elicit anti-idiotypic antibodies, or a combination.

Organ-Specific Diseases. In organ-specific autoimmunity, the antigens are available to the lymphoid system in low concentration only, and tolerance is not firmly established. The antibodies are organ specific. Because it is difficult to show that the patient's serum contains antibodies to autologous tissue, the serum is usually tested against homologous tissue.

The affected tissue is infiltrated by lymphocytes and plasma cells, and there is evidence that the CMI response plays an important role as well as the antibody (e.g., if the tissue antigen is injected into the skin, a delayed type of hypersensitivity response usually occurs).

Experimental lesions can be produced by the injection of antigen in Freund's adjuvant, and occasionally serum-complement levels are altered (sometimes reduced, sometimes elevated).

There is a family tendency to develop organ-specific autoimmune disease, of which the commonest examples are Hashimoto's thyroiditis, primary myxedema, thyrotoxicosis, pernicious anemia, Addison's disease, Goodpasture's syndrome, pemphigoid, sympathetic ophthalmia, optic neuritis, and phacogenic uveitis.

Non-Organ-Specific Diseases. In non-organ-specific autoimmunity, the antigens are fully accessible and tolerance is usually established; the antibodies are not organ-specific (e.g., rheumatoid factor is an IgM antibody against the patient's own IgG); and there may be a familial tendency to develop connective tissue disease.

The lesions are due to the deposition of antigen-antibody complexes and appear histologically as fibrinoid necrosis [330]. Increased T-lymphocyte responsiveness has occasionally been noted. Organ-specific and non-organ-specific diseases have the following in common: (1) increased serum-Ig levels (especially IgG and IgM); (2) ability of circulating autoantibodies to react with normal body constituents; (3) exacerbations and remissions; (4) a disease process that is not always progressive [331], and (5) selective deficiency of IgA [332].

The most often encountered non-organ-specific autoimmune diseases are systemic lupus erythematosus, discoid lupus, scleroderma, rheumatoid arthritis, and dermatomyositis. Some pathologic entities possess qualities of both types of diseases, organ-specific and non-organ-specific (e.g., Sjögren's syndrome).

TREATMENT. In organ-specific disease, appropriate treatment can be directed toward replacing specific hormone or hormones missing or destroyed (e.g., vitamin B_{12} in patients with pernicious anemia). In non-organ-specific autoimmune disease, treatment is directed toward suppressing the synthesis of the autoantibodies and treating the inflammatory response. Corticosteroids are often used for these purposes. Less often, immunosuppressives such as azathioprine, cyclophosphamide, and methotrexate are also used sometimes in conjunction with corticosteroids.

Immunosuppression. The desirability of eliminating the antigen, especially if it is identifiable and exogenous, cannot be overemphasized as a therapeutic maneuver to turn off the immune response. The induction of tolerance or the production of blocking antibodies may also interrupt the response, and desensitization, which uses IgG antibodies to block interaction between an allergen and IgE, is effective in many of the anaphylactic hypersensitivity reactions.

The depletion of unstimulated lymphocytes by one or more means—neonatal thymectomy, thoracic-duct drainage, radiation, or antilymphocyte serum (ALS)—may depress the immune response effectively. ALS is prepared by immunizing one species with the lymphocytes of another species, and then using the serum of the immunized animal to destroy the lymphocytes of the lymphocyte donor in vivo [333]. The exact mechanism of the action of ALS is not known.

The major effect of ALS is to depress the CMI response [334] by depressing the long-lived, recirculating, small T-lymphocytes. To a lesser extent the humoral immune response is also depressed [335].

Because ALS is in itself a heterogeneous antigen, it invokes many adverse reactions (e.g., serum sickness [336] and antigen-antibody glomerular basement membrane deposits [337]). The suppression of lymphocytes can also result in more infections (bacterial [338], viral [339], and fungal [340]) and in more neoplasms [341].

Immunosuppression by selective destruction of the dividing, differentiating, antigen-stimulated blast cell that has not yet begun to secrete antibody (prevents clonal expansion) can be accomplished by alkylating agents, purine and pyrimidine antagonists, folic acid analogs, some antibiotics, and alkaloids. These agents function as follows:

1. The alkylating agents block DNA replication in dividing cells, and mitosis stops [342]. It affects suppressor cells specific for the S phase of the growth cycle. Because of this profound effect on cell growth, a number of agents have been synthesized. The best known is cyclophosphamide, which is inherently inactive but is oxidized to an active metabolite by microsomal enzymes in the liver [343] (as is chlorambucil).
2. Of the purine antagonists, the most important are mercaptopurine, azathioprine, and thioguanine, all of which inhibit various steps in purine synthesis competitively and exert feedback inhibition on the earliest steps of the sequence [344]. NK cell function is depressed by these drugs [345].
3. The pyrimidine antagonists are principally the halogen-substituted analogs of uracil, deoxyuridine (IDU), and cytosine arabinoside. These halogenated pyrimidines are converted in vivo to metabolites that inhibit thymidine synthesis competitively and inhibit feedback at several steps in the chain of pyrimidine synthesis [346].
4. Folic acid is converted to tetrahydrofolate, which can convert deoxyuridylate to thymidylate. Thymidylate is the rate-limiting nucleotide in DNA synthesis. Any interruption in the supply of tetrahydrofolate will terminate DNA synthesis. Methotrexate acts by inhibiting the enzyme (folic reductase) that converts folic acid to tetrahydrofolate [347].
5. The antibiotics known to have immunosuppressive properties are mitomycin C, the actinomycins, azaserine, and chloramphenicol. Chlor-

amphenicol resembles part of the messenger RNA molecule and so competes with it for messenger-RNA binding sites on the ribosome [348].
6. The alkaloids, which are products of higher plants (e.g., colchicine and its analogs and the *Vinca* alkaloids), are potent mitotic inhibitors [349].
7. Cyclosporine is a powerful, relatively nontoxic immunosuppressant drug in human beings. Cyclosporine inhibits the proliferative activity of normal T-lymphocytes, the generation of cytotoxic T-lymphocytes, the expression of receptors for IL-1 and IL-2, and the secretion of IL-2 [350]. It does not prevent the T-cell independent activation of B cells.

Corticosteroids are discussed in detail earlier (page 47).

SPECIAL OCULAR CONSIDERATIONS

The general immunologic principles can be applied to specific ocular situations.

Anatomy and Physiology

The anatomy and physiology of the ocular tissue influence the host's immunologic responses.

The strong bony structure of the orbit protrudes, affording protection from trauma induced by large objects. The cilia are sensitive to contact with nonself objects, even air currents, initiating a rapid blink reflex. The eyelids thus protect the ocular adnexa mechanically. The skin of the eyelid is relatively impermeable to external substances and is basically populated by nonpathogenic, noninvasive bacteria. This normal flora of the lid skin and mucosal surfaces of the ocular adnexa contain aerobic and anaerobic organisms. *Propionibacterium acnes* is the most common of the obligate anaerobes and *Staphylococcus epidermidis* of the aerobic and facultative anaerobes [351]. These organisms can minimize the opportunity for pathogenic organisms to colonize. Certain acidic end products and antibioticlike substances [352] produced by the normal flora may be responsible for this effect. Interference with the normal flora may predispose the eye to colonization by the more virulent pathogens.

The intact surface of the cornea and conjunctiva, and the basement membranes of these mucosal epithelial surfaces, inhibits penetration and prevents deep spread of infectious agents.

BLOOD VESSELS AND LYMPHATICS. The lacrimal artery, the superior and inferior medial palpebral arteries, and the muscular branches of the ophthalmic artery (with their anterior ciliary branches) form the rich blood supply of the conjunctiva, eyelids, and lacrimal gland. The cornea and lens are avascular; the uveal tract and retina are both well supplied with blood vessels [353].

The eye's rich blood supply can be thought of as a natural immunologic defense. Ocular inflammation first dilates the blood vessels and then increases the leakage of serum and blood elements—macrophages,

PMNLs, lymphocytes, C-reactive protein, and immunoglobulins—into the extravascular spaces. These elements and the intact surface make up the first line of defense. The cornea and conjunctiva are capable of producing prostaglandins, thromboxanes [354], and leukotrienes C, D, and E [355]. The role of these substances in specific, and inflammation, in general, in the immune response is described earlier in the chapter.

Because the cornea is devoid of blood vessels, the cornea's immunologic mechanisms are modified by its poor recognition of antigens. This status can be altered if the cornea becomes vascularized, the stimulus for vascularization apparently being necrosis of tissue, possibly induced by toxins, proteases, or microorganisms.

In chronic corneal herpetic disease associated with vascularization, the lymphocytes become sensitized to the corneal tissue [356].

Corneal allografts placed in vascularized beds show increased recognition followed by increased rejection. In one series [357], hosts with avascular corneal beds rejected 3.5 percent of their grafts in an average of 10 months, whereas hosts with moderately vascularized corneal beds rejected 65 percent of their grafts within 2 months.

The lens is devoid of blood vessels and the immune system fails to recognize any of its organ-specific antigens. Should lens protein escape its isolation, the body may consider it nonself and produce autoantibodies to it as it would to a new or foreign antigen.

Lymphatics are present in the conjunctiva. The bulbar conjunctival lymphatics begin at the limbus in a series of arcades. There are two plexuses: (1) a superficial plexus composed of small vessels just beneath the vascular capillaries and (2) a deep plexus consisting of large vessels in the fibrous layer of the conjunctiva. These plexuses are interconnected and drain toward the palpebral commissures where they join the lymphatics of the lids.

The lymphatics draining the palpebral conjunctiva are arranged in pretarsal and posttarsal plexuses connected by cross channels. The posttarsal channels drain the conjunctival and tarsal glands; the pretarsal channels drain the skin and skin structure. Both plexuses on the lateral side drain into the preauricular and parotid lymph nodes (as can be seen, for example, in Parinaud's oculoglandular syndrome), and both plexuses on the medial side drain into the submandibular lymph nodes.

The normal, avascular cornea does not have lymphatic vessels, but if the cornea vascularizes, an ingrowth of cell-lined lymphatic channels occurs [358, 359]. Corneal and conjunctival immunologic reactions are often associated with immunologic activity in the draining lymph nodes [360].

No true lymphatic vessels exist inside the eye, the lymph usually follows the veins through the lamina cribrosa sclerae into the lymphatic spaces of the optic nerve and orbit. In spite of this lack of definite vessels, however, drainage to regional lymph nodes can occur after antigen injection into the vitreous, and immunologic reactions to the antigen may be demonstrable in the draining nodes [361]. The slow release of the antigen may enhance the immune response. The anterior chamber, however, seems to be an immunologically privileged site, not only because of the absence of lymphatic channels but because of an aberrant central processing of the antigenic stimulus (i.e., the antigen encounters the blood vessels prior to encountering a peripheral lymph node) [362].

TEAR FILM AND LACRIMAL APPARATUS. Tear production averages approximately 1μl/min under normal conditions of tear stimulation. With blinking, the tears drain nasally toward the two puncta. A continual tear flow across the surface of the eye washes away material such as microorganisms, foreign bodies, and desquamated epithelial cells [363]. When the surface of the eye is irritated, reflex tearing is induced. The excessive tears further dilute and wash away foreign substances. The neutral pH of the tear film may be important in neutralizing noxious chemical substances introduced onto the ocular adnexal surface.

In addition, the tears contain a number of substances that play an important role in defense of the outer eye. Lactoferrin, for example, is abundant in normal human tears. With a mean concentration of approximately 2 mg/ml it represents one of the main proteins in human tears [364]. Lactoferrin as well as many of the other tear proteins (tear-specific prealbumin, lysozyme, secretory immunoglobulin A [SIgA]) is synthesized and excreted by the lacrimal gland [365].

Lactoferrin is considered to play an important role in the nonspecific defense against a variety of bacteria [366]. It was initially thought that the antibacterial effect was due to the iron-binding capacity of lactoferrin. However, recent studies [367] indicate that lactoferrin also has a direct effect on certain strains of bacteria. It may also interact with specific antibody to produce an antibacterial effect more potent than either substance alone.

Lactoferrin plays a role in the regulation of the production of granulocyte- and macrophage-derived colony-stimulated factor [368]. Furthermore, it can inhibit the formation of the classical C3 convertase of the complement system, thus preventing the formation of the biologically active complement fragments C3a and C5a [369]. This activity may prevent complement activation in the tear film and thus decrease inflammation.

Lysozyme may account for as much as 30 percent of the tear protein. It can lyse bacteria cell walls of certain gram-positive organisms. In addition, lysozyme enhances bacteriolysis by SIgA in the presence of complement.

Another tear component, β lysin, ruptures bacterial cell membranes.

SIgA is present in tears in much higher concentrations than in the serum. SIgA may act to modulate the normal flora of the ocular adnexa allowing saprophytic growth, which prevents less-favorable flora from colonizing the surface. It also prevents adherence of bacteria to the mucosal surface [370], agglutinates bacteria, and can neutralize viruses and toxins [371]. Certain T-lymphocytes [372] and neutrophils [373] can interact with SIgA through cell surface receptors for the antibody.

The tear IgG increases notably during acute inflammation [374]. This increase is associated with the increased vascular permeability and is the result of serum IgG spilling into the tears. The tear IgG can neutralize viruses and toxins, lyse bacteria, enhance opsonization, and form immune complexes that would bind complement and result in immune adherence, chemotaxis of PMNLs, and release of anaphylatoxins [371].

Complement, properdin, and properdin factor B [375] are present in the tear film. The complement cascade can result in immune adherence and anaphylatoxin release, as previously noted, as well as the lysis and electrolytic death of bacteria.

A variety of other substances found in the tears may play a yet to be defined role in ocular mucosal inflammation and defense (i.e., interferon, prostaglandins, antibody, histamine, ceruloplasmin, and prealbumen) [376].

The mucin component of the tear film provides a hydrophilic surface over the cornea and conjunctiva, facilitating wetting by the aqueous tears. This mucin, when contaminated by the overlying lipid, may lose some of its surface-active properties and begin to accumulate in a viscous network [377]. This network entraps material and gradually engulfs them in a thick mucin thread in the inferior cul-de-sac. In addition, contained within the mucin network is an oxygen radical–producing system with antibacterial properties [378]. The mucin may concentrate IgA at the mucosal surface further enhancing its antibacterial effect [379].

The lipid component of the tear film stabilizes this film by retarding evaporation and containing the film at the lid margin.

MUCOSAL TISSUE. The submucosal tissue of the conjunctiva contains mast cells. In response to an allergen or injury these cells release histamine, platelet-activating factor, leukotrienes, heparin, and other pharmacologic mediators that can cause blood vessel dilation and increased vascular permeability. The transudate may contain substances that are effective in killing and halting the invasion of microorganisms [380].

The submucosal tissue also contains abundant numbers of plasma cells that can synthesize immunoglobulins, particularly IgA. The addition of the secretory component from the lacrimal gland epithelium results in the presence of SIgA in the tear film.

Foreign substances can be processed locally by the mucosal immune defense system. Tissue associated with this system is called MALT (as noted previously). This defense system is also seen in the bronchus (BALT) and gut (GALT). In the adnexa the conjunctival associated lymphoid tissues (CALT) are histologically distinct areas. The epithelium over these CALT sites show elongated microvilli with few microplicae. This appearance contrasts with the flat microplicae seen in adjacent areas. The underlying lymphoid nodules are multiple and packed with small and medium-sized lymphocytes [381, 382]. Larger lymphocytes undergoing mitoses are present and plasma cells are absent. Lymphocytes are also packed in the adjacent lymphatics.

Antigens are preferentially processed at these sites.

Another component of this system is the Langerhans' cell or dendritic cell. These cells are present mainly in the well-vascularized limbal region but may occur, albeit in small numbers, near the center of the cornea [383]. They play a major role in the processing of antigen presented by way of the epithelial surface and carry unique histocompatibility antigens (Ia) of importance in stimulating T- and B-lymphocytes. These cells bind antigens and carry them by way of the lymphatics to the draining lymph nodes, which leads to host sensitization [384]. These cells, the CALT system, or both also stimulate helper T cells, and B cells participate in humoral immune responses. The stimulated T- and B-lymphocytes in the regional lymph nodes then migrate through the bloodstream to the ocular adnexae. The T cells tend to home to submucosal sites in the conjunctiva, whereas B cells home to the lacrimal gland and accessory lacrimal gland epithelia. The B cells can produce immunoglobulins at these sites, particularly IgA [385]. Sensitized B cells from other MALT sites can also home to the lacrimal gland.

In different diseases, different populations of T cells can be seen (i.e., helper cells, suppressor cells) [386] in the conjunctival submucosal tissue.

NK cells may play a role in mucosal defense by destroying neoplastic and virus-infected cells.

Macrophages are situated in crucial areas (limbus) exposed to the circulation and there can trap immune complexes, possibly initiating interactions with T cells and cellular immune reactions [387].

The corneal epithelium, when damaged, can release a thymocyte-activating factor (CETAF) that can attract PMNLs, fibroblasts, and lymphocytes and cause the production of prostaglandin. This substance has interleukin-1–like properties [388].

The conjunctiva has a rich supply of immunoglobulins—IgA, IgG, and IgM—that probably come from the rich vascular supply, abundant plasma cells, and tear film. The central and peripheral corneal levels of IgG and IgA are the same, the IgG level is one-half the serum level, and the IgA is only one-fifth the serum level. IgM is found less often and has only rarely been detected in the central cornea [374]. The immunoglobulins are found principally in the stroma.

The iris is usually free of immunoglobulins. The usual double-walled vessels of the iris, with their tight junctions between the endothelial cells, may explain this lack. Although the stroma of the ciliary body and choroid contain all five immunoglobulins, the pigmented and nonpigmented epithelium of the ciliary body probably do not contain any.

In general, the retina has little or no immunoglobulins, but a few have occasionally been detected in the retina's rod and cone layer. The lens contains none at all [389].

There is some controversy as to the ability of the ocular tissues to produce notable amounts of antibody when challenged with a new antigen. We believe that a primary ocular challenge elicits its initial immune response at a distant site (e.g., a draining lymph node or a central organ such as the spleen). The sensitized effector cells (lymphocytes and plasma cells) then travel back to the ocular source of the antigen.

It has been shown in rabbits that the initial production of antibody to

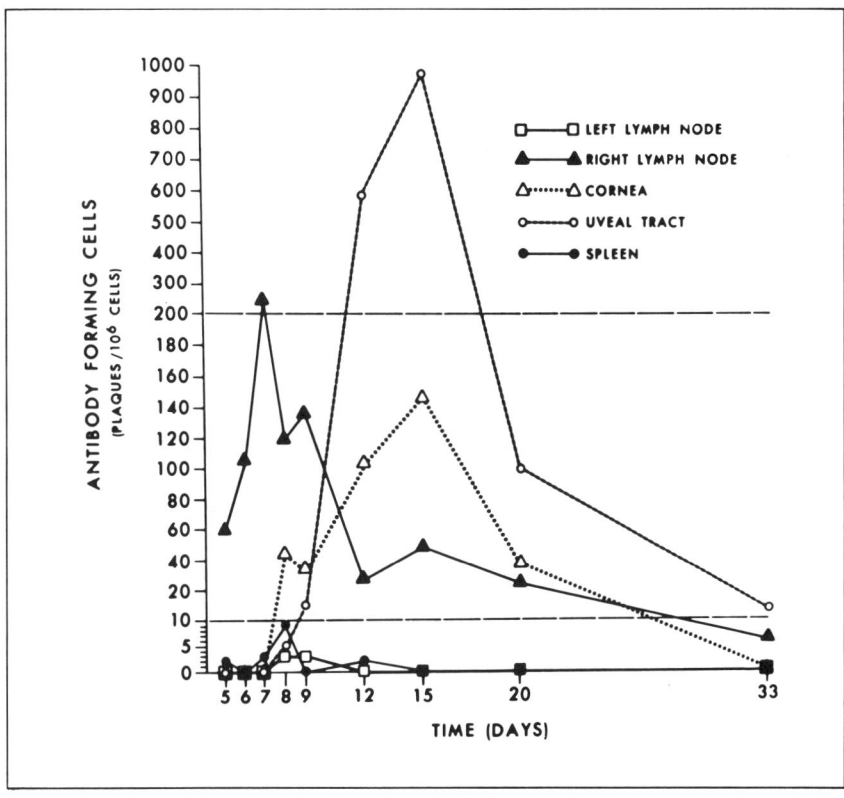

FIG. 1-28 Level of antibody-forming cells in draining lymph nodes, cornea, uveal tract, and spleen after injections of bovine gamma globulin into the rabbit cornea.

an intracorneal antigen occurs in the draining lymph nodes, preauricular or cervical [390]. Antibodies can be demonstrated after 5 or 6 days (Fig. 1-28). In the uveal tract and limbal tissue, detectable antibodies are first noted 9 or 10 days after intracorneal challenge, and they increase in number until days 13 to 15. This appearance of antibody and its increased level in the ocular tissue are associated with a concomitant, clinically observable, inflammatory immune response.

The antibodies that occur in the ocular tissue are specific for the inciting antigen and are probably formed elsewhere and travel to the ocular tissue. Indeed, the IgG-producing cells seen in the ocular tissue early after initial challenge are perivascular [391].

Silverstein [392] has shown that after an ocular immunologic challenge, exposure of the eyes of rabbits to roentgen rays does not affect the presence of antibody of the uveal or limbal tissue, but that exposure of the rest of the body to these rays does affect it.

At this point the lymphocytes (memory cells) sensitized to the original antigen reside in the ocular tissue, and if the antigen is reintroduced into the ocular tissue or elsewhere, these sensitized lymphocytes may produce antibody (principally IgG) [391] or lymphokines.

There is some conflicting evidence that the ocular tissues produce antibodies during an initial antigenic challenge [393] as well as after rechallenge.

Ocular Tissue Antigens

Corneal antigens are discussed in detail in Chapter 6, Corneal Graft Reaction.

At least nine antigens are present in the human lens [394]. Autologous lens proteins are only weakly antigenic, and even when they are liberated into the aqueous, they often fail to elicit an immune response. If they do elicit an immune response, it is usually humoral and not cellular [395]. Manski [395] believes that the majority of the antigenic determinants on the crystalline molecules participate in protein-protein interactions and are therefore not available for immune recognition. There are three types of lenticular protein: α, β, γ. Of these α protein is the most antigenic [396]. The lens capsule contains antigens such as those found in Descemet's membrane, the glomerular basement membrane, and vessels of the retina and uveal tract [397].

The vascular antigens of the retina are probably not peculiar to it because antibodies to retinal vessels cross-react with vessels in other body tissues [398]. The neural glial components of the retina are also antigenic. The specific retinal antigens, which are located largely in the photoreceptor layer [399], may play a role in the pathogenesis of several retinal disorders. In the pigment epithelium of the retina there may also be some specific antigens, and T-lymphocyte sensitization to them may play an important role in the pathogenesis of sympathetic ophthalmia [400].

In the uveal tract the antigens that are specific for the uvea are thought to be associated also with the pigment-containing cells. The uveal tract contains nonspecific antigens as well (e.g., plasma proteins and vascular elements). There are antigenic differences between the posterior and anterior uveas (possibly owing to their different embryologic origins), and these differences may account for the dissociation of choroiditis from iridocyclitis.

The antigenicity of the uveal tract is low, and the antibody responses of animals given homologous extracts disappear when the stimulus is withdrawn.

The antigenic determinants of the myelin in the optic nerve appear to be organ-specific, and a CMI response to them may cause an autoimmune optic neuritis.

Hypersensitivity Responses

TYPE I: ANAPHYLACTIC RESPONSE. As discussed earlier in this chapter, the antigen (allergen) in the anaphylactic response reacts with the Fab fragment of a specific class of antibody (IgE) that is bound to subepithelial mast cells or basophils through a special region of the Fc fragment. This reaction leads to degranulation of the mast cell or basophil and to the release of pharmacologic mediators. The edema and hyperemia of the tissue caused by these substances occur rapidly (e.g., in hay fever conjunctivitis and hay fever uveitis) [401]. Vernal keratoconjuncti-

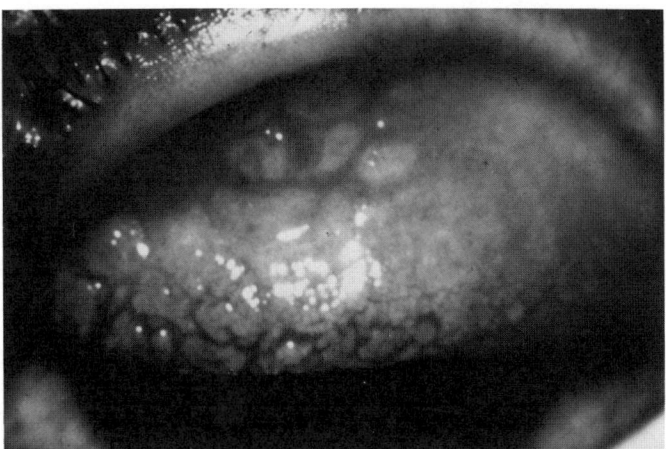

FIG. 1-29 Giant papillary response in the upper tarsus of a patient with vernal keratoconjunctivitis.

vitis and atopic keratoconjunctivitis differ from the acute hay-fever type of conjunctivitis in that round-cell infiltration prevails in the vernal and atopic diseases (Fig. 1-29). The reason for the accumulation of round cells is unclear but may be related to the role played by suppressor T cells or by the CMI reaction in this type of hypersensitivity. Bee-sting reactions of the ocular tissues and some drug reactions are other examples of this type of hypersensitivity response.

TYPE II: CYTOTOXIC RESPONSE. The binding of antibodies to an antigen on the cell surfaces causes a phagocytosis of the cell by (1) opsonic or immune adherence (C3b), (2) cytotoxicity by killer cells, and (3) lysis by the operation of the complement system.

Certain drugs may elicit a cytotoxic reaction of the ocular adnexal tissue by acting as haptens attached to cell membranes. Tissue necrosis can occur and produce severe inflammation and neovascularization, and there can be gross scarring of the conjunctival tissue.

Pemphigoid can cause scarring of the cornea and conjunctiva by producing antibodies to the basement membrane tissue, and pemphigus can produce antibodies to components of the epithelial tissue (Fig. 1-30).

The destruction of malignant melanoma of the choroid that has been exposed to autologous serum containing tumor-specific antibodies is a cytotoxic response. Some aspects of the immunologic response to sympathetic ophthalmia may be cytotoxic [402].

TYPE III: IMMUNE-COMPLEX RESPONSE. The density, size, and angulation of the limbal vasculature may contribute to the deposition of antigen, antibody, or immune complexes in the corneal periphery. Catarrhal ulcerations and peripheral corneal lesions in various immunologic diseases (e.g., Wegener's granulomatosis and polyarteritis nodosa) may

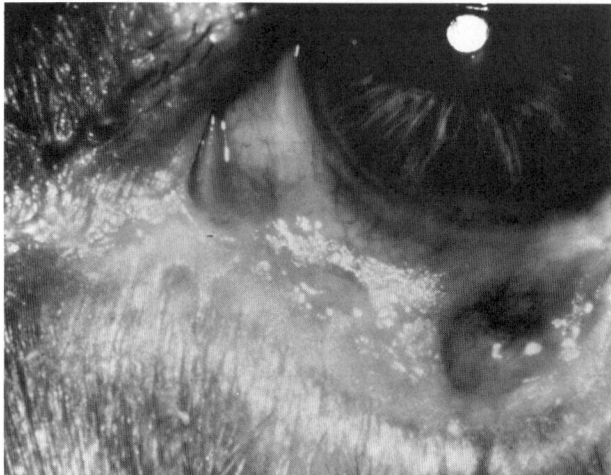

FIG. 1-30 Ocular cicatricial pemphigoid patient has symblepharon formation, shrink, and keratinization of the inferior cul-de-sac.

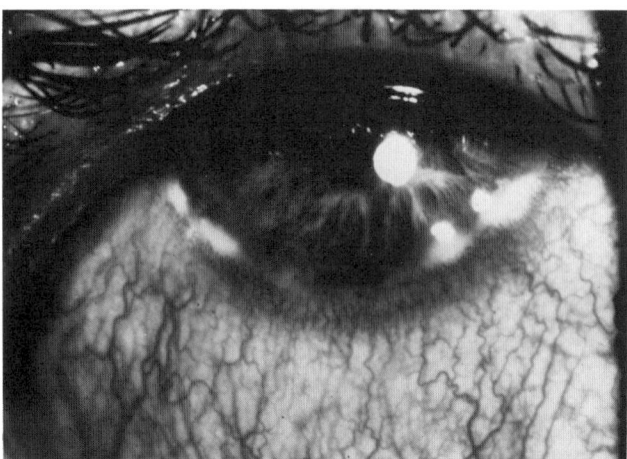

FIG. 1-31 Peripheral corneal infiltrates representing deposition of immune complexes in a patient with psoriatic arthritis.

be examples of ocular immune-complex disease (Fig. 1-31). If the immune complexes (or the vasculitis associated with the immunologic disease) occlude the limbal vasculature, the corneal periphery may ulcerate. This situation may occur in polyarteritis nodosa, Wegener's granulomatosis, and rheumatoid diseases. Occlusive vasculitis can also occur in the ganglion-cell layer of the retina in lupus erythematosus.

Recurrent immunogenic interstitial keratitis can be produced in guinea pigs by injecting intracutaneous and intravenous antigen [403].

Circulating immune complexes can increase ocular vascular permea-

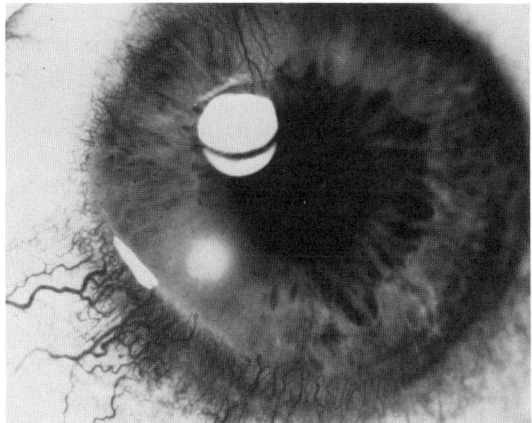

FIG. 1-32   Limbal phlyctenule.

bility in the rabbit [404]. Once vascular permeability is altered, the immune complexes can be deposited in the ocular tissue and can then bind complement and cause inflammation [405].

This phenomenon could explain the recurrence of uveitis after a quiescent period [406]. If there is nonimmunologic damage to ocular vessels such that increased vascular permeability precedes the formation of immune complexes in the host, deposition can occur and lead again to inflammation (the Auer reaction). Indeed, uveitis frequently occurs in patients who have diseases associated with circulating immune complexes (e.g., connective tissue disorders [407]), sarcoidosis [408], malignancies [409], and Crohn's disease [410]). Immune complexes can also be found in the aqueous humor in cyclitis [411].

TYPE IV: CELL-MEDIATED RESPONSE. The role of the T-lymphocytes in a variety of ocular conditions—phlyctenulosis, lens-induced endophthalmitis (as helper cells), contact dermatitis, allograft reactions, sympathetic ophthalmia, Vogt-Koyanagi-Harada syndrome, ocular tumors, ocular infections—is discussed in detail, as are all of the other types of hypersensitivity response, in subsequent chapters (Fig. 1-32).

It has been shown in guinea pigs that the classic CMI response—the tuberculin type and the cutaneous basophilic type—may take place in ocular tissues [412].

REFERENCES

1. Good, R. A., et al. Morphologic Studies on the Lymphoid Tissue Among Lower Vertebrates. In R. T. Smith, P. A. Miescher, and R. A. Good (Eds.), *Phylogeny of Immunity*. Gainesville, Fla.: University of Florida Press, 1966.
2. Papermaster B. W., Condie, R. M., and Good, R. A. Immune response in the California hagfish. *Nature* 196:355, 1962.
3. Finstad, J., and Good, R. A. Phylogenetic Studies of Adaptive Immune Re-

sponses in the Lower Vertebrates. In R. T. Smith, P. A. Meischer, and R. A. Good (Eds.), *Phylogeny of Immunity.* Gainesville, Fla.: University of Florida Press, 1966.

4. Cooper, M. D., Peterson, R. D. A., and Good, R. A. Delineation of the thymic and bursal lymphoid systems in the chicken. *Nature* 205:143, 1965.
5. Peterson, R. D. A., et al. The effect of bursectomy and thymectomy on the development of visceral lymphomatosis in the chicken. *J. Natl. Cancer Inst.* 32:1343, 1964.
6. Sela, M. Antigenicity: Some molecular aspects. *Science* 166:1365, 1969.
7. Holt, L. G. Quantitative studies in diphtheria prophylaxis. *Br. J. Exp. Pathol.* 32:151, 1951.
8. Thompson, R., and Olsen, H. Antibody production in rabbit's cornea. *J. Immunol.* 65:633, 1950.
9. Natali, P. G., et al. Ontogeny of human Ia antigens. *Cell. Immunol.* 73:385, 1982.
10. Thorsby, E. The human major histocompatibility system. *Transplant. Rev.* 18:51, 1974.
11. Pauling, L. A theory of the structure and process of formation of antibodies. *J. Am. Chem. Soc.* 62:2643, 1940.
12. Sprent, J. Circulating T and B lymphocytes of the mouse. *Cell Immunol.* 7:10, 1973.
13. Coutinho, A., and Forni, L. Antigen-specific and non-specific regulatory influences of antibody in immune responses are determined by variable region properties. *Ann. Immunol. (Paris)* 132C:131, 1981.
14. Tiselius, A., and Kabat, E. A. An electrophoretic study of immune sera and purified antibody preparations. *J. Exp. Med.* 69:119, 1939.
15. Edelman, G., et al. Reconstitution of immunologic activity by interaction of polypeptide chains of antibodies. *Proc. Natl. Acad. Sci. U.S.A.* 50:753, 1963.
16. Franek, F., and Nezlin, R. Recovery of antibody combining activity by interaction of different peptide chains isolated from purified horse antitoxins. *Folia Microbiol. (Praha)* 8:128, 1963.
17. Palmer, J., and Nisonoff, A. Reduction and reoxidation of critical disulfide bond in the rabbit antibody molecule. *J. Biol. Chem.* 238:2393, 1963.
18. Porter, P. R. Chemical structure of γ globulin and antibodies. *Br. Med. Bull.* 19:197, 1963.
19. Pichler, W. J., and Broder, S. Fc-IgM and FcIgG receptors on human circulating B lymphocytes. *J. Immunol.* 121:887, 1978.
20. Kolb, H., and Bosma, M. J. Clones producing antibodies of more than one class. *Immunology* 33:461, 1977.
21. Small, P. A., Jr., and Lamm, M. E. Polypeptide chain structure of rabbit immunoglobulins. *Biochemistry* 5:259, 1966.
22. Perlmann, P., Perlmann, H., and Wigzell, H. Lymphocyte mediated cytotoxicity in vitro. *Transplant. Rev.* 13:91, 1972.
23. Tomasi, T., et al. Characteristics of an immune system common to certain external secretions. *J. Exp. Med.* 121:101, 1965.
24. South, M. A., et al. The IgA system. *J. Exp. Med.* 123:615, 1966.
25. Tourville, D. R., et al. The human secretory immunoglobulin system. *J. Exp. Med.* 129:411, 1969.
26. Franklin, R. M., Kenyon, K. R., and Tomasi, T. B. Immunohistologic studies of human lacrimal gland. *J. Immunol.* 11:984, 1973.
27. Hong, R., Pollara, B., and Good, R. A. A model for colostral IgA. *Proc. Natl. Acad. Sci. U.S.A.* 65:602, 1966.

28. Tada, T., Ishizaka, K., and Henney, C. Gamma-E forming cells in human and monkey lymphoid tissues (abstract). Paper presented at American Association of Immunologists Annual Meeting. Atlantic City, N.J., April 1969.
29. Chokirker, W. B., and Tomasi, T. B., Jr. Gamma globulins. *Science* 142:1080, 1963.
30. Heremans, J. F. Immunoglobulin formation and function in different tissues. *Curr. Top. Microbiol. Immunol.* 45:131, 1968.
31. Tomasi, T. B. The gamma A globulins. *Hosp. Pract.* 2:25, 1967.
32. Alford, R. H., et al. Neutralizing and hemagglutination-inhibiting activity of nasal secretions following experimental human infection with A2 influenza virus. *J. Immunol.* 98:724, 1967.
33. Bellanti, J. A., et al. The nature of serum and nasal antibody in human and respiratory tularemia. *J. Immunol.* 98:171, 1967.
34. Smith, C. B., Bellanti, J. A., and Chanock, R. M. Immunoglobulins in serum and nasal secretions following infection with Type 1 parainfluenza virus and injection of inactivated vaccines. *J. Immunol.* 99:133, 1967.
35. Ishizaka, T., et al. $C^1 1$ fixation by human isoagglutinins. *J. Immunol.* 97:716, 1966.
36. Rome, D. S., et al. IgD on the surface of peripheral blood lymphocytes of human newborn. *Nature* 242:155, 1973.
37. Idem.
38. Idem.
39. Johansson, S. G. O. Serum IgND levels in healthy children and adults. *Int. Arch. Allergy Appl. Immunol.* 34:1, 1968.
40. Ishizaka, K., and Ishizaka, T. Human reagenic antibodies and immunoglobulin E. *J. Allergy* 42:330, 1968.
41. Finklestein, M. S., and Uhr, J. W. Specific inhibition of antibody formation by passively administered 19S and 7S antibody. *Science* 146:67, 1964.
42. Reinherz, E. O., and Schlossman, S. F. The differentiation and function of human T lymphocytes. *Cell* 19:821, 1980.
43. Parker, W. L., and Martz, E. Lectin-induced non-lethal adhesions between cytolytic T lymphocytes and antigenically unrecognizable tumor cells and nonspecific triggering of cytolysis. *J. Immunol.* 124:25, 1980.
44. Berke, G. Cytotoxic T-lymphocytes: How do they function? *Immunol. Rev.* 72:5, 1983.
45. Miller, J. F. A. P. Genetic Control of Lymphocyte Interaction. In Y. Yamamura and T. Tada (Eds.), *Progress in Immunology V.* New York: Academic Press, 1983, pp. 797–808.
46. Alexander, E. L., and Wetzel, B. Human lymphocytes. *Science* 188:732, 1975.
47. Dickler, H. B., Adkinson, N. F., and Terry, W. D. Evidence of individual human peripheral blood lymphocytes bearing both B and T cell markers. *Nature* 247:213, 1974.
48. Johnson, H. M., and Farrar, W. L. T cell proliferation. *Cell. Immunol.* 75:154, 1983.
49. Dumonde, D. C. Lymphokines. *Proc. R. Soc. Med.* 63:899, 1970.
50. Schrader, J. W., Clark-Lewis, I., Crapper, R. M., and Wong, G. H. P-Cell Stimulating Factor. In Y. Yamamura and T. Tada (Eds.), *Progress in Immunology V.* Academic Press, 1983, pp. 279–283.
51. Steward, W. E., II, Blalock, J. E., and Burke, D. C. Interferon nomenclature. *J. Immunol.* 125:2353, 1980.
52. Billiau, A. Pharmacokinetic and pharmacological aspects of interferon therapy in man. *Acta Microbiol. Acad. Sci. Hung.* 28:257, 1984.

53. De Maeyer, E., and De Maeyer-Guignard, J. Interferons as regulatory agents of the immune system. *Crit. Rev. Immunol.* 2:167, 1981.
54. Herberman, R. B., Ortaldo, J. R., and Rubenstein, M. Augmentation of natural and ADCC by pure leukocyte interferon. *J. Clin. Immunol.* 1:149, 1981.
55. Sherwin, S. A., Knost, J. A., and Fein, S. A multiple-dose phase 1 trial of recombinant leukocyte A interferon in cancer patients. *J.A.M.A.* 248:2461, 1982.
56. Welsh, R. M. Natural killer cells and interferon. *Crit. Rev. Immunol.* 5:55, 1984.
57. De Weck, A. L. The Biology of Lymphokines. In Y. Yamamura and T. Tada (Eds.), *Progress in Immunology V.* New York: Academic, 1983, pp. 307–314.
58. Watson, J. D., and Prestridge, R. L. Interleukin 3 and colony stimulating factors. *Immunol. Today* 4:276, 1983.
59. Greenberger, J. S., et al. Interleukin 3 dependent hematopoietic progenitor cell lines. *Fed. Proc.* 42:2762, 1983.
60. Gery, I., Gershon, R. K., and Waksman, B. H. Potentiation of the T lymphocyte response to mitogens. *J. Exp. Med.* 136:128, 1972.
61. Mizel, S. B., and Mizel, D. Purification to apparent homogeneity of murine interleukin-1. *J. Immunol.* 126:834, 1981.
62. Oppenheim, J. J., Scala, G., Kuang, Y., and Matsushima, K. The Role of Cytokines in Promoting Accessory-Cell Function. In Y. Yamamura and T. Tada (Eds.), *Progress in Immunology V.* Tokyo: Academic, 1983, pp. 285–294.
63. Simon, H. B. The immunology of exercise. *J.A.M.A.* 252:2735, 1984.
64. Ben-Zvi, A., Mizel, S. B., and Oppenheim, J. J. Generation of human peripheral blood stable E-rosette-forming T cells by interleukin-1. *Clin. Immunol. Immunopathol.* 19:330, 1981.
65. Farrar, W. L., Mizel, S. B., and Farrar, J. J. Participation of lymphocyte activating factor in the induction of cytotoxic T cell responses. *J. Immunol.* 124:1371, 1980.
66. Durum, S. K., and Gershon, R. K. Interleukin can replace the requirements for I-A-positive cells in the proliferation of antigen-primed T cells. *Proc. Natl. Acad. Sci. U.S.A.* 79:4747, 1982.
67. Gillis, S., Scheid, M., and Watson, J. Biochemical and biologic characterization of lymphocyte regulatory molecules. *J. Immunol.* 125:2570, 1983.
68. Mizel, S. B., Dayer, J. M., Krane, S. M., and Mergenhagen, S. E. Stimulation of rheumatoid synovial cell collagenase and prostaglandin production by partially purified lymphocyte activating factor. *Proc. Natl. Acad. Sci. U.S.A.* 78:2474, 1981.
69. Lachman, L. B. Human interleukin 1. *Fed. Proc.* 42:2639, 1983.
70. Paetkau, V., et al. Interleukin 2 in cell mediated immune responses. *J. Supramolec. Struct.* 13:271, 1980.
71. Mizel, S. B. Regulation of immune and inflammatory responses by interleukin 1. *Clin. Immunol. Newsl.* 3:123, 1982.
72. Gillis, S. Interleukin biochemistry and biology. *Fed. Proc.* 42:2635, 1983.
73. Hadden, J. W., and Coffey, R. G. Cyclic nucleotides in mitogen-induced lymphocyte proliferation. *Immunol. Today* 3:299, 1982.
74. Reinherz, E. L., et al. Abnormalities of T cell maturation and regulation in human beings with immunodeficiency disorders. *J. Clin. Invest.* 68:699, 1981.
75. Szewczuk, M. R., and Wade, A. W. Aging and the mucosal-associated lymphoid system. *Ann. N.Y. Acad. Sci.* 77:333, 1983.
76. Kishimoto, S., et al. Age-related changes in the subsets and functions of hu-

man T lymphocytes. *J. Immunol.* 121:1773, 1978.
77. Warren, S. L. A systematic approach to the evaluation of immunological disease patterns. *Ann. Allergy* 35:180, 1976.
78. Weigle, W. O. Recent observations and concepts in immunologic unresponsiveness and autoimmunity. *Clin. Exp. Immunol.* 9:437, 1971.
79. Weigle, W. O., Chiller, J. M., and Habicht, G. S. Effect of immunological unresponsiveness on different cell populations. *Transplant. Rev.* 8:3, 1972.
80. Melcher, F., Corbel, C., and Leptin, M. Requirements for B-Cell Stimulation. In Y. Yamamura and T. Tada (Eds.), *Progress in Immunology V.* New York: Academic Press, 1983, pp. 669–682.
81. Gershon, R. K. T Cell Control of Antibody Production. In M. D. Cooper and N. L. Warner (Eds.), *Contemporary Topics in Immunobiology.* New York: Plenum, 1974, p. 1.
82. Waldmann, T. A., and Broder, S. Suppressor cells in the regulation of the immune response. In R. Schwartz (Ed.), *Progress in Clinical Immunology* (Vol. III). New York: Grune & Stratton, 1977, p. 155.
83. Waldmann, T. A., et al. Role of suppressor T cells in pathogenesis of common variable hypogammaglobulinemia. *Lancet* 2:609, 1974.
84. Waldmann, T. A., et al. Defect in IgA secretion and in IgA specific suppressor cells in patients with selective IgA deficiency. *Trans. Assoc. Am. Physicians* 89:215, 1976.
85. Fujimoto, S., Greene, M., and Sehon, A. H. Regulation of the immune response to tumor antigens. *J. Immunol.* 116:791, 1976.
86. Rich, S., Carpino, M. R., Arhelger, C. Suppressor T cell growth and differentiation. *J. Exp. Med.* 159:1473, 1984.
87. Gilbert, K. M., and Hoffmann, M. K. Suppressor B lymphocytes. *Immunol. Today* 4:253, 1983.
88. Kiessling, R., Hansson, M., and Gronberg, A. Natural killer cells as regulators of malignant and normal cell growth. In Y. Yamamura and T. Tada (Eds.) *Progress in Immunology V.* New York: Academic, 1983, pp. 1181–1194.
89. Abo, T., and Balch, C. M. A differentiation antigen of human NK and K cells identified by a monoclonal antibody. *J. Immunol.* 127:1024, 1981.
90. Penschow, J., Mackay, I. R. NK and K cell activity of human blood. *Ann. Rheum. Dis.* 39:82, 1980.
91. Vose, B. M., Blackledge, G., Crowther, D., and Gallaher, J. Lectin-binding characteristics of human natural killer cells. *Immunology* 46:619, 1982.
92. Ortaldo, J. R., et al. Augmentation of human K-cell activity with interferon. *Scand. J. Immunol.* 12:355, 1980.
93. Miyasaka, N., Darnell, B., Baron, S., and Talal, N. Interleukin 2 enhances natural killing of normal lymphocytes. *Cell. Immunol.* 84:154, 1984.
94. Goto, T., Herberman, R. B., Maluish, A., and Strong, D. M. Cyclic AMP as a mediator of prostaglandin E–induced suppression of human natural killer cell activity. *J. Immunol.* 130:1350, 1983.
95. Petranyi, G. G., et al. Natural killer cells in man. In Y. Yamamura and T. Tada (Eds.), *Progress in Immunology V.* New York: Academic, 1983, pp. 1169–1180.
96. Herberman, R. B. Immune Surveillance Hypotheses. In Y. Yamamura and T. Tada (Eds.), *Progress in Immunology V.* New York: Academic, 1983, pp. 1157–1168.
97. Rowden, G., Phillips, T. M., and Lewis, M. G. Ia antigens on indeterminant cells of the epidermidis. *Br. J. Dermatol.* 100:531, 1979.

98. Muramatsu, S., et al. Accessory Cells In Immune Responses. In Y. Yamamura and T. Tada (Eds.), *Progress in Immunology V.* New York: Academic Press, 1983, pp. 989–999.
99. Stingl, G., et al. Immunologic functions of Ia bearing epidermal Langerhans' cells. *J. Immunol.* 121:2005, 1978.
100. Van Voorhis, W. C., Witmer, M. D., and Steiman, R. M. The phenotype of dendritic cells and macrophages. *Fed. Proc.* 42:3114, 1983.
101. Rosenthal, A. S. Regulation of the immune response. *N. Engl. J. Med.* 303:1153, 1980.
102. Spiegelberg, H. L. Fc receptors for IgE on macrophages and lymphocytes. *Fed. Proc.* 42:122, 1983.
103. Mackaness, G. R. Delayed Hypersensitivity and the Mechanism of Cellular Resistance to Infection. In B. Amos (Ed.), *Progress of Immunology.* New York: Academic, 1971, p. 413.
104. Wahl, S. M., et al. The role of macrophages in the production of lymphokines by T and B lymphocytes. *J. Immunol.* 114:1296, 1975.
105. David, J. R. Macrophage activation by lymphocyte mediators. *Fed. Proc.* 34:1730, 1975.
106. Scott, W. A., Rouzer, C. A., and Cohn, Z. A. Leukotriene C release by macrophages. *Fed. Proc.* 42:129, 1983.
107. Goodwin, J. S., and Ceuppens, J. Regulation of the immune response by prostaglandins. *J. Clin. Immunol.* 3:295, 1983.
108. Miller, M. E. The pathology of chemotaxis and random mobility. *Semin. Hematol.* 12:59, 1975.
109. Keller, H. U., Hess, M. W., and Cottier, H. The pathology of chemotaxis and random mobility. *Semin. Hematol.* 12:74, 1975.
110. Miller, M. E. Leukocyte movement. *J. Pediatr.* 83:1104, 1973.
111. Snyderman, R., and Stahl, C. Defective Immune Effector Function In Patients With Neoplastic and Immune Deficiency Diseases. In J. A. Bellanti and D. H. Dayton (Eds.), *The Phagocytic Cell in Host Resistance.* New York: Raven Press, 1975, p. 267.
112. Miller, M. E., Oski, F. A., and Harris, M. B. The lazy leukocyte syndrome. *Lancet* 1:565, 1971.
113. Clark, R. A., and Kimball, H. R. Defective granulocyte chemotaxis in the Chediak-Higashi syndrome. *J. Clin. Invest.* 50:2645, 1971.
114. Miller, M. E., et al. A new familial defect of neutrophil movement. *J. Lab. Clin. Med.* 82:1, 1973.
115. Altman, L. C., Snyderman, R., and Blaese, R. M. Abnormalities of chemotactic lymphokine synthesis and mononuclear leukocyte chemotaxis in Wiskott-Aldrich syndrome. *J. Clin. Invest.* 54:486, 1974.
116. Snyderman, R., et al. Deficient monocyte chemotactic responsiveness in humans with cancer. *Clin. Res.* 22:430, 1974.
117. Hill, H. R., and Quie, P. G. Defective Neutrophil Chemotaxis Associated with Hyperimmunoglobulinemia E. In J. A. Bellanti and D. H. Dayton (Eds.), *The Phagocytic Cell in Host Resistance.* New York: Raven, 1975, p. 249.
118. Hill, H. R., et al. Defect in neutrophil granulocyte chemotaxis in Job's syndrome of recurrent "cold" staphylococcal abscesses. *Lancet* 2:617, 1974.
119. Hill, H. R., and Quie, P. G. Raised serum IgE levels and defective neutrophil chemotaxis in 3 children with eczema and recurrent bacterial infections. *Lancet* 1:183, 1974.
120. Buckley, R. H., Wray, B. B., and Belmaker, E. Z. Extreme hyper-immuno-

globulinemia E and undue susceptibility to infections. *Pediatrics* 49:59, 1972.
121. Bagdade, J. D., Root, R. K., and Bulger, R. J. Impaired leukocyte function in patients with poorly controlled diabetes. *Diabetes* 23:9, 1974.
122. Muller-Eberhard, H. J. Complement and Phagocytosis. In J. A. Bellanti and D. H. Dayton (Eds.), *The Phagocytic Cell in Host Resistance.* New York: Raven, 1975, p. 87.
123. Stossel, T. P. Phagocytosis. *Semin. Hematol.* 12:83, 1975.
124. Klebanoff, S. J. Antimicrobial Systems of the Polymorphonuclear Leukocytes. In J. A. Bellanti and D. H. Dayton (Eds.), *The Phagocytic Cell in Host Resistance.* New York: Raven, 1975, p. 45.
125. Klebanoff, S. J. Antimicrobial mechanisms in neutrophilic polymorphonuclear leukocytes. *Semin. Hematol.* 12:117, 1975.
126. Wagoner, M. D. et al. Polymorphonuclear neutrophils delay corneal epithelial wound healing in vitro. *Invest. Ophthalmol.* 25:1217, 1984.
127. Spragg, J. The Plasma Kinin-Forming System. In G. Weissmann (Ed.), *Mediators of Inflammation.* New York: Plenum, 1974, p. 85.
128. Cochrane, C. G. The Hageman Factor. In G. Katona and J. R. Blengio (Eds.), *Inflammation and Anti-inflammatory Therapy.* New York: Spectrum, 1974, p. 119.
129. Nemerson, F. A., and Pitlick, F. A. The tissue factor pathway of blood coagulation. *Prog. Hemost. Thromb.* 1:1, 1972.
130. Kaplan, A. P., and Austen, K. F. The fibrinolytic pathway of human plasma. *J. Exp. Med.* 136:1376, 1972.
131. Muller-Eberhard, H. J. Complement. *Ann. Rev. Biochem.* 44:697, 1975.
132. Vogt, W. Activation, activities and pharmacologically active products of complement. *Pharmacol. Rev.* 28:125, 1974.
133. Naff, G. B., and Ratnoff, O. D. The enzymatic nature of C1r. *J. Exp. Med.* 128:571, 1968.
134. Muller-Eberhard, H. J., Dalmasso, A. P., and Calcott, M. A. The reaction mechanisms of C^13 in immune hemolysis. *J. Exp. Med.* 123:33, 1966.
135. Stroud, R. M., Austen, K. F., and Mayer, M. M. Catalysis of C^12 fixation by C^1a. *Immunochemistry* 2:219, 1965.
136. Mayer, M. M., et al. Kinetic studies on immune hemolysis. *J. Immunol.* 73:443, 1954.
137. Muller-Eberhard, H. J., Polley, M. J., and Calcott, M. A. Formation and functional significance of a molecular complex derived from the second and the fourth component of human complement. *J. Exp. Med.* 125:359, 1967.
138. Nilsson, U. R., and Muller-Eberhard, H. J. Studies on the modes of action of the fifth, sixth and seventh component of human complement in immune hemolysis. *Immunology* 13:101, 1967.
139. Yachnin, S. The hemolysis of red cells from patients with paroxysmal nocturnal hemoglobinuria by partially purified subcomponents of the third complement component. *J. Clin. Invest.* 44:1543, 1965.
140. Hadding, U., and Muller-Eberhard, H. J. The ninth component of human complement. *Immunology* 16:719, 1969.
141. Stolfi, R. L. Immune lytic transformation. *J. Immunol.* 100:46, 1968.
142. Muller-Eberhard, H. J. Complement. *Ann. Rev. Biochem.* 38:389, 1969.
143. Levy, L. R., and Lepow, I. H. Assay and properties of serum inhibitor of C^1 esterase. *J. Biol. Chem.* 236:1674, 1961.

144. Nelson, R. A., et al. Methods for the separation, purification and measurement of 9 components of hemolytic complement in guinea pig serum. *Immunochemistry* 3:111, 1966.
145. Tamura, N., and Nelson, R. A., Jr. Three naturally occurring inhibitors of components of complement in guinea pig and rabbit serum. *J. Immunol.* 99:582, 1967.
146. Lachmann, P. J. Conglutinin and immunoconglutinin. *Adv. Immunol.* 6:479, 1967.
147. Bakisch, V. R., Muller-Eberhard, H. J., and Cochrane, C. G. Isolation of fragment (C3a) of the third component of human complement containing anaphylatoxin and chemotactic activity and description of an anaphylatoxin inactivator of human serum. *J. Exp. Med.* 129:1190, 1969.
148. Gotze, O., and Muller-Eberhard, H. F. Mechanisms of lysis of nonsensitized cells by complement. *Fed. Proc.* 28:818, 1969.
149. Perlmann, P., et al. Cytotoxic effects of leukocytes triggered by complement bound to target cells. *Science* 163:937, 1969.
150. Klemperer, M. R., Rosen, F. S., and Donaldson, V. H. A polypeptide derived from the second component of human complement (C2) which increases vascular permeability. *Clin. Invest.* 48:44, 1969.
151. Shin, H. S., et al. Chemotactic and anaphylatoxic fragment cleaved from the fifth component of guinea pig complement. *Science* 162:361, 1968.
152. Egwang, T. G., and Befus, A. D. The role of complement in the induction and regulation of immune responses. *Immunology* 51:297, 1984.
153. Sundsmo, J. S. Leukocyte complement. *J. Immunol.* 131:886, 1983.
154. Morgan, E. L., Weigle, W. O., and Hugli, T. E. Anaphylatoxin-mediated regulation of human and murine immune responses. *Fed. Proc.* 43:2543, 1984.
155. Hugli, T. E. Biological Activities of Fragments Derived From Human Complement Components. In Y. Yamamura and T. Tada (Eds.), *Progress in Immunology V.* New York: Academic, 1983, pp. 419–426.
156. Donaldson, V. H., and Evans, R. R. A biochemical abnormality in hereditary angioneurotic edema. *Am. J. Med.* 35:37, 1963.
157. Pickering, R. M., et al. Deficiency of C1r in human serum. *J. Exp. Med.* 131:803, 1970.
158. Day, N. K., et al. C1r deficiency. *J. Clin. Invest.* 51:1102, 1972.
159. Ruddy, S., et al. Hereditary deficiency of the second component of complement (C2) in man. *Immunology* 18:943, 1970.
160. Alper, C. A., et al. Homozygous deficiency of C3 in a patient with reported infections. *Lancet* 2:1179, 1972.
161. Ziegler, J. B., et al. Restoration by purified C3b inactivator of complement-mediated function *in vivo* in a patient with C3b inactivator deficiency. *J. Clin. Invest.* 55:668, 1975.
162. Thompson, R. A., and White, R. H. R. Partial lipodystrophy and hypocomplementemic nephritis. *Lancet* 2:679, 1973.
163. Miller, M. E., and Nillson, U. R. A familial deficiency of the phagocytosis-enhancing activity of serum related to a dysfunction of the fifth component of complement (C5). *N. Engl. J. Med.* 282:354, 1970.
164. Miller, M. E., and Koblenzer, P. J. Leiner's disease and deficiency of C5. *J. Pediatr.* 80:879, 1972.
165. Rother, K., et al. Deficiency of the sixth component of complement in rabbits with an inherited complement defect. *J. Exp. Med.* 124:773, 1966.
166. Nillson, U. R., and Muller-Eberhard, H. F. Deficiency of the fifth compo-

nent of complement in mice with an inherited complement defect. *J. Exp. Med.* 125:1, 1967.
167. Schroeter, A. L., et al. Immunofluorescence of cutaneous vasculitis associated with systemic disease. *Arch. Dermatol.* 104:2, 1971.
168. Henson, P. M. Mechanisms of Mediator Release From Inflammatory Cells. In G. Weissmann (Ed.), *Mediators of Inflammation.* New York: Plenum Press, 1974, p. 9.
169. Lerner, R. G., Goldstein, R., and Cummings, G. Stimulation of human leukocyte thromboplastic activity by endotoxin. *Proc. Soc. Exp. Biol. Med.* 138:145, 1971.
170. Goldstein, I. M., and Weissman, G. Generation of C5-derived lysosomal enzyme releasing activity (C5a) by lysates of leukocyte lysosomes. *J. Immunol.* 113:1583, 1974.
171. Sly, R. M. Pathogenesis of asthma. *Ann. Allergy* 49:14, 1982.
172. Ninnemann, J. L. Prostaglandins and immunity. *Immunol. Today* 5:170, 1984.
173. Goldyne, M. E., and Stobo, J. D. Immunoregulatory role of prostaglandins and related lipids. *Crit. Rev. Immunol.* 12:189, 1981.
174. Ceuppens, J. L., and Goodwin, J. S. Endogenous prostaglandin E enhances polyclonal immunoglobulin production by tonically inhibiting T suppressor cell activity. *Cell. Immunol.* 40:41, 1982.
175. Prickett, J. D., Robinson, D. R., and Steinberg, A. D. Dietary enrichment with the polyunsaturated fatty acid, eicosapentaenoic acid, prevents proteinuria and prolongs survival in NZB/NZW F1 mice. *J. Clin. Invest.* 68:556, 1981.
176. Bhattacherjee, P. Prostaglandins and inflammatory reactions in the eye. *Methods Find. Exp. Clin. Pharmacol.* 2:17, 1980.
177. Kulkarni, P. S., and Srinivasan, B. D. The effect of intravitreal and topical prostaglandins on intraocular inflammation. *Invest. Ophthalmol. Vis. Sci.* 23:383, 1982.
178. Duffin, R. M., Weissman, B. A., Glasser, D. B., and Pettit, T. H. Flurbiprofen in the treatment of corneal neovascularization induced by contact lenses. *Am. J. Ophthalmol.* 93:607, 1982.
179. Smolin, G. Use of anti-inflammatory agents in destructive corneal disease. *Trans. Ophthalmol. Soc. U. K.* 98:406, 1978.
180. Garella, S., and Matarese, R. A. Renal effects of prostaglandins and clinical adverse effects of nonsteroidal antiinflammatory agents. *Medicine* 63:165, 1984.
181. Stern, R. S., and Bigby, M. An expanded profile of cutaneous reactions to nonsteroidal antiinflammatory drugs. *J.A.M.A.* 252:1433, 1984.
182. Trousdale, M. D., Dunkel, E. C., and Nesburn, A. B. Effect of flurbiprofen on herpes simplex keratitis in rabbits. *Invest. Ophthalmol. Vis. Sci.* 19:267, 1980.
183. Kehrl, J. H., and Fauci, A. S. The clinical use of glucocorticoids. *Ann. Allergy* 50:2, 1983.
184. Claman, H. N. How corticosteroids work. *J. Allergy Clin. Immunol.* 55:145, 1975.
185. Parker, C. W., Huber, M. G., and Baumann, M. L. Alterations in cyclic AMP metabolism in human bronchial asthma. *J. Clin. Invest.* 52:1342, 1973.
186. Mendelsohn, J., Mutler, M. M., and Boone, R. F. Enhanced effects of prostaglandin E and dibutyryl cyclic AMP on human lymphocytes in the presence of cortisol. *J. Clin. Invest.* 52:2129, 1973.

187. Webb, R. D. Steroids in allergic disease. *Med. Clin. North Am.* 65:1073, 1981.
188. Greeson, T. P., et al. Corticosteroid-induced vasocontriction studied by xenon 133-clearance. *J. Invest. Dermatol.* 61:242, 1973.
189. Germuth, F. G., Jr., et al. A unique influence of cortisone on the transit of specific macromolecules across vascular walls in immune complex disease. *Johns Hopkins Med. J.* 122:137, 1968.
190. Ward, P. A. The chemosuppression of chemotaxis. *J. Exp. Med.* 124:209, 1966.
191. Weissman, G., Sessa, G., and Bevans, V. Effect of DMSO on the stabilization of lysosomes by cortisone and chloroquin in vitro. *Ann. N.Y. Acad. Sci.* 141:326, 1967.
192. Rinehart, J. J., et al. Effects of corticosteroids on human monocyte function. *J. Clin. Invest.* 54:1337, 1974.
193. Cupps, T. R., and Fauci, A. S. Corticosteroid-mediated immunoregulation in man. *Immunol. Rev.* 65:133, 1982.
194. Coburg, A. J., et al. Disappearance rates and immunosuppression of intermittent intravenously administered prednisone in rabbits and human beings. *Surg. Gynecol. Obstet.* 131:933, 1970.
195. Stavy, L., Cohen, I. R., and Feldman, M. The effect of hydrocortisone on lymphocyte-mediated cytolysis. *Cell. Immunol.* 7:302, 1973.
196. Zweiman, B., Atkins, P. G., and Bedard, P. Corticosteroids' effect on circulating lymphocyte subsets. *J. Clin. Immunol.* 4:151, 1984.
197. Vann, D. C. Restoration of the *in vitro* antibody response of cortisone-treated spleen cells by T cells or soluble factors. *Cell. Immunol.* 11:11, 1971.
198. Wahl, S. M. Corticosteroid inhibition of chemotactic lymphokine production by T and B lymphocytes. *Ann. N.Y. Acad. Sci.* 256:375, 1975.
199. Kaplan, M. P., Lysz, K., Rosenberg, S. A., and Rosenberg, J. C. Suppression of interleukin 2 production by methylprednisolone. *Transplant. Proc.* 15:407, 1983.
200. Barlow, J. E., and Rosenthal, A. S. Glucocorticoid suppression of macrophage migration inhibition factor. *J. Exp. Med.* 137:1031, 1973.
201. Levine, B. B., Stember, R. H., and Fotino, M. Ragweed hay fever. *Science* 1978:1201, 1972.
202. Marsh, D. G., et al. Association of an HLA7 cross-reacting group with a specific reaginic antibody response in allergic man. *Science* 179:691, 1973.
203. Barrett, K. E., and Metcalfe, D. D. Mast cell heterogeneity. *J. Clin. Immunol.* 4:253, 1983.
204. McGlashan, D. W., Jr., et al. Comparative studies of human basophils and mast cells. *Fed. Proc.* 42:2504, 1983.
205. Hubscher, T., and Eisen, A. H. A Possible Immunopharmacological Role of Human Eosinophils in Allergic Reactions. In L. Goodfriend, A. H. Sehan, and R. P. Orange (Eds.), *Mechanisms in Allergy.* New York: Marcel Decker, 1973, p. 431.
206. Ishizaka, K., Ishizaka, T., Okudaira, H., and Bazin, H. Ontogeny of IgE-bearing lymphocytes in the rat. *J. Immunol.* 120:655, 1978.
207. Ishizaka, K. Regulation of the IgE antibody response. *Int. Arch. Allergy Appl. Immunol.* 66:1, 1981.
208. Gillon, J. Where do mucosal mast cells acquire IgE? *Immunol. Today* 2:80, 1981.
209. Parker, C. W. Intracellular Activation in Mast Cells and Lymphocytes. In Y. Yamamura and T. Tada (Eds.), *Progress in Immunology V.* New York: Academic Press, 1983, pp. 327–337.

210. Malley, A., Baecher, L., and Burger, D. The role of complement in allergen reagin mediated histamine release from monkey lung tissue. *Proc. Soc. Exp. Bio. Med.* 136:341, 1971.
211. Glauser, F. L., et al. The effect of endotoxin on the mast cell cAMP system. *Ann. Allergy* 38:104, 1977.
212. Siraganian, R. P., and Siraganian, P. A. Mechanism of action of concanavalin A on human basophils. *J. Immunol.* 114:886, 1975.
213. Vervlet, D., Vellieux, P., and Charpin, J. Potentiation of cutaneous reactivity and blood leukocyte histamine release by deuterium oxide in human beings. *Acta Allergol.* 31:367, 1976.
214. Ambache, N., and Brummer, A. C. A simple chemical procedure for distinguishing E from F prostaglandin with application to tissue extracts. *Br. J. Pharmacol. Chemother.* 33:162, 1968.
215. Belfort, R., et al. Indomethacin and the corneal immune response. *Am. J. Ophthalmol.* 81:650, 1976.
216. Wasserman, S. I. Mediators of immediate hypersensitivity. *J. Allergy Clin. Immunol.* 72:101, 1983.
217. Marom, Z., and Casale, T. B. Mast cells and their mediators. *Ann. Allergy* 50:367, 1983.
218. Kaliner, M., and Lemanske, R. Inflammatory responses to mast cell granules. *Fed. Proc.* 43:2846, 1984.
219. Abelson, M. B., and Udell, I. J. H_2-receptors in the human ocular surface. *Arch. Ophthalmol.* 99:302, 1981.
220. Goetzl, E. J., Payan, D. G., and Goldman, D. W. Immunopathogenetic roles of leukotrienes in human diseases. *J. Clin. Immunol.* 4:79, 1984.
221. Casale, T. B., and Marom, Z. Mast cells and asthma. *Ann. Allergy* 51:2, 1983.
222. Marom, Z., et al. Slow-reacting substances, leukotrienes C_4 and D_4, increase the release of mucus from human airways *in vitro*. *Am. Rev. Respir. Dis.* 126:449, 1982.
223. Farr, R. S. Platelet activating factor. *West J. Med.* 141:506, 1984.
224. Gleich, G. J., and Loegering, D. A. Immunobiology of eosinophils. *Ann. Rev. Immunol.* 2:429, 1984.
225. Hubscher, T. Role of the eosinophil in the allergic reactions. *J. Immunol.* 114:1379, 1975.
226. Rocklin, R. E. Modulation of cellular-immune responses *in vivo* and *in vitro* by histamine receptor-bearing lymphocytes. *J. Clin. Invest.* 57:1051, 1976.
227. Artis, W. M., Jones, H. E., and Balzkovec, A. A. Histamine inhibition of human lymphocyte transformation. *Fed. Proc.* 34(3):1002, 1975.
228. Verhaegen, H., DeCock, W., and Decree, J. Histamine receptor-bearing and peripheral T lymphocytes in patients with allergies. *J. Allergy Clin. Immunol.* 59:266, 1977.
229. Taylor, B., et al. Transient IgA deficiency and pathogenesis of infantile atopy. *Lancet* 2:111, 1973.
230. Jarett, E. E. E., and Hall, E. IgE suppression by maternal IgG. *Immunol.* 48:49, 1983.
231. Tada, T. Regulation of reaginic antibody formation in animals. *Prog. Allergy* 19:122, 1975.
232. Kishimoto, T., and Ishizaka, K. Regulation of antibody response *in vitro*. *J. Immunol.* 112:1685, 1974.
233. Waldmann, T. A., et al. Immunoglobulin E in immunologic deficiency diseases. *J. Immunol.* 109:304, 1972.
234. Buckley, R. H., Wray, B. B., and Belmaker, E. Z. Extreme hyperimmuno-

globulinemia E and undue susceptibility to infection. *Pediatrics* 49:59, 1972.
235. Katona, I. M., Tata, G., Scanlon, R. T., and Bellanti, J. A. Hyper IgE syndrome. *Ann. Allergy* 45:295, 1980.
236. Bier, D. J., et al. Abnormal histamine-induced suppressor-cell function in atopic subjects. *N. Engl. J. Med.* 306:454, 1982.
237. Damle, M. K., and Gupta, S. Autologous mixed lymphocyte reaction in man. *J. Clin. Immunol.* 1:241, 1981.
238. Coombs, R. R. A. Immunopathological mechanisms. *Proc. R. Soc. Med.* 67:525, 1974.
239. Irvine, W. J. Autoimmunity in endocrine disease. *Proc. R. Soc. Med.* 67:543, 1974.
240. Dacie, J. V., and Wolledge, S. M. Autoimmune hemolytic anemia. *Prog. Hematol.* 61:7, 1969.
241. Kerr, R. O., et al. Two mechanisms of eythrocyte destruction in penicillin-induced hemolytic anemia. *N. Engl. J. Med.* 287:1322, 1972.
242. Wintrobe, M. M. *Clinical Hematology* (5th ed.). Philadelphia: Lea & Febiger, 1961.
243. Cochrane, C. G. Contribution to Discussion. In I. H. Lepow and P. A. Ward (Eds.), *Inflammation—Mechanism and Control*. New York: Academic, 1972, p. 365.
244. Jasin, H. E., Lospalluto, J., and Ziff, M. Rheumatoid hyperviscosity syndrome. *Am. J. Med.* 49:484, 1970.
245. Dixon, F. J., et al. Pathogenesis of serum sickness. *Arch. Pathol.* 65:18, 1958.
246. Weigle, W. O., and Dixon, F. J. Relationship of circulating antigen-antibody complexes, antigen elimination and complement fixation in serum sickness. *Proc. Soc. Exp. Biol. Med.* 99:226, 1958.
247. Stavitsky, A. B., Hackel, D. B., and Heymann, W. Reduction of serum complement following *in vivo* antigen-antibody reaction. *Proc. Soc. Exp. Biol. Med.* 85:593, 1954.
248. Alper, C. A., and Rosen, F. S. Studies of the *in vivo* behavior of human C^{13} in normal subjects and patients. *J. Clin. Invest.* 46:2021, 1967.
249. Kohler, P. F., Hutt, M. P., and Riley, C. *In vivo* metabolism of C3 and C4 in hypocomplementemic chronic glomerulonephritis. *J. Clin. Invest.* 48:45a, 1969.
250. Paronetto, F., and Koffler, D. Immunofluorescent localization of immunoglobulins, complement and fibrinogen in human disease. *J. Clin. Invest.* 44:1657, 1965.
251. Tan, E. M., et al. DNA and antibodies to DNA in the serum of patients with systemic lupus erythematosus. *J. Clin. Invest.* 45:1732, 1966.
252. Fostiropoulos, G., Austen, K. F., and Block, K. J. Fatal hemolytic complement and second component of complement activity in serum and synovial fluid. *Arthritis Rheum.* 8:219, 1965.
253. Leddy, J. P. Immunological aspects of red cell injury in man. *Semin. Hematol.* 3:48, 1966.
254. Wemanbu, S. C. N., et al. Erythema nodosum leprosum. *Lancet* 2:933, 1969.
255. Ward, P. A., and Cochrane, C. G. Bound complement and immunologic injury of blood vessels. *J. Exp. Med.* 121:215, 1965.
256. Lawrence, H. S. The cellular transfer of cutaneous hypersensitivity to tuberculin in man. *Proc. Soc. Exp. Biol. Med.* 71:516, 1949.
257. Askernase, P. W., and Van Loveren, H. Delayed-type hypersensitivity. *Immunol. Today* 4:259, 1983.

258. David, J. R., et al. Delayed hypersensitivity *in vitro. J. Immunol.* 93:264, 1964.
259. David, J. R. Suppression of delayed hypersensitivity *in vitro* by inhibition of protein synthesis. *J. Exp. Med.* 122:1125, 1965.
260. Spitler, L. E., and Lawrence, H. S. Studies on lymphocyte culture. *J. Immunol.* 103:1072, 1969.
261. Granger, G. A. Mechanisms of lymphocyte-induced cell and tissue destruction *in vitro. Am. J. Pathol.* 59:469, 1970.
262. Smith, R. T., Baucher, J. A. C., and Adler, W. H. Studies of an inhibitor of DNA synthesis and a nonspecific mitogen elaborated by human lymphoblasts. *Am. J. Pathol.* 60:495, 1970.
263. Bennett, B., and Bloom, B. R. Reactions *in vivo* and *in vitro* produced by a soluble substance associated with delayed-type hypersensitivity. *Proc. Natl. Acad. Sci. U.S.A.* 59:756, 1968.
264. Onsrud, M. Enhancement of suppressor cell generation in human mixed lymphocyte cultures by interferon. *Int. Arch. Allergy Appl. Immunol.* 67:315, 1982.
265. Hokland, P., Berg, K. Interferon enhances the ADCC of human polymorphonuclear leukocytes. *J. Immunol.* 127:1585, 1981.
266. Trinchieri, G., and Santoli, D. Antiviral activity induced by culturing lymphocytes. *J. Exp. Med.* 147:1314, 1978.
267. Borashi, D., Soldateschi, D., and Tagliabue, A. Macrophage activation by interferon. *Eur. J. Immunol.* 12:320, 1982.
268. Waldorf, D. S., Wilkens, R. F., and Decker, J. L. Impaired delayed hypersensitivity in an aging population. *J. A. M. A.* 203:831, 1968.
269. Schultz, R. D. Assays of cellular immunity. *J. Am. Vet. Med. Assoc.* 181:1169, 1982.
270. De Weck, A. L. Contact Eczematous Dermatitis in Dermatology. In T. B. Fitzpatrick et al. (Ed.), *General Medicine.* New York: McGraw-Hill, 1971, p. 669.
271. Hjorth, N., and Fregert, S. Contact Dermatitis. In A. Rook, J. Ebling, and D. Wilkinson (Eds.), *Textbook of Dermatology.* London: Blackwell, 1972, p. 305.
272. Rudner, E. J., et al. The frequency of contact sensitivity in North America. *Contact Dermatol.* 1:277, 1975.
273. Brun, R. Epidemiology of contact dermatitis in Geneva. *Contact Dermatol.* 1:214, 1975.
274. De Panfilis, G., et al. Macrophage-T lymphocyte relationships in man's contact allergic reactions. *Br. J. Dermatol.* 109:183, 1983.
275. Aiba, S., Aizawa, H., Obata, M., Tagami, H. Dynamic changes in epidermal 1a-positive cells in allergic contact sensitivity reactions in mice. *Br. J. Dermatol.* 3:507, 1984.
276. Dvorak, H. F., Mihm, M. C., Jr., and Dvorak, A. M. Morphology of delayed-type hypersensitivity reactions in man. *Lab. Invest.* 34:179, 1976.
277. Bigley, N. J. (Ed.). *Immunologic Fundamentals.* Chicago: Year Book, 1975, p. 140.
278. Doherty, P. C., and Zinkernagel, R. M. T-cell mediated immunopathology in viral infections. *Transplant. Rev.* 19:89, 1974.
279. Zinkernagel, R. M., and Doherty, P. C. Immunological surveillance against altered self-components by sensitized T lymphocytes in lymphocytic choriomeningitis. *Nature* 251:547, 1974.
280. Doherty, P. C., and Zinkernagel, R. M. H-2 compatibility is required for T

cell mediated lysis of target cells infected with lymphocytic choriomeningitis virus. *J. Exp. Med.* 141:502, 1975.
281. Roger-Zisman, B., and Bloom, B. R. Immunologic destruction of herpes simplex virus I infected cells. *Nature* 251:542, 1974.
282. Merigan, T. C. Host defenses against viral disease. *N. Engl. J. Med.* 290:223, 1974.
283. Stevens, D. A., and Merigan, T. C. Interferon, antibody and other host factors in herpes zoster. *J. Clin. Invest.* 51:1170, 1972.
284. Remington, J. S. The compromised host. *Hosp. Pract.* 7:59, 1972.
285. Anderson, S. E., and Remington, J. S. Effect of normal and activated human macrophages on *Toxoplasma gondii. J. Exp. Med.* 131:1154, 1974.
286. Wing, E. J., and Remington, S. Cell-mediated immunity and its role in resistance in infection. *West. J. Med.* 126:14, 1977.
287. Kleinerman, E. S., Snyderman, R., and Daniels, C. A. Depressed monocyte chemotaxis during acute influenza infection. *Lancet* 2:1063, 1975.
288. Sullivan, L., et al. Measles infection of human mononuclear cells. *J. Exp. Med.* 142:773, 1975.
289. Yamamura, Y. A Brief Overview of Recent Progress in Tumor Immunotherapy. In Y. Yamamura and T. Tada (Eds.), *Progress in Immunology V.* New York: Academic, 1983, pp. 1129–1138.
290. Kerr, J. F. R., Wyllie, A. H., and Currie, A. R. Apoptosis. *Br. J. Cancer* 26:239, 1972.
291. Purtilo, D. T., and Linder, J. Oncological consequences of impaired immune surveillance against ubiquitous viruses. *J. Clin. Immunol.* 3:197, 1983.
292. Trentin, J. J., and Bryan, E. Immunization of hamsters and histoisogenic mice against transplantation of tumors induced by human adenovirus type 12. *Proc. Am. Assoc. Cancer Res.* 5:64, 1964.
293. Old, L. J., et al. Antigenic properties of chemically induced tumors. *Ann. N.Y. Acad. Sci.* 101:80, 1962.
294. Abelev, G. I. Production of embryonal serum and globulin by hepatomas. *Cancer Res.* 28:1344, 1968.
295. Gold, P., and Freedman, S. Specific carcinoembryonic antigens of the human digestive system. *J. Exp. Med.* 122:467, 1965.
296. Riesco, A. Five-year cancer cure. *Cancer* 25:135, 1970.
297. Cutler, S. J., et al. Further observations on prognostic factors in cancer of the female breast. *Cancer* 24:653, 1969.
298. Gold, P., and Freedman, S. Demonstration of tumor-specific antigens in human colonic carcinomata by immunological tolerance and absorption techniques. *J. Exp. Med.* 121:439, 1965.
299. Morton, D. L., et al. Demonstration of antibodies against human melanoma by immunofluroescence. *Surgery* 64:233, 1968.
300. Granger, G. A., and Kolb, W. P. Lymphocyte *in vitro* cytotoxicity. *J. Immunol.* 101:111, 1968.
301. Heise, E. R., and Weiser, R. S. Factors in delayed hypersensitivity. *J. Immunol.* 103:570, 1969.
302. Droller, M. J., Borg, H., and Perlmann, P. O. *In vitro* enhancement of natural and antibody-dependent lymphocyte mediated cytotoxicity against tumor target cells by interferon. *Cell. Immunol.* 47:248, 1979.
303. Attallah, A. M., Needy, C. F., and Noguchi, C. Enhancement of carcinoembryonic antigen expression by interferon. *Int. J. Cancer* 24:49, 1979.
304. Klimpel, G. R., Fleischmann, W. R., and Klimpel, K. D. Gamma interferon

and interferon α/β suppress murine myeloid colony formation. *J. Immunol.* 129:76, 1982.
305. Brysk, M. M., Tschen, E. H., and Hudson, R. D. The activity of interferon on ultraviolet light-induced squamous cell carcinomas in mice. *Am. Acad. Dermatol.* 27:61, 1981.
306. Sherwin, S. A., Knost, J. A., and Fein, S. Multiple-dose phase 1 trial of recombinant leukocyte A interferon in cancer patients. *J.A.M.A.* 248:2461, 1982.
307. Goodwin, J. S. Prostaglandins and host defense in cancer. *Med. Clin. North Am.* 65:829, 1981.
308. Fraumeni, J. F. Constitutional disorders of man leading to leukemia and lymphoma. *Natl. Cancer Inst. Monogr. Hemopoietic Neoplasms* 32:221, 1969.
309. Doak, P. B., et al. Reticulum cell sarcoma after renal homotransplantation and azathioprine and prednisone therapy. *Br. Med. J.* 4:746, 1968.
310. Harris, J., and Sinkovics, J. B. *The Immunology of Malignant Disease.* St. Louis: Mosby, 1970.
311. Rey, A., et al. Diminished IL-2 activity production in cancer patients bearing solid tumors and its relationship with natural killer cells. *Immunol. Lett.* 6:175, 1983.
312. Sjögren, H. O., et al. Suggestive evidence that blocking antibodies of tumor-bearing individuals may be antigen-antibody complexes. *Proc. Natl. Acad. Sci. U.S.A.* 68:1372, 1971.
313. Baldwin, R. W., et al. Immunity in the tumor-bearing host and its modification by serum factors. *Cancer* 34:1452, 1974.
314. Heppner, G. H., and Calabresis, P. Suppression by cytotoxin arabinoside of serum-blocking factors of cell-mediated immunity to syngeneic transplants of mouse mammary tumors. *J. Natl. Cancer Inst.* 48:1161, 1972.
315. Hellstrom, K. E., and Hellstrom, I. L. Lymphocyte mediated cytotoxicity and blocking serum activity to tumor antigens. *Adv. Immunol.* 18:209, 1974.
316. Nathanson, L., Hall, T. C., and Farber, S. Biological aspects of human malignant melanoma. *Cancer* 20:650, 1967.
317. Miller, R. A., Maloney, D. G., Warnke, R., and Levy, R. Treatment of B cell lymphoma with monoclonal antiidiotype antibody. *N. Engl. J. Med.* 306:517, 1982.
318. Hardy, M. A., et al. The effect of thymosin on human T cells from cancer patients. *Cancer* 37:98, 1976.
319. Currie, G. A., and Bagsgawe, K. D. The effect of *Corynebacterium parvum* on tumor invasion. *Br. Med. J.* 1:541, 1970.
320. Mathe, G. Attempts at Using Systemic Immunity Adjuvants in Experimental and Human Cancer Therapy. In Ciba Foundation Symposium, *Immunopotentiation.* Amsterdam: Associated Scientific Publishers, 1973.
321. Allison, A. C., and Davies, A. J. S. Requirement of thymus-dependent lymphocytes for potentiation by adjuvants of antibody formation. *Nature* 233:330, 1971.
322. Klein, E., et al. Immunotherapy for accessible tumors utilizing delayed hypersensitivity reactions and separated components of the immune system. *Med. Clin. North Am.* 60:389, 1976.
323. Ehrlich, P. On immunity with special references to cell life. *Proc. R. Soc. Lond.* 66B:424, 1900.
324. Bankhurst, A. D., Torriginai, G., and Allison, A. C. Lymphocytes binding

human thyroglobulin in healthy people and its relevance to tolerance for autoantigens. *Lancet* 1:226, 1973.
325. Hallgre, H. M., and Yunis, E. J. Suppressor lymphocytes in young and aged humans. *J. Immunol.* 118:2004, 1977.
326. Penhale, W. J., et al. Spontaneous thyroiditis in thymectomized and irradiated Wistar rats. *Clin. Exp. Immunol.* 15:225, 1973.
327. Talal, N. Disordered immunologic regulation and autoimmunity. *Transplant. Rev.* 31:240, 1976.
328. Talal, N., Dauphinee, M. J., Ahmed, A., and Christados, P. Sex Factors in Immunity and Autoimmunity. In Y. Yamamura and T. Tada (Eds.), *Progress in Immunology V.* New York: Academic Press, 1983, pp. 1589–1599.
329. Ishizaka, T., Campbell, D. H., Ishizaka, K. Internal antigenic determinants in protein molecules. *Proc. Soc. Exp. Biol. Med.* 103:5, 1960.
330. Klemperer, P., Pollack, A. D., and Baehr, G. Diffuse collagen disease. *J.A.M.A.* 119:331, 1942.
331. Roitt, I. *Essential Immunology* (2nd Ed.). London: Blackwell, 1974.
332. Fraser, K. J. IgA immunoglobulins and autoimmunity. *Lancet* 2:804, 1969.
333. Smolin, G., and Wilson, F. M., II. Antilymphocyte serum. *Surv. Ophthalmol.* 18:200, 1973.
334. Levey, R. H., and Medawar, P. B. Nature and mode of action of antilymphocytic antiserum. *Proc. Natl. Acad. Sci. U.S.A.* 56:1130, 1966.
335. Allison, A. C. Effects of antilymphocytic serum on bacterial and viral infections and virus oncogenesis. *Fed. Proc.* 29:167, 1970.
336. Huntley, R. T., et al. Use of antilymphocyte serum to prolong dog homograft survival. *Surg. Forum* 17:230, 1966.
337. Guttman, R. D., et al. Treatment with heterologous antithymus sera. *Transplantation* 5:1115, 1967.
338. Grogan, J. B. Effect of antilymphocyte serum on mortality of *Pseudomonas aeruginsa*–infected rats. *Arch. Surg.* 99:382, 1969.
339. Edelman, R., and Wheelock, E. F. Enhancement of replication of vesicular stomatitis virus in human lymphocyte cultures treated with heterologous antilymphocyte serum. *Lancet* 1:771, 1968.
340. Rifkind, D., et al. Systemic fungal infections complicating renal transplantation and immunosuppressive therapy. *Am. J. Med.* 43:28, 1967.
341. Rolland, J. M., and Nairn, R. C. Antilymphocyte serum. *Pathology* 4:85, 1972.
342. Bennett, L. L., Jr., et al. The primary site of inhibition by 6-mercaptopurine on the purine biosynthetic pathway in some tissues *in vivo*. *Cancer Res.* 23:1574, 1963.
343. Brock, N. Pharmacologic characterization of cyclophosphamide and cyclophosphamide metabolites. *Cancer Chemother. Rep.* 51:315, 1967.
344. Caskey, C. T., Ashton, D. M., and Wyngaarden, J. B. The enzymology of feedback inhibition of glutamine phosphoribosylpyrophosphate amidotransferase by purine ribonucleotides. *J. Biol. Chem.* 239:2570, 1964.
345. Dupont, E., Vandercruys, M., and Wybran, J. Deficient natural killer function in patients receiving immunosuppressive drugs. *Cell. Immunol.* 88:85, 1984.
346. Prussoff, W. H. Substitution of DNA with Base Analogs. In P. N. Campbell (Ed.), *Interaction of Drugs and Subcellular Components in Animal Cells.* London: Churchill, 1968.

347. Werkheiser, W. C. The biochemical, cellular and pharmacological action and effects of the folic acid antagonists. *Cancer Res.* 23:1277, 1963.
348. Coutsogeorgopoulos, C. On the mechanism of action of chloramphenicol in protein synthesis. *Biochem. Biophys. Acta* 129:214, 1966.
349. Bruchovsky, N., et al. Effects of vinblastine on the proliferative capacity of L cells and their progress through the division cycle. *Cancer Res.* 25:1232, 1965.
350. Helin, H. J., and Edgington, T. S. Cyclosporin A regulates monocytes/macrophage effector functions by affecting instructor T cells. *J. Immunol.* 132:1074, 1984.
351. McNatt, J., Allen, S. D., Wilson, L. A., and Dowell, V. R., Jr. Anaerobic flora of the normal human conjunctival sac. *Arch. Ophthalmol.* 96:1448, 1978.
352. Fredrickson, A. B. Behavior of mixed culture of microorganisms. *Ann. Rev. Microbiol.* 31:63, 1977.
353. Wolff, E. *Anatomy of the Eye and Orbit.* Philadelphia: Saunders, 1961.
354. Taylor, L., Menconi, M., Leibowitz, H. M., and Polgar, P. The effect of ascorbate, hydroperoxidases and bradykinin on prostaglandin production by corneal and lens cells. *Invest. Ophthalmol. Vis. Sci.* 23:387, 1982.
355. Kulkarni, P. S., and Srinivasan, D. B. Synthesis of slow reacting substance-like activity in rabbit conjunctiva and anterior uvea. *Invest. Ophthalmol. Vis. Sci.* 24:1079, 1983.
356. Henley, W. L., Okas, S., and Leopold, I. H. Clinical experiments in cellular immunity in eye disease. *Invest. Ophthalmol.* 12:520, 1973.
357. Ciba Foundation Symposium: *Corneal Graft Failure.* Amsterdam: Associated Scientific Publishers, 1973.
358. Collin, H. B. Lymphatic drainage of I^{131} albumin from the vascularized cornea. *Invest. Ophthalmol.* 9:146, 1970.
359. Smolin, G., and Hyndiuk, R. A. Lymphatic drainage from vascularized rabbit cornea. *Am. J. Ophthalmol.* 72:147, 1971.
360. Smolin, G., and Hall, J. M. The afferent arc of the corneal immunologic reaction. *Arch Ophthalmol.* 90:231, 1973.
361. Hall, J. M. Specificity of antibody formation after intravitreal immunization with bovine gamma globulin and ovalbumin. *Invest. Ophthalmol.* 10:775, 1971.
362. Kaplan, H. J., and Streilein, J. W. Analysis of immunologic privilege within the anterior chamber of the eye. *Transplant. Proc.* 9:1193, 1977.
363. Holly, F. J., and Lemp, M. A. Tear physiology and dry eyes. *Surv. Ophthalmol.* 22:69, 1977.
364. Kijlstra, A., Jeurissen, S. H. M., and Koning, K. M. Lactoferrin levels in normal human tears. *Br. J. Ophthalmol.* 67:199, 1983.
365. Janssen, P. T., and Van Bjisterveld, P. O. Origin and biosynthesis of human tear fluid proteins. *Invest. Ophthalmol. Vis. Sci.* 24:623, 1983.
366. Arnold, R. R., Cole, M. F., and McGhee, J. R. A bactericidal effect for human lactoferrin. *Science* 197:263, 1977.
367. Arnold, R. R., et al. Bactericidal activity of human lactoferrin. *Infect. Immun.* 35:792, 1982.
368. Badgy, G. C., et al. Interaction of lactoferrin monocytes and lymphocyte subsets in the regulation of steady-state granulopoiesis *in vitro. J. Clin. Invest.* 68:56, 1981.
369. Kijlstra, A., Jeurissen, S. H. M. Modulation of classical C_3 convertase of complement by tear lactoferrin. *Immunology* 47:263, 1982.

370. Gibbons, R. J. Bacterial adherence to the mucosal surfaces and its inhibition by secretory antibodies. *Adv. Exp. Med. Biol.* 45:315, 1974.
371. Tomasi, T. B. *The Immune System of Secretion.* Englewood Cliffs, N.J.: Prentice-Hall, 1976, pp. 109–112.
372. Strober, W., Hague, H. E., Lum, L. G., and Henkart, P. A. IgA-F_c receptors on mouse lymphoid cells. *J. Immunol.* 121:2140, 1978.
373. Van Epps, D. E., and Williams, R. C., Jr. Suppression of leukocyte chemotaxis by human IgA myeloma components. *J. Exp. Med.* 144:1227, 1976.
374. Allansmith, M. R., and McLelland, B. Immunoglobulins in the human cornea. *Am. J. Ophthalmol.* 80:123, 1975.
375. Bluestone, R. Lacrimal immunoglobulins and complement quantified by counter-immunoelectrophoresis. *Br. J. Ophthalmol.* 59:279, 1975.
376. Abelson, M. B., and Lamberts, D. W. *Dry Eye Update.* N.J.: Excerpta Medica, 1983, pp. 2–4.
377. Adams, A. D. The morphology of human conjunctival mucus. *Arch. Ophthalmol.* 97:730, 1979.
378. Proctor, P., Kirkpatrick, D., and McGinness, J. A. Superoxide producing system in the conjunctival mucus thread. *Invest. Ophthalmol. Vis. Sci.* 16:762, 1977.
379. Franklin, R. M., and Rice, C. D. Autoimmune Diseases of the Conjunctiva. In G. R. O'Connor (Ed.), *Immunologic Diseases of the Mucous Membranes.* New York: Masson, 1980, pp. 109–118.
380. Allansmith, M. R. Defense of the ocular surface. *Int. Ophthalmol. Clin.* 12:93, 1979.
381. Chandler, J. W., and Axelrod, A. J. Conjunctiva-Associated Lymphoid Tissue. In G. R. O'Connor (Ed.), *Immunologic Diseases of the Mucous Membranes.* New York: Masson, 1980, pp. 63–70.
382. Franklin, R. M., and Remus, L. E. Conjunctival-associated lymphoid tissue. *Invest. Ophthalmol. Vis. Sci.* 25:181, 1984.
383. Vantrappen, L., Geboes, K., Missotten, L. et al. Lymphocytes and Langerhans' cells in the normal human cornea. *Invest. Ophthalmol. Vis. Sci.* 26:220, 1985.
384. Chandler, J. W., and Gillette, T. E. Immunologic defense mechanisms of the ocular surface. *Ophthalmology* 90:585, 1983.
385. Jackson, D. E., Lally, E. T., Nakamura, M. C., and Montgomery, P. C. Migration of IgA bearing lymphocytes into salivary glands. *Cell. Immunol.* 63:203, 1981.
386. Bhan, A. K., Fujikawa, L., and Foster, C. S. T-cell subsets and Langerhans' cells in normal and diseased conjunctiva. *Am. J. Ophthalmol.* 94:205, 1982.
387. Uananue, E. R. Regulatory Functions of Mononuclear Phagocytes. In Y. Yamamura and T. Tada (Eds.). *Progress in Immunology V.* New York: Academic, 1983, pp. 973–983.
388. Grabner, G., Luger, T. A., Smolin, G., and Oppenheim, J. J. Corneal epithelial cell-derived thymocyte-activating factor. *Invest. Ophthalmol. Vis. Sci.* 23:757, 1982.
389. Allansmith, M. R., and O'Connor, G. R. Immunoglobulins. *Surv. Ophthalmol.* 14:367, 1970.
390. Smolin, G., Hall, J., and Stein, M. Afferent arc of the corneal immunologic reaction. *Can. J. Ophthalmol.* 7:336, 1972.
391. Shimada, K., and Silverstein, A. M. Local antibody formation within the eye. *Invest. Ophthalmol.* 14:573, 1975.

392. Silverstein, A. M. Ectopic Antibody Formation in the Eye. In A. E. Maumenee and A. M. Silverstein (Eds.), *Immunopathology of Uveitis.* Baltimore: Williams & Wilkins, 1964, p. 83.
393. Smith, R. E., Jensen, A. D., and Silverstein, A. M. Antibody formation by single cells during experimental immunogenic uveitis. *Invest. Ophthalmol.* 8:373, 1969.
394. Maisel, H., and Goodman, M. Analyses of mammalian lens protein by electrophoresis. *Arch. Ophthalmol.* 71:671, 1964.
395. Manski, W. Immunologic Studies on Normal and Pathologic Lenses. In Ciba Foundation Symposium (Ed.), *The Human Lens in Relation to Cataract.* Amsterdam: Associated Scientific Publishers, 1973.
396. Keda, H. Experimental endophthalmitis phacoanaphylactica in rabbits sensitized with the purified alpha crystallin. *Folia Ophthalmol. Jpn.* 12:304, 1961.
397. Nazaki, M., Foster, L., and Sery, T. W. Uveal and other ocular tissue reactions to heterologous anti-lens capsule antibodies. *Invest. Ophthalmol.* 2:641, 1963.
398. Roberts, D. Studies on the antigenic structure of the eye using the fluorescent antibody technique. *Br. J. Ophthalmol.* 41:338, 1957.
399. Barbanov, B. M., and Mikhailov, A. T. Immunoelectrophoretic analyses of water-soluble antigens of the chick retina. *Bull. Exp. Biol.* 8:73, 1970.
400. Marak, G. Immunopathology of Sympathetic Ophthalmia. In *Proceedings of the First International Symposium on Immunity and Immunopathology of the Eye.* Basel: Karger, 1976.
401. Coles, R. S. Treatment of Uveitis. In F. H. Theodore and A. Schlossman (Eds.), *Ocular Allergy.* London: Baillière, Tindall & Cox, 1958, pp. 334.
402. Rahi, A. H. S. Autoimmune reactions in uveal melanoma. *Br. J. Ophthalmol.* 55:793, 1971.
403. Kopeloff, L. M. Recurrent immunogenic interstitial keratitis. *Arch. Pathol. Lab. Med.* 10:74, 1976.
404. Howes, E. L., Jr., and McKay, D. G. Circulating immune complexes. *Arch. Ophthalmol.* 93:365, 1975.
405. Wong, V. G., Anderson, R., and O'Brien, R. J. Sympathetic ophthalmia and lymphocyte transformation. *Am. J. Ophthalmol.* 72:960, 1971.
406. Gamble, C. N., Aronson, S. B., and Brescia, F. B. Experimental uveitis. *Arch. Ophthalmol.* 84:321, 1970.
407. Lurhuma, A. Z., et al. Detection of circulating antigen-antibody complexes by their inhibitory effect on the agglutination of IgG-coated particles by rheumatoid factor or C1q. *Clin. Exp. Immunol.* 25:212, 1976.
408. Hedfors, E., and Norberg, R. Evidence for circulating immune complexes in sarcoidosis. *Clin. Exp. Immunol.* 16:421, 1974.
409. Sjögren, H. O., et al. Suggestive evidence that the "blocking antibodies" of tumor bearing individuals may be antigen-antibody complexes. *Proc. Natl. Acad. Sci. U.S.A.* 68:1372, 1971.
410. Doe, W. F., Booth, C. C., and Brown, D. L. Evidence for complement-binding immune complexes in adult coeliac disease, Crohn's disease, and ulcerative colitis. *Lancet* 1:402, 1973.
411. Dernouchamps, J. P., et al. Immune complexes in the aqueous humor and serum. *Am. J. Ophthalmol.* 84:24, 1977.
412. Friedlaender, M. H., et al. Histopathology of delayed hypersensitivity reaction in the guinea pig uveal tract. *Invest. Ophthalmol. Vis. Sci.* 17:327, 1978.

2   IMMUNOLOGIC TESTING PROCEDURES

In order to confirm the immunologic origin of a specific disease of the eye, laboratory tests are often performed. Depending on the nature of the patient's condition, these tests may or may not be useful.

GENERAL CONSIDERATIONS

The investigator must consider many factors before launching a full-scale, expensive investigation.

Usefulness of Immunologic Testing

A patient whose symptom complex and previous medical history suggest the possibility of immunologic disease of the eye can and should be subjected to immunologic testing. Such testing will only rarely detect the *cause* of a particular patient's problem; it will often confirm the *category* of immunologic disease from which he or she is suffering. "Blanket" testing of individuals suffering from ocular inflammatory disease is both expensive and wasteful. Many tests described in this chapter are new and experimental; to recommend their general application to all patients with presumptive immunologic disease of the eye would be pure folly. One must be guided by the symptom complex of the patient into a limited program of testing that has some probability of "payoff." For example, the finding of rheumatoid factor in the serum of a patient with nodular scleritis may confirm the rheumatoid nature of his disease, even in the absence of overt joint disease. Such a test is of value because it reveals the prognosis of the patient's eye disease and gives the therapist some idea of what kind of treatment might be useful.

By contrast, testing for anti-*Toxoplasma* antibodies in the serum of a patient with inflammatory disease affecting the anterior segment of the eye alone appears useless. Although the test may be positive at a high titer, it is not likely to shed any light on the cause of the patient's disease, because *Toxoplasma* has never been shown to cause inflammatory disease of the anterior segment alone [1]. Many patients with eye lesions unrelated to toxoplasmosis have a positive *Toxoplasma* dye test. Those with high titers may have active, though asymptomatic, systemic disease. But if such patients have iritis alone (without a concomitant retinal lesion), they are unlikely to have ocular toxoplasmosis. This example is just one illustration of what is meant by useless immunologic testing.

Relationship of Immunologic Tests to Bodily Disease

Blood tests and skin tests mirror systemic disease much more often than they mirror specific ocular disease. Although the eye may participate in the expression of a disease of immunologic origin, the results of immunologic testing may be disappointing if the eye is the only symptomatic organ of the body. This situation makes sense if one remembers that the eye weighs only a few grams and that the fragment of ocular tissue affected by a given inflammation may weigh less than a milligram. If this weight is contrasted with the 70 kg that represents the average bodily mass, it can be appreciated that inflamed ocular tissue may represent only a minor antigenic stimulus for the body as a whole. Generally speaking, serum antibody levels reflect the activities of lymphoid organs such as the lymph nodes and spleen much more than they reflect immunologic activity in an inflamed eye. An absolutely negative serum test, on the other hand, may rule out certain diseases of the eye. Although two exceptions have been reported [2, 3], a patient with an absolutely negative *Toxoplasma* dye test is highly unlikely to have ocular toxoplasmosis. Similarly, a patient with cysts of the ciliary body, a finding characteristic of multiple myeloma, would be very unlikely to have that disease if his serum immunoglobulin pattern is normal.

TESTS FOR ANTIBODY

Antibody responses reveal an exposure of the patient to previous infectious or allergic insults.

Infectious Diseases

In many cases, such as those concerned with toxoplasmosis, the initial exposure to the infectious pathogen will have produced few, if any, symptoms.

TOXOPLASMA DYE TEST. This test, originally described by Sabin and Feldman [4] in 1948, measures the ability of antibodies to make holes in the surface membrane of Toxoplasma organisms. To do this, antibodies must work in concert with an "accessory factor," thought to be identical with complement [5], as found in normal serum. Once these holes are made in the surface membrane of the organism, osmolysis of its cytoplasm occurs, and the parasite then no longer stains with methylene blue dye. The titer of a given serum is the reciprocal of that dilution in which 50% or more of the organisms being examined fail to stain with the dye. Actually, it is not necessary to use methylene blue for the final readout of the test. Under the influence of the antibodies and "accessory factor," the parasites swell and their cytoplasm becomes clear, making it possible to count the numbers of affected organisms by ordinary light microscopy or, preferably, by phase microscopy.

In order to perform the *Toxoplasma* dye test one must maintain living *Toxoplasma* organisms in the laboratory. This testing is ordinarily accomplished by serial intraperitoneal inoculations of parasite suspensions. Depending upon the number of organisms injected and their virulence, laboratory mice are usually killed by the infection within 5 to 7 days. Therefore subinoculation at least twice a week is usually necessary to keep the mice alive and to provide suspensions of living organisms for the dye test. This procedure is expensive, troublesome, and potentially dangerous for laboratory workers. Therefore, alternatives that utilize nonliving antigens are constantly being sought.

It must be remembered that the titers of dye-test antibodies may be very low in individuals whose sole clinical manifestations of toxoplasmosis are ocular in nature. A case described by Zscheile [6] illustrates this point very well. In this particular patient the retinas of both eyes were shown to be heavily parasitized by *Toxoplasma gondii*, yet the patient's dye test was positive only in undiluted serum (1:1). In response to the question: What is a significant titer of antibodies in patients suspected of ocular toxoplasmosis? we can state that any titer of antibodies is significant if the patient manifests a fundus lesion that is compatible with ocular toxoplasmosis. Under these conditions, no titer is too low to be considered meaningful.

Under certain circumstances dye-test antibodies will be present in greater concentration in the aqueous humor than in serum. This suggests that dye-test antibodies may be formed by plasma cells in the anterior uveal tract in response to intraocular infection. In order to prove that the antibodies are actually being formed within the eye, one must show more antibody per milligram of immunoglobulin in the aqueous humor than in simultaneously sampled blood serum. Desmonts and co-workers [7] have demonstrated this finding in large numbers of patients with presumed ocular toxoplasmosis and have gone so far as to state that they can differentiate primary attacks of ocular toxoplasmosis from recurrent disease on the basis of an aqueous:serum ratio.

OTHER TESTS FOR TOXOPLASMOSIS. Numerous other procedures, most of them utilizing nonliving antigens, have been developed for the serodiagnosis of toxoplasmosis. These alternative procedures include a hemagglutination test [8, 9], an indirect fluorescent antibody test [10] (Fig. 2-1), a flocculation test [11], a direct agglutination test [13], a precipitin test [12], a complement-fixation test [14], a plate hemolysin test [15], and an enzyme-linked immunosorbent assay [16]. Each of these tests was standardized against the Sabin-Feldman dye test at the time of its original description, and in most cases the correlation of titers has been excellent. The precipitin test and the complement-fixation test represent conspicuous exceptions. They become positive several months after the dye test becomes positive; but these types of antibody also dis-

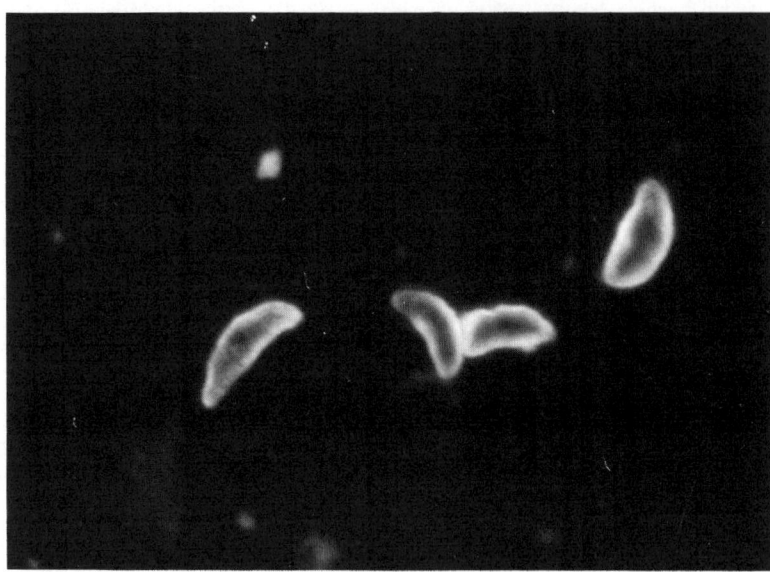

FIG. 2-1 Indirect fluorescent antibody test for toxoplasmosis. Note brilliant fluorescence of fluorescein-tagged antihuman IgG on the surface of the cell membrane. Ultraviolet light. ($\times$ 1200)

appear earlier than dye-test antibodies, i.e., generally before 2 years have elapsed. When positive, these tests are thought to reflect active multiplication of the organism within the body.

When Jackson et al. [15] described the plate hemolysin test (Fig. 2-2), they thought it would provide a device for the rapid mass screening of certain populations for the presence of anti-*Toxoplasma* antibody. While it is true that many sera can be tested simultaneously on a single agar plate by this method, the test has not fulfilled its original promise. Under the best of conditions the antigen-coated sheep erythrocytes that this test utilizes remain intact for only 3 to 5 days. Since mail between two cities is often longer in transit than 5 days, the problem of supplying test plates to remote testing centers looms large.

It seems likely that the enzyme-linked immunosorbent assay ("ELISA test") will ultimately replace all other tests for *Toxoplasma* antibodies. This test uses nonliving antigens, which are fixed to an insoluble matrix (a cellulose disk or a test tube wall). If a serum containing antibodies is incubated with this matrix, antibodies will unite with the antigen. All unbound immunoglobulins are then washed off the matrix. In the next stage of the test, alkaline phosphatase-labeled goat antihuman globulin serum is added to the matrix. It fixes to the Fc portion of the human immunoglobulin molecule. Again, all excess enzyme-labeled antihuman globulin is washed off. Finally, the substrate paranitrophenyl phosphate, is incubated with the matrix. When the phosphate moiety is cleaved from the molecules, paranitrophenol appears. This substance is yellow and

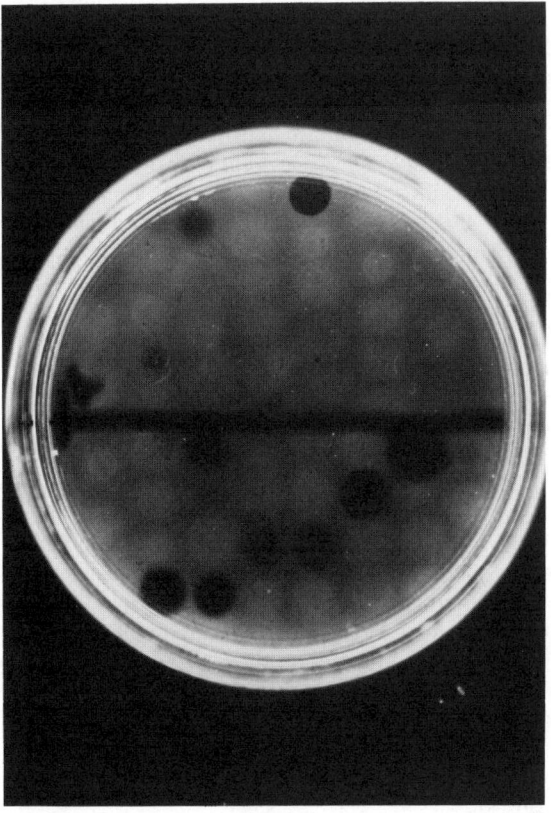

FIG. 2-2 Plate hemolysin test for toxoplasmosis. Note clear round spots representing zones of red-cell lysis at each point where a drop of positive serum has been applied.

can be measured on a spectrophotometer. It is clear that the results of this test are highly parallel to those of the dye test. It seems likely that it will replace it, for it is much safer and more convenient to use a nonliving antigen than a living, potentially infectious parasite. As more and more commercial kits for other antigens are made up, it also seems likely that the ELISA test will replace many other cumbersome serologic procedures. Any antigen that can be fixed to an insoluble matrix without denaturation becomes a good candidate for the ELISA test.

VDRL AND FTA-ABSORPTION TESTS. Syphilis is known to produce a number of highly destructive inflammatory lesions of the eye. In many clinics a luetic serology test is performed routinely when the patient enters. Within recent years, routine testing of the leutic serology has been abandoned in many centers, and this omission is a serious error. Even more serious, many Venereal Disease Research Laboratory (VDRL) tests are reported as negative when they are in fact *positive at low titer*. The following case will illustrate the folly of this reporting.

A 41-year-old black man with blurred vision and minimal redness of the left eye of 7 days' duration was studied in our Uveitis Survey Clinic. When the referring ophthalmologist first examined him, the patient had a coarse horizontal nystagmus with the fast component to the left, and a visual acuity of 20/40 in the right eye and 20/200 in the left. Neither pupil reacted to light. The left cornea showed several geographic areas of infiltration with both deep and superficial vessels invading the stroma. The anterior chamber showed 1+ cells and flare. A few small, pigmented, healed chorioretinal lesions were present in both fundi. A diagnosis of interstitial keratitis was made, and the pupillary abnormalities and nystagmus suggested neurosyphilis. The patient denied that either he or his parents had ever had syphilis and stated that his own serologic tests for syphilis had been negative on four previous occasions: on joining the Army, on release from the Army, before his first marriage, and before his second marriage.

The patient's left eye was treated with fluorometholone (FML) drops twice a day. His vision improved dramatically (to 20/30) within 24 hours, and both the central portion of his corneal opacity and the mild cellular reaction in his anterior chamber cleared. Since the cause of his eye condition was in doubt, however, he was sent to the Uveitis Survey Clinic for further study.

On examination in our clinic we found a visual acuity of 20/40 O.D. and 20/25 O.S. (The patient told us that his left eye had always had the better vision.) In addition to the interstitial keratitis, nystagmus, and nonreactive pupils, we noted that the patient had a saddlenose deformity and Hutchinsonian teeth. His upper medial incisors were small, tapered, and concave on their inferior edges—all signs strongly suggestive of congenital syphilis. Additional probing into the medical history uncovered the fact that the patient had received a brief course of penicillin therapy for a bacterial pneumonia while in the Army 10 years previously.

Our laboratory studies included the fluorescent treponemal antibody (FTA)-absorption test for lues and the VDRL test. A telephone report from the laboratory two days after the tests informed us that the VDRL was negative, the FTA-absorption test still pending. Three days later we received a report that the FTA-absorption test was positive, and that the VDRL was also positive at a titer of 1:4. Since then the patient has had a spinal tap and is receiving penicillin therapy for neurosyphilis. We feel that he is a classic case of congenital syphilis with interstitial keratitis and cerebral involvement.

How was this patient's diagnosis missed on four previous occasions, and how did he almost elude diagnosis in our clinic? The answer is that the VDRL test alone was performed on all previous occasions, and that it is the custom of many serology laboratories to dilute the serum 1:8 or 1:16 before running the test in order to eliminate the myriad of false positives that would be reported on patients with low levels of VDRL antibodies. Such patients do not have syphilis; many of them have collagen-vascular diseases such as dermatomyositis, lupus, or rheumatoid arthritis. It is only when the FTA-absorption test is positive that laboratories do titered VDRL tests. Thus, the diagnosis was missed on four occasions. The extent to which our patient's previous penicillin therapy affected his VDRL titer, if at all, is unknown. The FTA-absorption test will always remain positive despite previous penicillin therapy. Thus, we recommend performance of both the FTA-absorption test and the VDRL test whenever syphilis is suspected.

Smith [17] as well as other authors [18, 19] are responsible for directing the attention of the ophthalmic community to the possibility that *T. pallidum* may be the source of chronic ocular inflammatory disease in individuals who have negative or only weakly positive blood tests for syphilis. Smith claimed that pathogenic *T. pallidum* could be detected in the aqueous humor of such patients, and he subsequently attempted to transmit treponemal infections from humans to experimental animals. This effort met with only limited success, and it raised the question of whether the treponemas that he detected in the aqueous humor might have been nonpathogenic organisms such as *Treponema microdentium*. Since the time of Smith's original discovery, carefully absorbed fluorescein-tagged antisera have been used to detect *T. pallidum* in the aqueous humor. The number of positive isolations has subsequently decreased remarkably, indicating that Smith's original studies may have detected nonpathogenic treponemes.

CHLAMYDIAL ANTIBODY TESTS. Infections with the rickettsia-like organisms of the genus *Chlamydia* may produce trachoma and inclusion conjunctivitis, and they have been associated with Reiter's syndrome. The principal test that has been used to detect serum antibodies against the chlamydial agents is the complement-fixation reaction. However, this group-specific test does not detect the difference between lymphogranuloma venereum, for example, and trachoma. Furthermore, low titers of complement-fixing antibodies may have little significance (only titers of 1:16 or above are generally considered to be indicative of active infection.)

Wang and Grayston [20] devised a microimmunofluorescence test for antibodies to the chlamydial agents that appears to be type-specific. In this test microsuspensions of elementary bodies are mixed with the patient's serum. After the excess antibody is removed, fluorescein-tagged antihuman immunoglobulin is added, and the elementary bodies are examined under ultraviolet light. This test allows for the differentiation of certain serotypes of chlamydial agents. Serotypes A, B, and C, for example, are associated with hyperendemic trachoma; inclusion conjunctivitis is associated with serotypes D through K. All laboratory-confirmed cases of inclusion conjunctivitis have been antibody-positive. The test appears to be both sensitive and specific.

CANDIDA SEROLOGY. *Candida* endophthalmitis has become a highly significant problem in ophthalmology over the past two decades. This increased incidence is related to (1) the extensive use of indwelling plastic catheters for intravenous hyperalimentation, (2) the use of massive doses of broad-spectrum antibiotics, and (3) the use of contaminated injection equipment by drug abusers. *Candida* is an ever-present opportunistic organism. The development of delayed hypersensitivity to this fungus early in life generally affords protection against the organism. However, a massive, intravenous inoculum of the organism or conditions of immunologic compromise may allow infection to become established in such sites as the retina. Edwards et al. [21] have reviewed the subject extensively. Under conditions of massive infection, agglutinins, and precipitating antibodies may be stimulated [22]. The latter, though present at low titer, may be detected with great efficiency by the technique of counterimmunoelectrophoresis [23]. This procedure is essentially a modification of the agar diffusion test in which antigen and antibody are propelled toward each other in an electrophoretic field. The pH of the buffer used to dissolve the agar can be adjusted in such a way as to make both antigen and antibody mobile. At the position in the agar where the optimal concentration of both antibody and antigen is reached, precipitation will occur in a band or fine line. Although more sophisticated antibody tests for the detection of *Candida* infection are now available (e.g. the ELISA test [24]), it seems likely that the demonstration of circulating antigen [25] will prove more useful in the early detection of disseminated infection.

HISTOPLASMA SEROLOGY. Patients with the presumptive ocular histoplasmosis syndrome (POHS) are thought to develop their ocular lesions as a late sequela of systemic infection with *Histoplasma capsulatum*. While it is likely that organisms are present in the original focal granulomas that develop in the choroid, they apparently do not remain in the lesions for more than a few weeks. Serologic tests for histoplasmosis have been disappointing, as far as the diagnosis of the ocular lesions is concerned. Schlaegel and O'Connor [26] have found the complement-fixation test for yeast-phase *H. capsulatum* positive in only one-third of their cases of presumptive ocular histoplasmosis, and Krill et al. [27] reported similar results. The histoplasmin skin test appears to be a much more reliable indicator of immunologic reactivity to *H. capsulatum*, but here again, 11% of eye patients suffering from POHS appear to be skin-test negative [26].

CYTOMEGALOVIRUS SEROLOGY. The importance of cytomegalovirus retinopathy has come to the fore during the era of organ transplantation. This infection has also been seen with distressing frequency among patients with the newly described acquired immune deficiency syndrome or AIDS (See Chapter 7). While it is true that certain cases had been described previously in connection with other immunosuppressive states (such as neoplasms of the lymphoid system [28]), the greatest efflorescence of this disease has occurred in association with the use of immunosuppressive agents. While virus-laden cells can be detected by cytologic examination of the urine sediment, serologic tests can also be performed to confirm the presence of the disease. A complement-fixation test at a titer greater than 1:20 is thought to be indicative of active infection, particularly if rising titers can be subsequently documented. Lower titers are of no significance since cytomegalovirus, like *Candida*, is a common opportunistic pathogen.

Recently, Cappel et al. [29] have described an enzyme-linked immunosorbent assay for cytomegalovirus that detects both IgG and IgM antibodies. The presence of IgM signals a recently acquired infection and may have special value in tracing the course of the disease.

Cytomegalovirus infection, like toxoplasmosis, may be a congenital disease. Many women harbor the organism in their genital tracts without knowing of their infection. When the disease is acquired in utero, the fetus may be seriously harmed. Cerebral damage may occur and paraventricular calcification may be seen on roentgenograms of the skull. Chorioretinitis often develops at the same time. Infants affected by the disease will generally have IgM antibodies in their circulation at birth, while infants that are not affected may show only IgG antibodies received from their mothers by passive transfer through the placenta.

TOXOCARA SEROLOGY. Infestations of the eye with the third-stage larvae of *Toxocara* sp. may produce one of these principal manifestations: (1) a pseudoglioma of the posterior pole, (2) a diffuse endophthalmitis, or (3) a peripheral uveitis with a pars plana exudate. Although visceral larva migrans and ocular toxocariasis are caused by the same organism, they evoke different responses in the body. Visceral larva migrans causes eosinophilia and is generally accompanied by systemic antibody responses. Ocular toxocariasis generally causes no eosinophilia and its victims show only mild antibody responses in the absence of visceral involvement.

Patients with *Toxocara* infections may show isohemagglutinins against blood group substances A and B [30]. This finding, however, is not thought to mirror ocular infection. Hemagglutination tests [31] using antigen-coated sheep erythrocytes have been used for *Toxocara* serology, but unless the sera are carefully absorbed of anti-*Ascaris* antibodies, the test may give false-positive results.

An enzyme-linked immunosorbent assay (ELISA) has been devised for *Toxocara* serology. Reports by Cypess et al. [32] and Glickman et al. [33] indicate that it is both sensitive and highly specific. Because the test uses only 10 μl of sample, it is possible to test aspirated aqueous humor or vitreous humor for its antibody content. Biglan [34] has recently made use of this factor in confirming a case of ocular toxocariasis. The isolation and characterization of excretory-secretory antigens from *Toxocara* [35] and the detectability of IgM antibodies directed against these antigens [36] may increase our ability to make a diagnosis by the examination of ocular fluids.

Noninfectious Diseases

Immunologic abnormalities in a given individual may reflect genetic, metabolic, or allergic disorders.

EVALUATION OF IMMUNOGLOBULINS. The range of normal values for the levels of serum immunoglobulins in the human has been determined [37]. Normansell [38] has recently reviewed the merits and limitations of the various chemical, electrophoretic, and immunologic methods of doing this. The vast majority of patients with immunologic abnormalities affecting the eye alone will show normal serum values. Patients with systemic abnormalities that reflect immunologic disease may show abnormally high levels of certain immunoglobulins. Thus patients with rheumatoid arthritis are likely to show high levels of IgM, and patients with atopic disease may show elevated levels of IgE. Certain patients with autoimmune diseases may show a selective IgA deficiency, while patients with sarcoidosis may show high levels of IgG. Gross estimates of the serum proteins, as performed by moving boundary electrophoresis or paper strip electrophoresis, are not, in general, very useful. If an exaggerated peak is seen in one of the serum protein components, it may, however, alert the physician to other abnormalities. Thus a sharply delimited, high peak in the gamma globulin region may prompt further investigation into the possibility of a myeloma.

ELECTROPHORESIS AND IMMUNOELECTROPHORESIS. Since each of the immunoglobulins is a member of a unique protein class, based on the number and arrangement of amino acids in its heavy chain, it is not surprising that each immunoglobulin type has its own characteristic electrophoretic mobility. At pH 8.6, most immunoglobulins will wander in an electrophoretic field toward the anode (+), while IgG is virtually immobile at this pH; i.e., it is at its isoelectric point. The immunoglobulins in serum, in aqueous humor, or in cerebrospinal fluid can thus be separated from each other by electrophoresis. The individual bands or spots of immunoglobulins can be distinguished from one another on a strip of cellulose acetate that has been moistened with a suitable buffer and placed in an electrophoretic field, provided that the proteins are immediately fixed in a solution such as trichloroacetic acid after separation and then stained with a dye such as Amido Black at the end of the procedure. A thin strip of agarose gel can be used as an alternative electrophoretic medium. The density and width of the bands can then be determined by an optical density scanner and, after reference is made to a standard serum, an appropriate value can be determined for each immunoglobulin.

Since the isoelectric points of the various immunoglobulins are rather close to each other, there is usually a good deal of overlap among these bands. Therefore, this method for the determination of immunoglobulin levels is not often used in practice. One relies, instead, upon a combination of other techniques to be described subsequently.

Each of the immunoglobulins has its own specific characteristics as an antigen, and when it is injected into another species, it evokes the formation of specific antibodies directed against the Fc portion of the immunoglobulin molecule. Precipitating antibodies, so developed, can detect the location of a specific human immunoglobulin on an agar plate or cellulose acetate strip by forming a discrete band or arc of precipitate (Fig. 2-3). Thus immunoglobulins that have been separated by electrophoresis can be precipitated by antibodies directed against them, and these arcs of precipitate can be stained with Amido Black or Ponceau R.

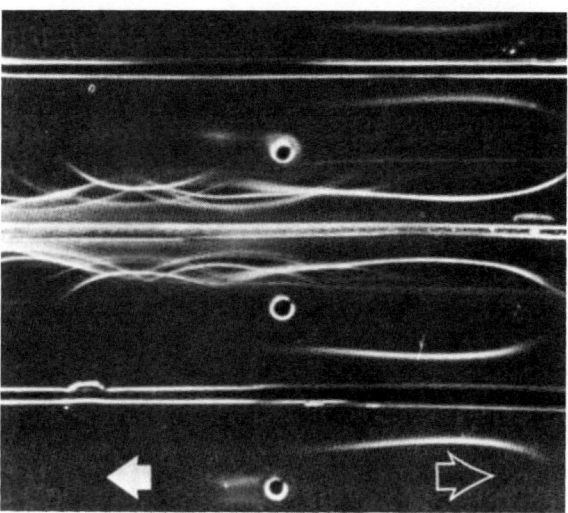

FIG. 2-3 Immunoelectrophoresis on a thin layer of agarose gel. *Solid white arrow* denotes migration toward the anode; *linear white arrow,* migration toward the cathode. Arcs of precipitated protein are viewed in oblique light against a dark background. (Reproduced with permission from I. L. Weissman, L. E. Hood, and W. B. Wood. *Essential Concepts in Immunology.* Menlo Park, Ca., Benjamin/Cummings, 1978)

Unusually prominent arcs signal the presence of elevated amounts of antibody, and again, the density of a particular band can be scanned by optical means.

RADIAL DIFFUSION. Mancini et al. [39] are responsible for the development of a technique that is most widely used for the quantitation of immunoglobulins. It depends, once more, upon the precipitation of a particular immunoglobulin by specific antibodies from a heterologous source, e.g., rabbit antibodies directed against human IgG. The success of the test depends upon the availability of highly purified human immunoglobulins with which to immunize the rabbit in the first place. Once the antibodies have been raised in the rabbit, they are incorporated into warm, slightly molten agar in thin sheets. A hole or "well" made in this sheet can then act as a diffusion source for the specimen that is to be tested. When the patient's serum is put into this well, the proteins contained therein will diffuse in all directions through the agar medium. A ring of precipitate will develop in the agar at a point where the concentration of human IgG reaches a "ratio of optimal proportions" with the corresponding anti-IgG in the agar. Within certain limitations, the diameter of the circle of precipitate so produced will be proportional to the amount of IgG in the patient's serum, a larger circle always corresponding to an increased amount of IgG. A known concentration of human IgG in a standard test solution is always used for calibration of a given test plate, and tests on specimens are always run in duplicate or triplicate so that the final result can be based on the mean of several diameter measurements. The major advantage of the Mancini technique is that it can be performed on rather small quantities of fluid. Moreover, Simmons [40] has shown how the technique can be modified in a way that allows for the detection of plasma proteins present in extremely low concentrations, as in the case of ocular fluids.

IgE DETERMINATIONS. Immunoglobulin E, or "reaginic antibody," is ordinarily the immunoglobulin that is present in least quantity in human serum. Normal values usually run about 0.003 mg/dl of serum. While the serum level of IgE may be elevated in atopic disease or in individuals suffering from massive parasite infestation, the levels of IgE in most patients are too small to detect by radial diffusion techniques of the type described by Mancini. Instead, one is obliged to use a radioimmunoassay test to quantitate these very small amounts of immunoglobulin. In this instance, anti-IgE antibodies, raised in another species, are suspended in an agar layer. The IgE to be assayed is allowed to diffuse through the agar layer (for a specified period) from a well or cup made in the agar. The resultant ring of precipitate is too faint to be seen. However, after all uncombined reactants have been washed out, the ring of precipitate may be reacted with ^{125}I-labelled anti-IgG. After removing all uncombined radiolabelled material, the agar layer is exposed to stripping film or painted with a photographic emulsion. The ring thus visualized is measured according to the Mancini principle. This method, described by Gleich et al. [41], has been used by Brauninger and Centifano [42] to quantitate the amount of IgE in tears. Other methods of assay include a solid phase radioimmunoassay (RIST) in which antibody against IgE is coupled to CNBr-activated cellulose or Sephadex [43]. The IgE to be measured competes with a ^{125}I-labelled IgE that is added to the column in known quantity. The IgE to be measured is thus inversely proportional to the amount of radioactive IgE that is bound.

ALLERGEN-SPECIFIC IgG. The same methods that have been used to measure IgE content can be used for the determination of allergen-specific IgG. It is clear that immunoglobulins such as IgG are present in large quantities in the serum, but only a relatively small portion of the total population of IgG molecules is committed to react with certain allergens (antigens). If one can obtain a highly purified sample of that antigen and tag it with a tracer such as ^{125}I, it should be possible to identify that portion of the total IgG population that is committed to react with the allergen. This procedure has been used by Adkinson and Lichtenstein [44] in their assessment of certain allergic states.

AUTOANTIBODIES. It seems clear that certain inflammatory diseases of the eye reflect the interaction between tissue antigens from the patient and antibodies directed against those auto-antigens. Even in allegedly normal individuals, antibodies against lens antigens can be detected in the serum by hemagglutination techniques [45]. Here, sheep red blood cells coated with soluble lens antigens are incubated with the patient's serum at 37°C. The tubes containing these suspensions are then refrigerated overnight, and the pattern in which the sheep erythrocytes settle out at the bottom of the test tube is observed. A widespread, reticulated pattern represents a positive test. A compact button represents a negative test. The titer is generally taken as the reciprocal of that dilution of the serum which produces a "2+ ring." Marak et al. [46] have recently produced evidence indicating that lens-induced uveitis is an immune complex disease. Under these circumstances, tolerance to native lens antigens is lost, and antibodies are formed against these proteins.

Aronson et al. [47] have demonstrated the existence of precipitating antibodies against uveal tissue antigens in the serum of individuals suffering from long-standing diffuse uveitis. For this purpose, a precipitin test in agar was used. A similar test was used by Jones [48] to demonstrate antibodies against lacrimal gland antigens among individuals with Sjögren's disease.

RHEUMATOID FACTOR. Perhaps the most important of the autoantibodies is "rheumatoid factor," an IgM (or IgA or IgG) antibody directed against the patient's own IgG. Under certain circumstances IgG antibody formation may be evoked in response to altered native tissues such as the synovial lining or scleral collagen. It appears that infection or trauma may play some role in this process, but in any case, the patient's own IgG molecules become pathologically adherent to these altered tissues. Macroglobulin antibodies directed against the Fc portion of the patient's IgG are generated in certain individuals with a genetic predisposition to rheumatoid disease. These macroglobulin antibodies can be detected in a number of ways. Human IgG can be coated onto latex particles. When a suspension of these particles is mixed with serum containing rheumatoid factor, agglutination will occur. Although gross clumps of these particles are usually visible to the naked eye, the suspensions are generally examined under a light microscope in order to determine the titer of the reaction. The same is true of the so-called F-II hemagglutination test [49] for rheumatoid factor. Here, sheep erythrocytes are coated with human IgG, and again, the agglutination of the red cells is monitored by gross and microscopic examination.

ANTIBODIES TO NUCLEIC ACID CONSTITUENTS. Individuals suffering from the ocular complications of juvenile rheumatoid arthritis may show the presence of antinuclear antibodies in their serum. Schaller et al. [50] have indicated that over 80% of patients with this malady will show the presence of antinuclear antibodies at one time or another during the course of their disease. The test is an indirect fluorescence reaction in which the patient's serum is reacted with fixed human white blood cells on a slide. After a certain reaction period has elapsed, all excess serum is washed off, and the preparation is then covered with fluorescein-tagged antihuman IgG. Fluorescence of the nuclear structures of the leukocytes indicates an adherence of the patient's antibodies to nuclear proteins. The test correlates well with the "L.E. prep" in patients with lupus erythematosus, but its exact significance in juvenile rheumatoid arthritis is unknown.

COMPLEMENT COMPONENTS AND LEVELS. It now appears certain that many acute inflammatory reactions that occur in the eye are mediated by the precipitation of immune complexes in the eye and the concomitant binding of complement to those complexes. This combination of immunologic events triggers the formation of platelet thrombi in certain of the ocular blood vessels, attracts polymorphonuclear leukocytes to the site of immune complex deposition, and results in the release of certain kinins and vasoactive amines that bring about the dilatation of blood vessels and the leakage of serous fluid into the ocular tissues.

Collagen-vascular diseases such as rheumatoid arthritis cause destructive changes in both the joints and the sclera. In the synovial fluid, it is clear that a sudden decline in the complement level may signal the onset of an acute attack of arthritis, indicating the binding of complement, particularly $C'3$ to immune complex deposits. It is doubtful that alterations in serum levels of complement can be accurately correlated with the formation of scleral nodules, the counterpart of synovial inflammation in rheumatoid conditions.

On the other hand, levels of circulating complement may show dramatic fluctuations in diseases such as Behçet's syndrome, which is almost certainly an immune-complex–mediated disease. Although levels of circulating complement components may be initially high in Behçet's syndrome [51], serum levels of complement may decline rather rapidly immediately before or concomitant with an attack of this disease [52]. Presumably the massive amounts of immune complexes that become precipitated in the target organs immediately before an attack bind complement to a degree that lowers the serum levels of complement, particularly $C'3$.

TESTS FOR IMMUNE COMPLEXES. Several laboratory tests have become available for the assay of immune complexes in serum and in other body fluids such as the synovial fluid and aqueous humor. These tests have been used in studies of uveitis and ocular tumors in an attempt to elucidate the role that immune complexes play in the pathogenesis of the disease or in the protection of the body against the disease.

C1q Binding Test. The first component of complement to be bound to an immune complex is C1q, an umbrella-shaped molecule that makes its attachment to the Fc portion of an antigen-bound antibody molecule. This attachment appears to be a prerequisite for all subsequent events that occur in the complement cascade. C1q can be isolated and labelled with radioisotopes such as ^{125}I. By adding labelled C1q to a solution containing immune complexes, and by analyzing the radioactivity in the washed precipitate that is subsequently isolated by centrifugation, it is possible to estimate the number of immune complexes in the test sample [53]. The test is done in several ways, one of which involves a solid phase immunoassay. In this test, antigen-antibody complexes in the test solution are bound to the wall of a tube or to a plastic disc. ^{125}I-C1q is then added, and after a suitable reaction period, all unbound C1q is then washed off. The test tube or disc is then assayed for its radioactivity. ^{125}I is a relatively weak gamma emitter with a half-life of 60 days. It has generally replaced ^{131}I, a much stronger gamma emitter with a half-life of 8 days in tests of this sort.

Raji Cell Technique. Raji cells are malignant cells of lymphoid origin (Burkitt's lymphoma) that have receptors for the third component of complement (C'3) on their surface membranes. Circulating complexes of antibody and antigen combine readily with C'3 under most circumstances, and the fact that C'3 is already joined to the complex makes it possible to enumerate the number of such complexes in a given volume of serum or aqueous humor. Theofilopoulos et al. [54] have described a technique utilizing this principle. When Raji cells are exposed to the serum (or aqueous humor), i.e., the specimen to be analyzed under tissue culture conditions, the C'3 component of the antigen-antibody-complement complex becomes fixed to the surface membrane of the cell. If ^{125}I-labelled goat anti-human Fc globulin is now added to the washed cells, the labelled antibody will attach to the Fc portion of the adherent antigen-antibody complex. When cells so labelled are subsequently washed and centrifuged, the pelleted cells will bear radioactive labels in direct proportion to the number of immune complexes in the specimen. The radioactivity of the cells can be measured in a gamma counter and the results referred to a standard curve. This technique has the added advantage that extremely small quantities of fluid may be analyzed.

Polyethylene Glycol Technique. Another standard method for the determination of immune complex levels utilizes the observation that the complexes are relatively insoluble in polyethylene glycol (PEG). Brandslund et al. [55] have utilized this principle, together with their consumption of complement, to devise a rapid and highly accurate test for the determination of immune complex levels.

SKIN TESTS. The intradermal injection of standard amounts of microbial or nonmicrobial antigens has been successfully used as a test of delayed hypersensitivity to these antigens. Characteristically, an indurated erythematous skin lesion appears at the site of the inoculation 48 hours after injection. It is generally agreed that dermal reactions of this type represent delayed hypersensitivity to the antigen in question and that this reaction is basically a function of T lymphocytes. Histologic sections of positive skin-test sites show accumulations of lymphocytes and macrophages. Blood vessels in the immediate area of the skin test may show hypertrophy of the endothelial cells, an unusually wide lumen, and penetration of the vessel wall by lymphocytes that first attach themselves to the endothelium and then migrate through the junctions between these cells. When the level of hypersensitivity is very high, positive skin-test reactions occasionally produce necrotizing reactions at the injection site. Such reactions are accompanied by polymorphonuclear leukocyte infiltration and occasionally by hemorrhage.

Toxoplasmin. Toxoplasmin is an aqueous extract of lysed *Toxoplasma* organisms. Van Metre et al. [56] have shown an extremely high correlation between skin-test positivity to toxoplasmin and the existence of focal necrotizing retinochoroiditis, the hallmark of ocular toxoplasmosis. There was also a very high level of dye-test positivity among the same patients. The existence of a positive skin test merely indicates that the patient in question has had previous exposure to *Toxoplasma gondii* and has developed delayed hypersensitivity to the organism. It cannot be correlated with the stage or prognosis of the eye disease.

As a screening test, the toxoplasmin skin-test reaction is valuable; it serves virtually the same purpose as a survey for dye-test antibodies. It is regrettable, therefore, that toxoplasmin is no longer available in the United States. Because *Toxoplasma* is an obligate intracellular, it must be propagated upon living cells. Since the extract of *Toxoplasma* organisms that is used for the skin test is likely to be contaminated with the products of these cells, it is incumbent upon the manufacturer to show that the cells are not incidentally contaminated with viruses or other oncogenic agents. This kind of control is difficult and expensive and, since the market for toxoplasmin is relatively small, candidate manufacturers of this product in the United States have not felt that it was commercially feasible to continue the production of it.

Tuberculin (Mantoux). The tuberculin skin test is of great value in ophthalmology. The use of a purified protein derivative (PPD) of the tubercle bacillus gives a highly specific reaction indicative of previous exposure to the organism. The intensity of the induration and erythema is thought to reflect the degree of hypersensitivity manifested by the patient, and where tuberculosis is suspected as the possible cause of ocular inflammation, the extent of the reaction may influence the ultimate decision to treat with antituberculous drugs.

The most reliable product for the tuberculin skin test appears to be a Tween-stabilized extract of *Mycobacterium tuberculosis,* which comes in three different strengths: 1 TU (i.e., 1 U.S. tuberculin unit), 5 TU, and 250 TU. For the initial intracutaneous tuberculin test it is customary to use 5 TU. The 1 TU is reserved for individuals suspected of being highly sensitized. Larger initial doses may, in this case, result in severe skin reactions with necrosis. The preparation containing 250 TU per test dose of 0.1 ml should be used exclusively for the testing of individuals who fail to react to a previous injection of either 1 or 5 TU.

In proven cases of ocular tuberculosis, such as the one described by Darrell [57], the skin-test reaction to the lowest dosage of tuberculin was negative. Only at higher test doses did the patient react. It is important, therefore, to test the patient at all strengths of tuberculin before concluding that he is tuberculin negative. In most of the industrialized nations the incidence of tuberculin positivity has decreased markedly over the past three decades. This makes tuberculin positivity, when detected, even more noteworthy. Among tuberculin-positive patients with refractory uveitis, in whom no other etiology could be found, Schlaegel and O'Connor [58] have occasionally found treatment with antituberculous drugs to be effective, even in the absence of pulmonary findings in these patients.

Histoplasmin. Delayed hypersensitivity to extracts of *Histoplasma capsulatum* can be demonstrated by skin tests in most subjects who live or have lived in an endemic area. In the United States, geographic areas supplied by tributaries of the Mississippi River are most affected, although there are also important endemic areas in the southeastern states. The majority of patients with the "presumed ocular histoplasmosis syndrome (POHS)" will show dermal hypersensitivity to this antigen, although Schlaegel and O'Connor [59] state that 11% of patients with the typical findings of POHS can be expected to be histoplasmin negative.

Some authors, such as Schlaegel and O'Connor [59], believe that they have seen a worsening of the macular manifestations of ocular histoplasmosis with hemorrhage and edema following the intradermal administration of histoplasmin. This finding is similar to the "focal syndromic reaction" described by Campinchi [60] and others. Under these circumstances, histoplasmin diluted 1:100 is sometimes given instead of the full strength skin-test material as an initial inoculation. If it is negative, it may be followed by a full-strength skin test. The immunologic basis of these "focal syndromic reactions" is not known. It may be that antigen-antibody complexes become localized in a lesion that has already been compromised by a breakdown of vascular integrity.

Coccidioidin. Reactions to aqueous extracts of *Coccidioides immitis* may be seen among individuals living in Arizona and California as well as in certain other areas of the southwestern United States. Ocular involvement with this fungus is relatively rare, yet it may produce disseminated lesions in the retina and choroid among patients subject to hematogenous dissemination of the organism, and it has occasionally been known to cause local granulomata of the anterior segment of the eye in otherwise normal individuals [61].

The skin-test reaction in such individuals has been universally positive. There appears to be a small amount of nonspecific cross-reactivity between coccidioidin and histoplasmin. This factor must be taken into account, particularly among individuals who have never lived in the "*Histoplasma* belt" but who, nevertheless, manifest a positive skin test to histoplasmin.

Capacity to Express Delayed Hypersensitivity Reflected in Skin Testing. The general capacity of a patient to express delayed hypersensitivity is of importance in certain disease states such as suspected sarcoidosis. Among sarcoid patients, there is a deficiency of T-cell immunity, which does not permit them to express delayed hypersensitivity. In order to test for the presence or absence of this type of background immunity, a battery of skin tests is generally applied to the skin of the forearm. This battery includes antigens to which the patient would almost certainly have been exposed at some time in the past: mumps, *Candida*, *Trichophyton*, and streptokinase-streptodornase. An absence of delayed hypersensitivity to all of these common antigens would give evidence of an immunologic deficiency. This deficiency is expressed naturally among patients with sarcoidosis, but might also be seen in patients under treatment with immunosuppressive drugs.

IN VITRO TESTS FOR DELAYED HYPERSENSITIVITY. Certain aspects of T-cell immunity can be tested only under laboratory conditions.

Lymphocyte Transformation In Vitro. The lymphocyte population of a given sample of patient's blood can be effectively separated from other cellular elements by a technique known as differential density centrifugation. Heparinized blood is added to the mixture of Ficoll-Hypaque adjusted to concentrations that allow a layer of virtually pure lymphocytes to be isolated from the centrifuge tube [62]. These lymphocytes can then be washed and suspended in a suitable tissue-culture medium. When antigens to which the patient has developed an immunologic response are added to the tissue culture medium, a blastogenic change will occur in certain of these lymphocytes. This lymphoblast transformation expresses a reversion to an embryonal form of the lymphocyte, a change that prepares it for cell division. The lymphocytoblast is a large cell with abundant basophilic cytoplasm and a large nucleolated nucleus. Although it can usually be detected in any cell population by its morphology alone, the incorporation of radioactive thymidine (^{3}H-thymidine) into the nuclear structure of the cell signals a definite lymphocytoblastic change (Fig. 2-4). This transformation occurs almost exclusively among T-cells and is thought to represent one of the earliest phases of delayed hypersensitivity reactions.

The production of lymphocytoblasts in response to a specific antigen such as tuberculin indicates a basic ability to respond to that antigen. The degree of responsiveness (or lack of responsiveness) to a specific antigen should always be compared with the response of the patient to polyclonal mitogens such as phytohemagglutinin, concanavalin A, or pokeweed mitogen. These substances produce nonspecific blastogenic responses in lymphocytes and indicate a background of general responsiveness to mitogenic stimuli. In the case of either specific or nonspecific mitogenic stimulation, the cells are allowed to react with the mitogen for periods ranging from 72 to 120 hours before the tritium-labeled thymidine is added to the tissue-culture vessel. Ultimately the unbound radioactive label is washed off, and the cells are placed in scintillation vials with a measured amount of scintillation fluid. The vials are counted in a scintillation counter and the results are expressed as counts per minute. To show a significant stimulation effect, the radioactivity of stimulated cells should, in general, be at least twice that of nonstimulated cells. Applications of this technique to the study of chronic retinal diseases can be found in the work of Brinkman and Broekhuyse [63]. Nussenblatt et al. [64], using the same technique, demonstrated evidence of autoimmunity to retinal S-antigen in patients suffering from chronic retinal inflammations such as ocular toxoplasmosis.

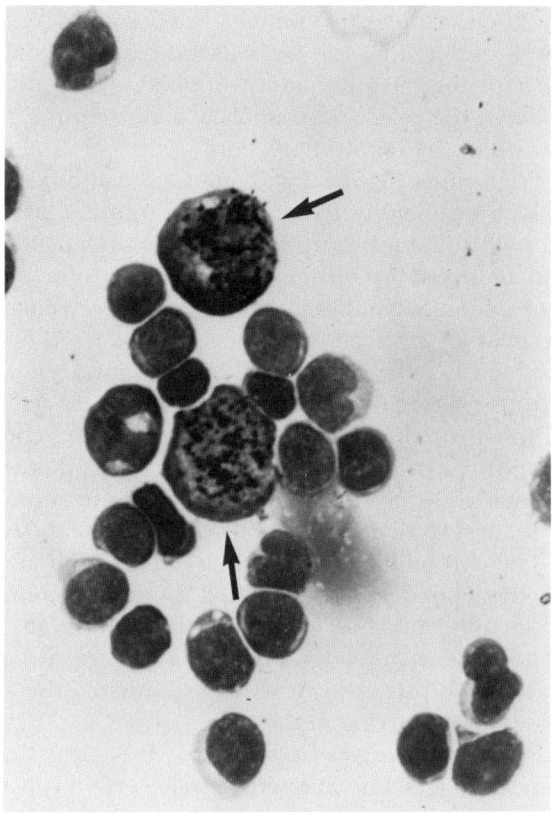

FIG. 2-4 Lymphocytoblast transformation among cultured lymphocytes stimulated with *Toxoplasma* antigen. *Arrows* denote large blast forms containing black dots. These dots represent sites of uptake of tritiated thymidine. Giemsa, × 1000

Antibody-Dependent Cytotoxicity. Certain types of T lymphocytes have Fc receptors on their surface membranes that can bind specific antibodies. It appears that this combination of antibody molecules with lymphocytes is necessary for the killing of certain cells, thus, the origin of the name "antibody-dependent cytotoxicity." The phenomenon of antibody-dependent cell-mediated toxicity is known to occur in herpetic infections of the eye, for example, and may be an important mechanism for the destruction of virus-laden cells [65]. It seems that when a cell becomes infected with herpes virus, its surface membrane becomes modified in such a way as to express herpetic antigens. These antigenic sites can bind to the Fab portion of an antibody molecule. If the antibody is attached to a T lymphocyte, lysis of the cell can be brought about.

There are many ways to detect whether the surface membrane of a cell has been broken down. Cells can, for example, be examined under light microscopy in the presence of trypan blue. Cells with damaged membranes will take up the dye; intact cells will not. Lysed cells will swell and their cytoplasmic contents will become progressively more transparent, an effect that can be detected easily by phase-contrast microscopy. Perhaps the most frequently applied quantitative method is that which involves the release of radioactive chromium, ^{51}Cr. This method is described in the following section.

^{51}Chromium Release Test. Under the conditions of this test, the target cells are generally treated with a solution of $Na^{51}CrO_4$. Chromate is thought to be taken up by an energy-independent process into the cell and reduced. According to Sanderson [66], 20% of the chromium is found complexed to cell organelles and the remainder is probably bound to small organic cations. When a cell is lysed by one of several possible mechanisms, the chromium bound to intracellular structures is released into the external milieu where it can be detected by a gamma counter. In this procedure the cells under study must be washed free of all unbound ^{51}Cr prior to the addition of agents that will cause lysis. Similarly, all intact cells must be removed by centrifugation prior to the conclusion of the test so that only the ^{51}Cr released by the lysis of cells is counted.

The chromium release technique is highly useful in quantitating antibody-dependent cell-mediated immunity, complement-dependent antibody-mediated lysis, or cell-mediated immunity directed against certain target cells. It provides a quantitative measure of immunologically mediated lytic processes in vitro. Presumably the same kinds of lytic processes are occurring in the target tissues.

Products of Activated Lymphocytes. It is clear that lymphocytes, primed to react to a certain antigen, secrete certain substances into the extracellular environment within a short time after making contact with that antigen. Such substances, referred to collectively as "lymphokines," are the soluble mediators of cellular immunity. They are nonantibody in nature and appear in chromatographic and electrophoretic fractions that are quite distinct from those of the classical immunoglobulins. It has been suggested that lymphokines might act by regulating lymphoid cell traffic through critical regions of lymphatic and microvascular systems and by expediting cellular cooperation between sensitized T cells and other cells participating in immune responses. Lymphokines are generally thought to be anionic glycoproteins of molecular weight ranging between 30,000 and 100,000. They are precipitable in 40- to 90%-saturated ammonium sulfate solution, and after suitable dialysis to remove the ammonium sulfate, they can be stored for weeks or months in the freeze-dried state at $-20°C$.

Macrophage Migration Inhibition Factor (MIF). This classic lymphokine inhibits the outward migration of macrophages from glass tubes into which they are loosely packed. For purposes of the test, macrophages are generally harvested from the peritoneal cavities of normal guinea pigs 2 to 3 days after the intraperitoneal injection of sterile mineral oil. The cell suspensions are then centrifuged at 450 g at 4°C to pack the cells, and the cells are washed twice more with cold sterile Hanks' balanced salt solution. Finally, they are suspended in Eagle's minimal essential me-

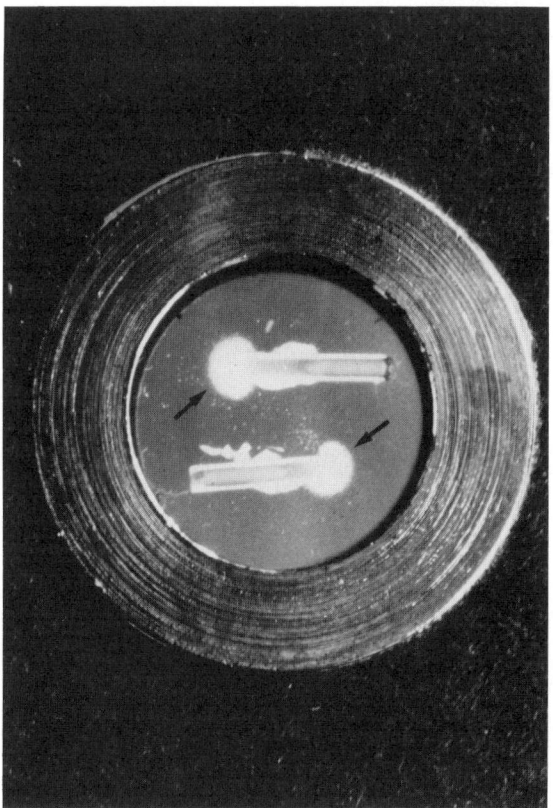

FIG. 2-5 Migration inhibition factor (MIF) test performed in a Sykes-Moore culture chamber. *Arrows* denote migration of macrophages in a fanlike pattern from the open ends of the capillary tubes.

dium (MEM) and loaded into glass capillary tubes 1.0 to 1.2 mm in internal diameter, one end being plugged with molten paraffin. The tubes are centrifuged at 250 g for 5 minutes. The capillary tubes are then cut at the cell-liquid interface and put into tissue culture chambers containing nutrient medium. The Sykes-Moore chamber (Fig. 2-5) has classically been used for this purpose. Prior to the addition of the culture medium, the capillary tube is fixed to the bottom coverslip with a small amount of sterile silicone grease. Control tubes are incubated with supernates of human lymphocytes cultured for 24 hours without antigen. Tubes used for the analysis of the lymphokine are incubated with the supernatant fluid of lymphocytes that had been cultured in the presence of a specific antigen for a similar period.

The assembled chambers are incubated at 37°C overnight. After 15 to 18 hours of incubation, the areas of cell migration are photographed and the areas of cell migration are determined by planimetry. Alternatively, the migration areas may be measured by weighing cutouts of photographed or traced camera lucida images on ruled paper. Significant inhibition of macrophage migration is thought to occur when lymphokine-containing cultures show areas of migration that are at least 20% less than those of the control cultures.

A useful modification of this test consists of the mixture of human lymphocytes with guinea pig macrophages in capillary tubes. Upon the addition of the appropriate antigen, inhibition of macrophage migration is observed and quantitated as indicated previously.

Leukocyte Migration Inhibition Factor (LIF). Cells from the buffy coat of heparinized whole blood are generally used for this assay. Three main types of tests have been developed for this procedure. The first, described by Søberg and Bendixen [67], measures the area of cells migrating out of a capillary tube into a tissue culture chamber containing nutrient medium and antigen. Observation and quantitation are performed in a manner similar to that for the MIF test. An important modification, described by Clausen [68], utilizes an agarose well assay. Granulocytes placed in such wells generally migrate outward in a uniform pattern beneath the agarose layer; but in the presence of antigen, migration is significantly inhibited. At the conclusion of the experiment, the agar layer can be fixed, dried, and stained with dyes such as hematoxylin. The diameter of the area of cell migration can then be measured under suitable magnification. This technique has been largely replaced by the micro-agarose droplet technique described by Harrington and Stastny [69]. The latter, requiring substantially less leukocytes and antigen and technically simpler, has been used to test a wide range of antigen concentrations on a single sample of patient cells.

In the LIF test normal granulocytes are inhibited in their motion by lymphokines released from antigen-stimulated lymphocytes. Using purified granulocytes from normal donors, Maurer et al. [70] described a two-step procedure in which the lymphocytes of the patient (or test animal) are first stimulated with the antigen in question; the supernatant fluid from this cell culture is then added to the suspension of granulocytes from the normal donor. Migration of the latter cells is significantly inhibited by the lymphokine if the patient's lymphocytes are normally reactive.

Henley [71] and colleagues found a high correlation between positive LIF tests and presumed autoimmune diseases of the retina and choroid when the leukocytes obtained from the buffy coats of the patients were exposed to aqueous extracts of human retina or choroid. Caution must be used in the interpretation of some of these results, however. Although MIF production is thought to be highly correlated with delayed hypersensitivity, as manifested by positive skin-test responses, Senyk and Hadley [72] could not correlate skin-test response to common antigens such as *Candida* with LIF tests to the same antigen.

MONOCLONAL ANTIBODIES. The discovery of a technique for the production of massive amounts of antibody directed against a single antigenic determinant has proved highly advantageous in the diagnosis and treatment of certain ocular diseases. Individual plasma cells produce antibody characterized by a specific affinity for only one antigen. If an individual plasma cell can be isolated and fused with a malignant myeloma cell, a tumor that produces antibody of a single specificity can be created in vitro. Köhler and Milstein [73] discovered a technique for doing this in 1975.

An infection such as herpes zoster may initiate the production of multiple different antibodies, each one being directed against a different specific glycoprotein elaborated by the virus. Thus Grose et al. [74] were able to produce monoclonal antibodies against three different glycoproteins of the varicella-zoster virus.

Lymphocytes with different glycoprotein antigens on their surface membranes can now be differentiated from one another by using fluorescein- or peroxidase-labelled monoclonal antibodies [75], and this is the basis for defining the abnormal ratios of OKT_4^+ cells to OKT_8^+ cells in AIDS patients (Chap. 7). In the same way, the different kinds of lymphocytes and monocytes that infiltrate the choroid in sympathetic ophthalmia can now be differentiated from one another [76].

MISCELLANEOUS TESTS. Serum factors other than antibodies have recently been found to be important in the diagnosis of various inflammatory conditions.

Serum Lysozyme. Lysozyme is one of a number of enzymes released by activated macrophages. Serum levels of this enzyme appear to be elevated in certain chronic granulomatous diseases such as sarcoidosis and leprosy where macrophages accumulate at the sites of diseased tissue, seemingly unable to complete the task for which they were mobilized. Pascual et al. [77] found elevated levels of lysozyme in the serum of patients with confirmed sarcoidosis, and Weinberg and Tessler [78] showed that patients with active sarcoid uveitis as well as active systemic disease had mean serum levels of 24.2 ± 11.1 µg/ml, as compared with normal values of 0 to 10 µg/ml. Even among patients with presumptive ocular sarcoidosis but no documented evidence of active systemic disease, the mean serum level was 17.1 ± 4.1 µg/ml. Patients with inactive disease who were taking systemic corticosteroid therapy appeared to have normal levels of lysozyme in the serum. This test appears to offer some promise as an aid to the diagnosis of ocular sarcoidosis in the absence of overt systemic disease, but it is elevated in many granulomatous diseases.

Serum Angiotensin Converting Enzyme (ACE). This enzyme is also released into the bloodstream under conditions of increased macrophage activity, but elevated levels are seen in only a few known diseases, e.g., sarcoidosis, leprosy, and Gaucher's disease. The angiotensin converting enzyme assay was described by Lieberman [79] in 1974 as a new confirmatory test for sarcoidosis. Later Weinreb et al. [80] showed that the serum ACE level was significantly elevated in patients with systemic sarcoidosis and in patients with granulomatous uveitis but no other signs of sarcoidosis. Using a normal mean value of 22 ± 6.3 nanomols/ml/min,

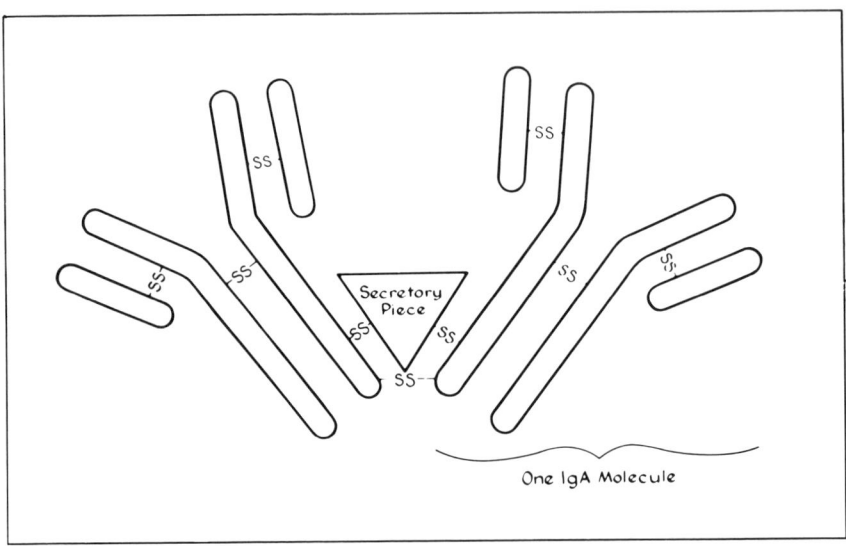

FIG. 2-6 Diagrammatic representation of secretory IgA molecule. (From M. R. Allansmith, and G. R. O'Connor. Immunoglobulins: structure, function, and relation to the eye., *Surv. Ophthalmol.* 14:367, 1970. Copyright © 1980 The Williams & Wilkins Co., Baltimore. Reproduced with permission.)

they showed that these two groups had significantly higher amounts of ACE in their serum than a control group of non-sarcoid uveitis patients ($p < 0.005$).

Elevated levels of ACE are found in leprosy [81], in Gaucher's disease [82], and in primary biliary cirrhosis [83]. Therefore, the test cannot be considered as absolutely specific for sarcoid. Nevertheless, the test provides a valuable marker for ocular sarcoidosis, particularly when combined with positive results from the physical examination of the eye and with positive results from gallium scanning [84]. Patients currently under treatment with corticosteroids show consistently lower levels than patients receiving no therapy [80].

Tests on Tears and Aqueous Humor

TEAR IgA AND IgG. Normal tears contain small but significant amounts of IgG and IgA. McClellan et al. [85] showed that the normal IgG value is approximately 14 mg/dl and that the IgA level is 17 mg/dl. A very small amount of IgE is present in normal tears as well (0.025 mg/dl). All of these values can be increased appreciably under conditions of inflammation, particularly in anaphylactoid reactions that increase the permeability of conjunctival blood vessels. IgA is normally present in a dimeric form called "secretory IgA" that is actually heavier than the sum of two IgA units owing to the addition of a "J piece" and a "secretory component" in the process of its formation (Fig. 2-6). By means of studies utilizing fluorescein-tagged antisecretory component, Gillette et al. [86]

have shown that secretory IgA is elaborated in both the main lacrimal glands and the accessory lacrimal glands of the conjunctiva. This material is believed to function as a kind of "immunologic paint," protecting the mucosal surfaces by combining with microbes and preventing their attachment to susceptible cells. Although IgA does not fix complement, it does allow for the agglutination and disposal of microorganisms on the surface of the mucosae. Centifano and Kaufman [86a] and others have stated that IgG is in competition with IgA and may, under certain circumstances, be detrimental to its function. Herpesviruses, for example, when combined with IgG may still enter susceptible cells. Depending upon the amount of IgG released into the conjunctival sac upon irritation of the eye (with the subsequent increase of permeability of the conjunctival vessels), IgG may win out over IgA in its competition for the microbe.

IgM is normally not present in the tears. Under conditions of a marked increase in the permeability of the conjunctival vessels, it too may appear in the tears [85]. IgM is very efficient as an agglutinator of organisms and as a binder of complement, but normally it plays little role in conjunctival defenses unless a bacterial conjunctivitis has been present for a number of days and the permeability of the conjunctival vessels has been seriously altered.

The question of whether hemolytic complement is present in tears has been the subject of some debate. Yamamoto and Allansmith [87] found evidence of both the classic hemolytic complement system and the alternate pathway of complement in human tears and confirmed the earlier work of Chandler et al. [88]. Kijlstra and Veerhuis [89], on the other hand, failing to find evidence of hemolytic complement in tears, looked for factors that might deactivate complement. Later studies by them [90] showed that lactoferrin, an iron-binding protein present in many external secretions as well as in the granules of polymorphonuclear leukocytes, inactivated the $C'3$ convertase of complement in normal tears. It now seems clear that both complement and lactoferrin are present in tears in easily measurable quantities and that both contribute to the bactericidal qualities of the tear film.

IMMUNOGLOBULINS IN AQUEOUS HUMOR. The direct analysis of immunoglobulins contained in the ocular fluids may shed some light on the nature of inflammatory processes that are occurring in the eye.

SPECIFIC IMMUNOGLOBULINS. Immunoglobulins are ordinarily present in only very small quantities in the aqueous humor. Allansmith et al. [91] state that IgG is present in quantities approaching 7 mg/dl and IgA is present at a level of about 1 mg/dl. Under conditions of increased permeability of the anterior uveal vessels (e.g., uveitis, persistent corneal ulceration, and blunt trauma to the eye), the levels of immunoglobulins in the aqueous may approach those of the circulating plasma. Other plasma components such as albumin and fibrinogen may also be present. Indeed, under certain circumstances, a fibrin clot may form in the anterior chamber.

AQUEOUS/SERUM RATIO IN DIAGNOSIS. Witmer [92] and others have shown that immunoglobulins may be synthesized locally in the eye. Plasma cells in the iris and ciliary body are probably responsible for the lion's share of this synthesis, and it is generally assumed that these plasma cells are responding to some specific infectious or antigenic insult. Therefore, if one could detect the specific nature of the antibodies being produced, one might obtain specific leads as to the etiology of a given uveal inflammation.

The situation is complicated by the fact that the same antibodies that one detects in the aqueous humor are often present in the circulating plasma as well. If the permeability of the blood-aqueous barrier is increased, large amounts of immunoglobulin may enter the aqueous humor from the bloodstream. If one can demonstrate more specific antibody per unit of immunoglobulin in the aqueous humor than in the corresponding plasma, one could theoretically say that the particular antibody under discussion is being manufactured locally within the eye. If a particular antibody test, e.g., the ELISA test for toxoplasmosis, can be adapted to the aqueous humor, as has been accomplished by Rollins et al. [93] in rabbits, it should be possible to test both aqueous humor and serum simultaneously for antibody. If the amount of IgG in each of these fluids is then separately determined, it should be possible to state whether more specific antibody is present in the aqueous humor than could be accounted for on the basis of altered vascular permeability alone. Certain European authors have laid great store by these examinations. As stated earlier in this chapter, Desmonts [7] believes that he can make a definite serologic diagnosis of ocular toxoplasmosis on the basis of the aqueous/serum ratio alone.

This type of testing presumes that normal aqueous circulation dynamics are in effect. Under certain circumstances, spurious results could be obtained. For example, a phthisical eye or prephthisical eye usually shows a good deal of protein in the aqueous humor. This protein is stagnant and thus does not return to the circulation by the usual channels. Tests on the aqueous humor of such a patient might be expected to give spuriously low ratios, for the nonspecific IgG level (the denominator) might be abnormally high in comparison to the specific antibody activity. Conversely, tests on secondary aqueous, i.e., aqueous removed within hours after a previous paracentesis, might contain abnormally high amounts of specific antibody if the patient's circulating plasma happened to contain very large amounts of specific antibody at the time of the aqueous tap.

IMMUNE COMPLEXES IN AQUEOUS HUMOR. In many disease states it is likely that antibody found in the aqueous humor will already have become complexed with antigen. Depending upon the ratios of antigen to antibody, this situation may even make it impossible to detect specific antibody reactivity in certain of these molecules, because the antigen-reactivity sites on the antibody molecule will have become occupied.

As stated in the earlier discussions on immune complexes (p. 116), it is possible to detect these substances by a number of techniques, most of which are concerned with their complement-binding capacity. Dernouchamps et al. [94] have demonstrated the presence of high levels of immune complexes in Fuchs' heterochromic cyclitis, and Char et al. [95] have shown the same thing in patients with idiopathic anterior and diffuse uveitis. Until the antigenic component of these complexes has been analyzed, it will probably not be possible to interpret the presence of these complexes very meaningfully. Suffice it to say that they are present in the aqueous humor of a good many patients suffering from uveitis. Their role in the pathogenesis of uveal inflammation remains to be determined.

COMPLEMENT IN AQUEOUS HUMOR. Mondino and Rao [96] have been able to measure hemolytic complement in the aqueous humor of normal subjects, although the quantities appear to be minute. Inflamed eyes, on the other hand, were shown to contain considerable quantities of both IgG and complement components. The ratio of IgG to $C'3$ failed to change appreciably under conditions of uveal inflammation. Thus the consumption of complement could not be demonstrated in the aqueous humor, whereas the consumption of complement can easily be demonstrated in joint fluid in conditions such as rheumatoid arthritis. This is obviously an area where further study is indicated. For one thing, a much broader range of patients with uveal inflammation must be studied.

In another study, Mondino and Rao [97] were not able to demonstrate factor B, an essential component of the alternate complement pathway, in the aqueous humor of normal patients. They were, however, able to detect factor B in the aqueous humor of patients with anterior chamber inflammation. Since the alternate pathway of complement activation is often used by the body for defense against bacterial infection, indirect evidence of bacterial infection in certain cases of uveitis may be at hand.

REFERENCES

1. O'Connor, G. R. Ocular Toxoplasmosis. In E. A. Klein (Ed.), *Symposium on Medical and Surgical Diseases of the Retina and Vitreous.* St. Louis: Mosby, 1983. P. 115.
2. Franceschetti, A., and Engelbrecht, E. Mise en évidence de toxoplasmes dans un cas de choriorétinite séro-negative. *Ophthalmologica* 147:273, 1964.
3. Wilfuhr, G., and Hudemann, H. Weitere Ergebnisse über Erregernachweiss bei Toxoplasmose durch Tierversuch. *Z. Kinderheil.* 74:320, 1954.
4. Sabin, A. B., and Feldman, H. A. Dyes as microchemical indicators of a new immunity phenomenon affecting a protozoan parasite (Toxoplasma). *Science* 108:660, 1948.
5. Schreiber, R. D., and Feldman, H. A. Identification of the activator system for antibody to Toxoplasma as the classical complement pathway. *J. Infect. Dis.* 141:366, 1980.
6. Zscheile, F. P. Recurrent toxoplasmic retinitis with weakly positive methylene blue dye test. *Arch. Ophthalmol.* 71:645, 1964.
7. Desmonts, G. Definitive serologic diagnosis of ocular toxoplasmosis. *Arch. Ophthalmol.* 76:839, 1966.
8. Balfour, A. H., et al. An evaluation of the ToxHA test for the detection of antibodies to Toxoplasma gondii in human serum. *J. Clin. Pathol.* 33:644, 1980.

9. Balfour, A. H., et al. Comparative study of three tests (Dye-Test, Indirect Hemagglutination Test, Latex Agglutination Test) for the detection of antibodies to Toxoplasma gondii in human sera. *J. Clin. Pathol.* 35:228, 1982.
10. Gordon, M. A., et al. Automated immunofluorescence test for toxoplasmosis. *J. Clin. Microbiol.* 13:283, 1981.
11. Siim, J. C., and Lind, K. A Toxoplasma flocculation test. *Acta Pathol. Microbiol. Scand.* 50:445, 1960.
12. Desmonts, G., et al. Direct agglutination test for diagnosis of Toxoplasma infection. *J. Clin. Microbiol.* 11:562, 1980.
13. O'Connor, G. R. Precipitating antibody to Toxoplasma: a follow-up study on findings in the blood and aqueous humor. *Am. J. Ophthalmol.* 44:75, 1957.
14. Filice, G., et al. A new complement fixation test for toxoplasmosis: Comparison with other serological methods. *Boll. Ist. Sieroter. Milan* 60:129, 1981.
15. Jackson, W. B., O'Connor, G. R., and Hall, J. M. Plate hemolysin test for the rapid screening of toxoplasma antibodies. *Appl. Microbiol.* 27:896, 1974.
16. Konishi, E., et al. Reproducible enzyme-linked immunosorbent assay with a magnetic processing system for diagnosis of toxoplasmosis. *J. Clin. Microbiol.* 17:225, 1983.
17. Smith, J. L. *Spirochetes in Late Seronegative Syphilis, Penicillin Notwithstanding.* Springfield, IL.: Thomas, 1969. P. 44.
18. Ryan, S. J., Nell, E. E., and Hardy, P. H. A study of aqueous humor for the presence of spirochetes. *Am. J. Ophthalmol.* 73:250, 1972.
19. Whitfield, R., and Wirostco, E. Uveitis and intraocular treponemes. *Arch. Ophthalmol.* 84:12, 1970.
20. Wang, S. P., and Grayston, J. T. Immunologic relationship between genital TRIC, lymphogranuloma venereum, & related organisms in a new microtiter indirect immunofluorescence test. *Am. J. Ophthalmol.* 70:367, 1970.
21. Edwards, J. E., et al.: Ocular manifestations of Candida septicemia: Review of seventy-six cases of hematogenous Candida endophthalmitis. *Medicine* 53:47, 1974.
22. Filice, G., Ya, B., and Armstrong, D. Immunodiffusion and agglutination tests for Candida in patients with neoplastic disease. *J. Infect. Dis.* 135:349, 1977.
23. Glew, R. H., et al. Serologic tests in the diagnosis of systemic candidiasis: enhanced diagnostic accuracy with crossed immunoelectrophoresis. *Am. J. Med.* 64:586, 1978.
24. Szepes, E., et al. Enzyme-linked immunosorbent assay (ELISA) for detection of antibodies against *Candida albicans*. *Mykosen* 26:42, 1983.
25. Gentry, L. O., et al. Latex agglutination test for detection of Candida antigen in patients with disseminated disease. *Eur. J. Clin. Microbiol.* 2:122, 1983.
26. Schlaegel, T. F., and O'Connor, G. R. Fungal Uveitis. In T. F. Schlaegel (Ed.), *Current Aspects of Uveitis.* Boston: Little, Brown, 1977. P. 12.
27. Krill, A. E., et al. Multifocal inner choroiditis. *Trans. Am. Acad. Ophthalmol. Otolaryngol.* 73:222, 1969.
28. Peace, R. J. Cytomegalic inclusion disease in adults: complication of neoplastic disease of hemopoietic and reticulo-histiocytic systems. *Am. J. Med.* 24:48, 1958.
29. Cappel, R., DeCuyper, F., and de Braekeleer, J. Rapid detection of IgG and IgM antibodies for cytomegalovirus by the enzyme linked immunosorbent assay (ELISA). *Arch. Virol.* 58:253, 1978.
30. Huntley, C. C., Lyerly, A. D., and Patterson, M. V. Isohemagglutinins in parasitic infections. *J.A.M.A.* 208:1145, 1969.

31. Kagan, I. G., Normal, L., and Allain, D. S. Studies on the serology of visceral larva migrans. I. Hemagglutination and flocculation tests with purified *Toxocara* antigens. *J. Immunol.* 83:297, 1959.
32. Cypess, R. H., et al. Larva-specific antibodies in patients with visceral larva migrans. *J. Infect. Dis.* 135:633, 1977.
33. Glickman, L., et al. Toxocara-specific antibody in the serum and aqueous humor of a patient with presumed ocular and visceral toxocariasis. *Am. J. Trop. Med. Hyg.* 28:29, 1979.
34. Biglan, A. W., Glickman, L. T., and Lobes, L. A. Serum and vitreous Toxocara antibody in nematode endophthalmitis. *Am. J. Ophthalmol.* 88:898, 1979.
35. Maizels, R. M., et al. Characterization of surface and excretory-secretory antigens of *Toxocara canis* infective larvae. *Parasite Immunol.* 6:23, 1984.
36. Matsura, K., et al. Detection of specific IgM antibodies to toxocaral E-S antigens: Effect of absorption of sera with protein A sepharose. *Zentralbl. Bakteriol. Microbiol. Hyg.* [A] 255:549, 1983.
37. Gilliland, B. C. Immunologic quantitation of serum immunoglobulins. *Am. J. Clin. Pathol.* 68:664, 1977.
38. Normansell, D. E. Quantitation of serum immunoglobulins. *C.R.C. Crit. Rev. Clin. Lab. Sci.* 17:103, 1982.
39. Mancini, G., Carbonara, A. O., and Heremans, J. F. Immunochemical quantitation of antigens by single radial immunodiffusion. *Immunochemistry* 2:235, 1965.
40. Simmons, P. Quantitation of plasma proteins in low concentrations using RID. *Clin. Chim. Acta* 35:53, 1971.
41. Gleich, G. E., Averbeck, A. K., and Sedlund, H. A. Measurement of IgE in normal and allergic serum by radioimmunoassay. *J. Lab. Clin. Med.* 77:690, 1971.
42. Brauninger, G. E., and Centifano, Y. M. Immunoglobulin E in human tears. *Am. J. Ophthalmol.* 72:558, 1971.
43. Giallongo, A., et al. Enzyme and radioimmunoassays for specific murine IgE and IgG with different solid-phase immunosorbents. *J. Immunol. Methods* 52:379, 1982.
44. Adkinson, N. F., and Lichtenstein, L. M. Assessment of allergic states; IgE methodology and the measurement of allergen-specific IgG antibody. In F. H. Bach and R. A. Good (Eds.), *Clinical Immunobiology.* New York: Academic, 1976. P. 305.
45. Misra, R. N., et al. Antilens antibody in normal persons and in different clinical conditions. *Indian J. Ophthalmol.* 29:203, 1981.
46. Marak, G. E., Font, R. L., and Alepa, F. P. Experimental lens-induced granulomatous endophthalmitis: passive transfer with serum. *Ophthalmol. Res.* 8:117, 1976.
47. Aronson, S. B., et al. The occurrence of an autoanti-uveal antibody in human uveitis. *Arch. Ophthalmol.* 72:621, 1964.
48. Jones, B. R. Lacrimal and salivary precipitating antibodies in Sjögren's syndrome. *Lancet* 2:773, 1958.
49. Heller, G., et al. The hemagglutination test for rheumatoid arthritis. II. The influence of human plasma factor II (gamma globulin) on the reaction. *J. Immunol.* 72:66, 1954.
50. Schaller, J., et al. Antinuclear antibodies in patients with iridocyclitis and JRA. *Arthritis Rheum.* 16:130, 1973.
51. Kogure, M., Shimada, K., and Hara, H. G. Complement titer in patients with Behçet's disease. *Acta Soc. Ophthalmol. Jpn.* 75:1260, 1971.

52. Shimada, K., et al. Reduction of complement in Behçet's disease and drug allergy. *Med. Biol.* 52:234, 1974.
53. Zubler, R. H., and Lambert, P. H. The ^{125}I-C1q binding test for the detection of soluble immune complexes. In B. R. Bloom, and J. R. David (Eds.), *In vitro Methods in Cell-Mediated and Tumor Immunity.* New York: Academic, 1976. P. 565.
54. Theofilopoulos, A. N., Wilson, C. B., and Dixon, F. J. The Raji cell immunoassay for detecting immune complexes in human serum. *J. Clin. Invest.* 57:169, 1976.
55. Brandslund, I., et al. Detection and quantitation of immune complexes with a rapid polyethylene glycol precipitation complement consumption method (PEG-CC). *Methods Enzymol.* 74(c):551, 1981.
56. Van Metre, T. E., Know, D. L., and Maumenee, A. E. The relation between toxoplasmosis and focal exudative retinochoroiditis. *Am. J. Ophthalmol.* 58:6, 1964.
57. Darrell, R. W. Acute tuberculous panophthalmitis. *Arch. Ophthalmol.* 78:51, 1967.
58. Schlaegel, T. F., and O'Connor, G. R. Tuberculosis and syphilis. *Arch. Ophthalmol.* 99:2206, 1981.
59. Schlaegel, T. F., and O'Connor, G. R. Fungal Uveitis. In *Current Aspects of Uveitis.* Boston: Little, Brown, 1977. P. 123.
60. Campinchi, R. Uveitis of Tuberculous Origin. In R. Campinchi, et al. (Eds.), *Uveitis, Immunologic and Allergic Phenomena.* Springfield, IL.: Thomas, 1973. P. 366.
61. Pettit, T. H., Learn, R., and Foos, R. Y. Intraocular coccidioidomycosis. *Arch. Ophthalmol.* 77:655, 1967.
62. Boyum, A. Isolation of mononuclear cells and granulocytes from human blood. *Scand. J. Clin. Lab. Invest.* 21(Suppl. 97):77, 1968.
63. Brinkman, C. J. J., and Broekhuyse, R. M. Cell-mediated immunity after retinal detachment, as determined by lymphocyte stimulation. *Am. J. Ophthalmol.* 85:260, 1978.
64. Nussenblatt, R. B., et al. Cellular immune responsiveness of uveitis patients to retinal S-antigen. *Am. J. Ophthalmol.* 89:173, 1980.
65. Kohl, S., et al. Murine antibody-dependent cellular cytotoxicity to herpes simplex virus-infected target cells. *J. Immunol.* 123:25, 1979.
66. Sanderson, A. R. Applications of isoimmunocytolysis using radiolabelled target cells. *Nature* 204:250, 1964.
67. Søborg, M., and Bendixen, G. Human lymphocyte migration as a parameter of hypersensitivity. *Acta Med. Scand.* 181:247, 1967.
68. Clausen, J. E. Tuberculin-induced migration inhibition of peripheral leucocytes in agarose medium. *Acta Allergol.* 26:56, 1971.
69. Harrington, J. J., and Stastny, P. Macrophage migration from an agarose droplet. Development of a micromethod for assay of delayed hypersensitivity. *J. Immunol.* 110:752, 1973.
70. Maurer, B. A., et al. Indirect capillary tube leukocyte migration inhibition assay for cell-mediated immunity to human tumor-associated antigens. In B. R. Bloom, and J. R. David (Eds.), *In Vitro Methods In Cell-Mediated and Tumor Immunity.* New York: Academic, 1976. P. 613.
71. Henley, W. L., Leopold, I. H., and Okas, S. Leukocyte migration inhibition in chorioretinitis. *Infect. Immun.* 9:839, 1974.
72. Senyk, G., and Hadley, W. K. *In vitro* correlates of delayed hypersensitivity

in man. Ambiguity of polymorphonuclear neutrophils as indicator cells in leukocyte migration test. *Infect. Immun.* 8:370, 1973.
73. Köhler, G., and Milstein, C. Continuous cultures of fused cells secreting antibody of predefined specificity. *Nature* 256:495, 1975.
74. Grose, C., et al. Monoclonal antibodies against the three major glycoproteins of varicella-zoster virus. *Infect. Immun.* 40:381, 1983.
75. Talle, M. A., et al. Patterns of antigenic expression on human monocytes, as defined by monoclonal antibodies. *Cell. Immunol.* 78:83, 1983.
76. Jakobiec, F. A., et al. Human sympathetic ophthalmia: An analysis of the inflammatory infiltrate by hybridoma-monoclonal antibodies, immunochemistry, and correlative electron microscopy. *Ophthalmology* 90:77, 1983.
77. Pascual, R. S., Gee, B. L., and Finch, S. C. Serum lysozyme in diagnosis and evaluation of sarcoidosis. *N. Engl. J. Med.* 289:1074, 1973.
78. Weinberg, R., and Tessler, H. Serum lysozyme in sarcoid uveitis. *Am. J. Ophthalmol.* 82:105, 1976.
79. Lieberman, J. Elevation of serum angiotensin converting enzyme (ACE) level in sarcoidosis. *Am. J. Med.* 59:365, 1975.
80. Weinreb, R. N., et al. Angiotensin-converting enzyme in sarcoid uveitis. *Invest. Ophthalmol.* 18:1285, 1979.
81. Lieberman, J., and Rea, T. Serum angiotensin converting enzyme in leprosy and coccidioidomycosis. *Ann. Intern. Med.* 87:422, 1977.
82. Lieberman, J., and Beutler, E. Elevation of serum angiotensin converting enzyme in Gaucher's disease. *N. Engl. J. Med.* 294:1442, 1976.
83. Studdy, P., et al. Serum angiotensin converting enzyme (SACE) in sarcoidosis and other granulomatous disorders. *Lancet* 2:1331, 1978.
84. O'Connor, G. R. Ocular Sarcoidosis. In E. A. Klein (Ed.), *Symposium on the Medical and Surgical Diseases of the Retina and Vitreous.* St. Louis: Mosby, 1983. P. 218.
85. McClellan, B. H., et al. Immunoglobulins in tears. *Am. J. Ophthalmol.* 76:89, 1973.
86. Gillette, T. E., et al. Histologic and immunohistologic comparison of main and accessory lacrimal tissue. *Am. J. Ophthalmol.* 89:724, 1980.
86a. Centifano, Y. M., and Kaufman, H. E. Secretory immunoglobulin A and herpes keratitis. *Infect. Immun.* 2:778, 1970.
87. Yamamoto, G. K., and Allansmith, M. R. Complement in tears from normal humans. *Am. J. Ophthalmol.* 88:758, 1979.
88. Chandler, J. W., et al. Quantitative determinations of complement components and immunoglobulins in tears and aqueous humor. *Invest. Ophthalmol.* 13:151, 1974.
89. Kijlstra, A., and Veerhuis, R. The effect of an anticomplementary factor on normal human tears. *Am. J. Ophthalmol.* 92:24, 1981.
90. Kijlstra, A., et al. Modulation of classical C3 convertase of complement by tear lactoferrin. *Immunology* 47:263, 1982.
91. Allansmith, M. R., et al. Immunoglobulins in the human eye. Location, type, and amount. *Arch. Ophthalmol.* 89:36, 1973.
92. Witmer, R. H. Antibody formation in rabbit eye studied with fluorescein-labelled antibody. *Arch. Ophthalmol.* 53:811, 1955.
93. Rollins, D. F., et al. Detection of toxoplasmal antigen and antibody in ocular fluids in experimental ocular toxoplasmosis. *Arch. Ophthalmol.* 101:455, 1983.
94. Dernouchamps, J. P., et al. Immune complexes in the aqueous humor and serum. *Am. J. Ophthalmol.* 84:24, 1977.

95. Char, D. H., et al. Immune complexes in uveitis. *Am. J. Ophthalmol.* 87:678, 1979.
96. Mondino, B. J., and Rao, H. Hemolytic complement activity in aqueous humor. *Arch. Ophthalmol.* 101:465, 1983.
97. Mondino, B. J., and Rao, H. Complement levels in normal and inflamed aqueous humor. *Invest. Ophthalmol. Vis. Sci.* 24:380, 1983.

3 ATOPIC DISEASES AFFECTING THE EYE

GENERAL CONSIDERATIONS OF ATOPY

Atopy plays an important role in a large number of ocular diseases. A general understanding of atopy is essential prior to a discussion of specific ocular entities.

Definition of Atopy

In 1923 Coca and Cook [1] used the word *atopy,* meaning "strange reactivity," to refer to the reactions of persons with hereditary backgrounds of allergic disease who showed (1) immediate flare and wheal skin reactivity to *skin-sensitizing antibodies* (now called immunoglobulin E or IgE), and (2) the Prausnitz-Küstner reaction. This reaction is the result of the atopic patient's ability to transfer reactivity to the skin of a normal patient by the intradermal injection of his or her IgE-containing serum [2]. Unlike other immunoglobulins, which diffuse, IgE attaches to skin cells. To make the Prausnitz-Küstner test, the appropriate allergen is injected into the site of the IgE skin attachment 48 hours after the serum injection, and a wheal and flare appear immediately. (This test is used less often now than formerly because of the danger of transferring serum hepatitis.)

Clinical examples of atopy are seasonal and perennial rhinitis, bronchial asthma, food allergy, urticaria, nonhereditary angioedema, and atopic conjunctivitis, uveitis, and dermatitis. Atopy was originally defined as occurring only in human beings, but several clinical conditions highly suggestive of atopy occur in dogs, cattle, and other species [3, 4].

Incidence, Heredity, and Onset of Atopy

It is estimated that approximately 10 percent of the population show hereditary allergic manifestations, with the incidence higher in young boys than in young girls. The inherited factor is the tendency for allergies to develop that are not evident at birth, may not appear for years, and may lead to any of the atopic diseases. About half of all atopic persons first show allergic manifestations during the first decade of life. Those homozygous for the allergy gene tend to develop the allergic diseases early, and heterozygous persons, with one normal and one allergy gene, tend to develop them late. The majority of heterozygous persons are apparently normal throughout life but may transmit the factor to their children [5]. The greater the prevalence of allergic disease in the family or the greater its severity, the earlier the onset of allergic manifestations in the progeny. Early onset is associated, in turn, with severe, long-lasting disease. On the average, 40 to 70 percent of asthmatic children and adults, and 35 to 80 percent of hay fever patients, have family histories of allergic disease [6]. Vasomotor rhinitis, hay fever atopic dermatitis, and asthma are all genetically related [7].

The number of pairs of genes participating in the heredity of allergy is in dispute. Weiner and colleagues [5] state that it is only a single pair and that the allergic factor is an incomplete recessive gene. Because only a small percentage of persons heterozygous for the allergy gene ever develop allergic disease, it seems likely that the degree of antigenic exposure is often important. Although sensitization does not regularly follow exposure, many allergists recommend that children with a known tendency to atopy, or a strong family history of atopy, be kept from contact with recognized potential allergens so as to reduce the likelihood of sensitization.

The association of specific histocompatibility antigen with atopic disease is discussed in detail in Chapter 1.

Pathogenesis of Sensitization in Atopy

The specific allergen and the body's response to it are the important factors in the sensitization process.

ALLERGENS. Antigens that are innocuous to most of the population may cause disease when an atopic person is exposed to them by inhalation or ingestion. On the other hand, atopic persons are often insensitive to allergens to which they are heavily exposed even when these same allergens cause severe reactions in other atopic persons. Why atopic persons become sensitive to certain allergens on exposure and not to others remains a mystery.

Inhaled allergens comprise wind-borne plant pollens, mold spores, and insect parts, all of which can be spread in sufficient quantities to cause atopic disease (e.g., hay fever, asthma) in susceptible persons. Of these inhaled allergens, which affect the ocular nasal and lung tissues, plant pollens are the principal offenders. A small number of species are anemophilous, that is, depend on wind for pollination and produce large amounts of light, dry pollen, which is easily borne long distances by air currents. For a pollen to be considered the etiologic agent of a respiratory or ocular allergy, it must fulfill Thommen's postulates: (1) The pollen must be wind-borne; (2) the pollen must occur in large quantities; (3) the plant must be widespread; and (4) the pollen must contain hay fever excitant [8].

The few plant pollens that cause hay fever have definite seasonal characteristics related to their times of pollination. Ragweed, which is the commonest cause of hay fever in North America, contains a large number of antigens [9]. It has been estimated that a single plant produces a billion grains of pollen, which can be blown tremendous distances and have been found at altitudes of 14,000 feet and as far as 400 miles out at sea.

Grasses that pollinate in late spring or early summer are the second most common cause of hay fever in North America. A high degree of cross-reaction occurs between the different grass pollens. Like ragweed pollen, they are antigenically complex.

Tree pollens, molds, fungi, parts of insects, and animal dander are also allergenic. Human dander, which has also produced skin reactions in some atopic patients [10], is probably an autoallergen, and the atopic person may produce IgE antibodies to many other such autoallergens.

House dust, which often aggravates perennial rhinitis and asthma, is a mixture of animal and human dander; bacteria; molds; products of the degeneration of fibrous material; and remains of foods, plants, and insects. Certain mites, for example, particularly *Dermatophagoides*, are a major allergen in house dust [11].

Ingested allergens cause allergic manifestations almost immediately or from 2 to 12 hours after their ingestion. The commonest allergenic foods are milk, eggs, and cereals, with fish, shellfish, nuts, and spices next in order, and fruits and vegetables cited occasionally. Milk is a complex liquid containing at least 16 antigens [12] of which the most often implicated in atopic disease are α lactalbumin, β lactalbumin, casein, and bovine serum albumin. The active allergens in milk can pass unchanged through the gastrointestinal tract into breast milk, sensitizing breast-fed infants and causing allergic symptoms. They may also sensitize the infant by passing through the placenta into the fetus. In these ways an infant with an atopic background may develop an allergy to milk. To obviate this possibility, some pediatricians suggest that severely atopic mothers eliminate potent allergenic foods (milk, eggs, wheat) during pregnancy.

Metabisulfite (an oxidant) is added to most foods and can cause mast cell degranulation.

In atopic persons, ingested allergens may cause asthma, rhinitis, conjunctivitis (exceedingly rarely), atopic dermatitis (eczema), urticaria, and gastrointestinal symptoms.

HYPERSENSITIVITY RESPONSES. The type I hypersensitivity reaction (anaphylaxis) is characteristic of atopy. There is one report of allergic rhinitis owing to cell-mediated immune (CMI) hypersensitivity.

The type I hypersensitivity reaction is discussed in detail in Chapter 1. In atopy levels and activity of suppressor T cells are decreased, and T-helper to T-suppressor ratios of 4 : 1 can exist. B-cell activity is enhanced with the production of IgE. In addition the responsiveness of the β-adrenergic receptor is decreased, and autoantibodies may be present to this receptor [13, 14]. The level of these autoantibodies correlates with the responsiveness of the receptor [15]. Cyclic adenosine monophosphate

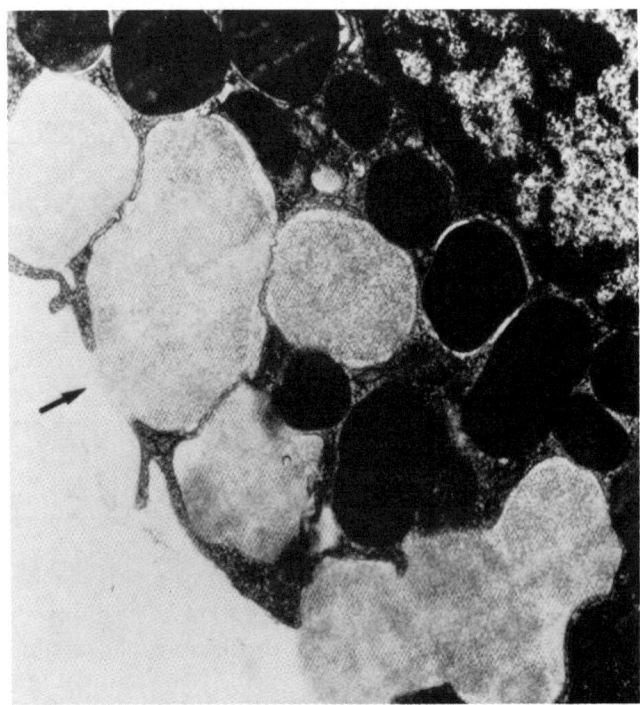

FIG. 3-1   Mast-cell degranulating and releasing substances that cause symptoms of allergy.

(cAMP) responses are depressed [16], and phosphodiesterase activity is elevated. All of these alterations lead to a tendency of the mast cells, both interstitial and mucosal, to degranulate and release the substances that cause the symptoms of allergy (Fig. 3-1).

In atopy, cell-mediated immunity, T-cell responsiveness to mitogens, and antibody-dependent monocyte-mediated cytotoxicity [17] may be depressed, natural killer (K) cell activity enhanced, and levels of interferon depressed. Patients with hyperimmunoglobulin E syndromes may have similar alterations in their immune status, and association of these syndromes with vernal conjunctivitis is interesting [18].

It is now generally accepted that immediate hypersensitivity states, such as hay fever, asthma, and food allergies, are associated with humoral skin-sensitizing antibodies (mainly IgE, very rarely IgG), which are produced spontaneously by the allergic person in response to either inhalation or ingestion of a given allergen.

IgE levels in relation to atopic disease in young children have been studied extensively [19, 20]. An accurate way to measure IgE levels is by the radioallergosorbent test. A level above 100 μm/ml at any age, or above 20 μm/ml in infancy, is strongly suggestive of atopic disease. The half-life of IgE in the serum is 2 to 3 days whereas it may be 3 weeks

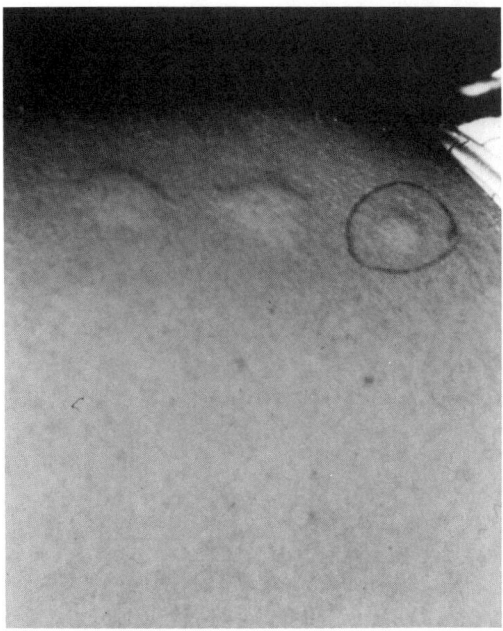

FIG. 3-2 Flare and wheal reaction to injected allergens.

when attached to a mast cell. But although assays are useful in the management of pediatric allergy (e.g., there is a definite association between serum IgE levels and atopic dermatitis) [21], they do not constitute a major diagnostic tool when other special tests are available.

Diagnosis Nasal smears are valuable and become more so with increasing age [22]. They are in fact a most helpful adjunct to family history, clinical picture, and the result of skin tests to common allergens, forming with them the major basis for diagnosis. The positivity of a number of skin tests increases with age (Fig. 3-2).

The diagnosis of atopic disease in very young children is much more difficult than in children more than 4 years old or in adults. Traditionally the disease progresses from infantile eczema through childhood asthma to hay fever. In one series [23], however, rhinorrhea, which is often associated with conjunctivitis, was the commonest early symptom.

TREATMENT OF ATOPY. The discussion in this section focuses on the general principles underlying the treatment of atopic disease. The special treatment of ocular conditions is discussed in detail later in the chapter. Coverage of the therapy of type 1 hypersensitivity reactions is provided in Chapter 1, and, that material will for the most part not be repeated here.

General Measures. A number of prophylactic measures can be taken to attempt to alleviate or prevent atopic disease; some or all of these measures should be used if a child has a family history of widespread atopy or of unusually severe atopy, or if a child has already shown signs of atopy. Breast-feeding infants may prevent sensitizing some of these children to cow's milk. Allergic mothers can avoid allergenic foods during pregnancy so that allergens do not reach and sensitize the fetus in utero. In an effort to prevent colds, the child should be protected against exposure to sick children and adults as well as changes in weather. Drugs should be taken only with the physician's knowledge because normally harmless medication may be injurious to the atopic child.

In general, the atopy-prone or atopic child should avoid (1) musty places, (2) swimming in chlorinated pools (the use of nose clips can reduce the danger), (3) perfumes and heavily scented toiletries, (4) spices and highly seasoned food, (5) frequent trips to zoos or barns, and (6) exposure to pets. It may sometimes be psychologically undesirable to avoid these places, activities, and substances, but the parent should be aware of the advantages and disadvantages of doing so.

Rarely, even exercise can induce an adverse allergic reaction [24].

AVOIDANCE OF EXPOSURE TO SPECIFIC ALLERGENS. The first step in treating allergy is instructing the patient to avoid exposure to offending agents. As a rule the patient is sensitive to many allergens, and the problem of avoiding them is difficult.

Techniques designed for carefully cleaning the house may be helpful to reduce exposure to house dust. When a brief exposure to excessive dust is anticipated (e.g., sweeping or working in an attic or basement), a face mask should be used. Insect powders and sprays and irritating fumes (from gasoline or leaky gas stoves) should be avoided. An exhaust fan in the kitchen may be helpful. Electrostatic precipitators clean the air of 99.5 percent of particulates during a single passage of air through the precipitating device [25]. The use of fungicidal agents in the house may also be at least partially protective in especially humid climates.

If the person is sensitive to a particular pollen, it may be possible to take a vacation in an area relatively free from the pollen during the usual time of pollen exposure at home. This measure will be feasible only if the troublesome period is relatively short (i.e., 3 weeks or so). If the period is much longer, it may be worthwhile to consider a change of job to a pollen-free (or relatively pollen-free) area if the breadwinner or member of the family is severely atopic. This drastic step may be effective and the only satisfactory solution to a serious problem.

Persons sensitive to certain foods must avoid them in whatever form they appear. For example, the list of ingredients on packaged foods should be read carefully to ensure that the food does not include an allergen that must be avoided. The commonest allergens are wheat, milk, and eggs. Diets that avoid these offenders can be tested on allergic infants before resorting to an allergy survey. Goat's milk can be given instead of cow's milk, and commercial products containing soy flour (provided adequate vitamin supplements are also given) can be substituted for milk.

PSYCHOTHERAPY. Although emotional difficulty alone does not produce allergic symptoms, emotions can apparently influence the clinical course and prognosis of these symptoms, possibly by affecting suppressor T-cell activity. For this reason it is important to investigate the allergic patient's mental health. If the patient is troubled, simple, brief, and informal psychotherapy is usually all that is needed. If the patient is to recount his psychiatric history, he must have confidence in his physician and be given ample time and opportunity to confide; successful psychotherapy of children may require the child's cooperation and that of the family and teachers. In severe and complicated cases, the services of a psychiatrist may be needed.

The relationship between allergic disease and the patient's mental health is complex to say the least. Although emotional problems may precipitate atopic symptoms, it is also true that the disease itself may affect the patient's self-image and relation to environment.

Specific Drug Therapy. The relationship of cAMP to the release of the vasoactive amines that cause the allergic symptoms is discussed in Chapter 1. Many of the agents used to increase the cellular levels of cAMP (e.g., β_2-receptor stimulators, prostaglandin-receptor stimulators, inhibitors of phosphodiesterase) will alleviate allergic symptoms. Other agents (e.g., antihistamines) actually competitively inhibit one of the vasoactive amines. Some of the β_2-receptor stimulators (e.g., epinephrine) can cause vasoconstriction of the conjunctival vessels and bronchodilation, both of which reduce the symptoms of atopy. Aerosol administration provides the greatest selectivity and effectiveness for β_2-agonists in asthma [26]. Metaproterenol is effective by this route. β_2-agonists (i.e., terbutaline, albuterol, fenoterol) have not been used topically or orally for ocular atopic diseases.

The phosphodiesterase inhibitors that have been used to increase the levels of cellular cAMP are papaverine, theophylline, aminophylline, caffeine, possibly cromolyn sodium (disodium cromoglycate; DSCG), and a group of new agents [27, 28]. The antiallergenic effect of DSCG is also related to the calcium influx. By inhibiting the calcium "gate" the mast cell is stabilized. Eosinophil migration, the effect of 48/80, and the neurogenic reflex may all be blocked by DSCG. The toxicity of DSCG is low, and no neoplastic or teratogenic effects have been noted. Reported adverse effects, which are rare and associated with systemic administration, include anaphylaxis, generalized acute dermatitis, acute myositis, gastroenteritis, and acute chemosis. Topically, stinging pain has been noted as well as an extremely rare allergic reaction.

DSCG is effective in seasonal rhinitis and less so in perennial rhinitis. A 4 percent solution of Nasalchrom is available for these conditions. DSCG is also effective in extrinsic (allergic) asthma and less effective in intrinsic (nonallergic) asthma. The recommended dose of DSCG for treating asthma is the inhalation of the micronized powder contained in one 20-mg capsule four times daily [29]. DSCG is of no benefit in vasomotor or nonallergic rhinitis.

Antihistamines are the steric analogs of histamine. It is believed that they act by competing with histamine for the cellular receptors (H_1), thereby blocking the action of histamine. That also reduces capillary permeability. Antihistamines do not neutralize histamine in either the tissues or the bloodstream. Their anticholinergic activity is relatively weak, but patients using them have complained of dry mouth, difficulty voiding, and impotence [30]. Dry eyes have been noted with systemic use of antihistamine-decongestant combinations [31]. Antihistamines are not effective in bronchial asthma, perhaps because they inhibit the action of the catecholamines and because mediators other than histamine are liberated.

There are five major groups of antihistamines: (1) ethylenediamines (tripelennamine [Pyribenzamine] and methapyrilene [Histadyl]) are potent and moderately sedative; (2) ethanolamines (diphenhydramine [Benadryl], carbinoxamine maleate [Clistin], and doxylamine succinate [Decapryn]) are highly potent and sedative; (3) alkylamines (chlorpheniramine maleate [Chlor-Trimeton], dexchlorpheniramine maleate [Polaramine], brompheniramine maleate [Dimetane], and triprolindine [Actidil]) are mildly potent and sedative; (4) phenothiazines (promethazine [Phenergan], chlorpromazine [Thorazine], and trimeprazine tartrate [Temaril]) are highly sedative; and (5) cyclizines (meclizine [Bonine], cyclizine [Marezine], and hydroxyzine [Atarax]) are used for motion sickness, and hydroxyzine is effective against pruritus [32].

The sedative effect of the antihistamines may be harmful (e.g., if taken before or while driving an automobile) [33] or beneficial (e.g., if sleeplessness is a consequence of the discomforts of allergic symptoms). Only when an antihistamine has little penetration to the central nervous system, as does terfenadine, may some real improvement in decreasing the sedative effect be anticipated. Patients vary considerably in their susceptibility to the several effects of antihistamines, and it is often useful to try several drugs sequentially in a range of doses to discover the drug and dose that are optimally effective.

Topically applied antihistamines penetrate the surface tissues well [34].

Cimetidine is less effective than antihistamines in moderating the pruritus associated with atopic skin diseases. In addition, cimetidine has more side effects (some serious) than antihistamines [35]. A combination of antihistamine and cimetidine may be effective for topical use in ocular allergy because H_1 and H_2 receptors are present in the conjunctiva.

Atropine and similar drugs lower the levels of guanosine monophosphate (GMP), thereby inhibiting the release of the vasoactive amines. They also dry up the mucous membranes and are usually used in low doses in combination with antihistamines and decongestants.

Nonsteroidal anti-inflammatory drugs (NSAID) have been used to treat allergies. In general, aspirin has been found to be ineffective in treating atopic diseases [36]. In vitro testing of eosinophil migration revealed little effect with aspirin or indomethacin but a major inhibitory effect with BW 755C, a lipoxygenase inhibitor [37].

Corticosteroids have also been used to treat allergies. Corticosteroids increase the production of cAMP by PGE and PGF, potentiate the catecholamines, reduce the histamine content of guinea pig tissue, cause vasoconstriction, reduce vascular permeability, reduce neutrophil (basophil) chemotaxis, and stabilize lysosomes. All these effects are important in counteracting or preventing the allergic symptoms caused by release of the vasoactive amines. Corticosteroids are discussed in detail in Chapter 1.

Corticosteroids in adequate doses are highly efficient in their effect on allergic diseases. For example, relief of allergic rhinitis is almost complete in 12 to 36 hours. The glucocorticoids with the least mineralocorticoid activity, of which prednisone is typical, are the most useful in treatment, and for topical application, the highly soluble dexamethasone is much used. The acetate form gives the greatest bioavailability [38].

For a variety of reasons, however, the dangers implicit in the indiscriminate use of these drugs and the importance of using them conservatively should be impressed on the patient. Only minimal doses should be used for the shortest possible periods. Alternate-day therapy and tapering the dose should be accomplished as soon as possible. DSCG has been used in patients with severe bronchial asthma in attempts to reduce or discontinue the use of corticosteroids. Corticosteroids should never be used when there are well-established contraindications, nor should they be used routinely in the care of allergic patients for whom they are no substitute for a thorough evaluation and workup. In any case, the less dangerous therapeutic procedures previously noted should first be given exhaustive trials.

In the following special circumstances, corticosteroids may be indicated for the treatment of allergy: (1) as a temporary measure in acute, severe, transient disorders, such as poison oak dermatitis; (2) to control otherwise uncontrollable, disabling disease, such as intractable bronchial asthma, atopic dermatitis, or exfoliative dermatitis; (3) as a lifesaving procedure in status asthmaticus and in allergic emergencies (drug and insect allergic reactions); (4) as a crutch while intensive medical and allergic studies are being conducted; and (5) if other forms of therapy are inadequate. This short-term treatment may tide a patient over a difficult period and give him much-needed confidence in his physician.

Wound healing is retarded by the corticosteroids. Steroids with androgenic properties (i.e., nandrolone) and NSAID do not retard skin repair and regeneration [39].

T-lymphocyte deficiency, and more specifically suppressor-cell deficiency, may have a cause-and-effect relationship to atopic diseases. As a result, trials with transfer factor have been made in the treatment of severely atopic patients [40, 41]. In one trial, one unit of transfer factor, corresponding to 400 ml of blood, was administered subcutaneously weekly for 10 weeks. After 3 weeks of treatment, clinical improvement was striking and there was an increase in the number of both the demonstrable rosette-forming lymphocytes in the blood and circulating T and B cells. Serum levels of IgE also fell markedly. Although only a few patients have been treated with transfer factor thus far, further experiments designed to stimulate T cells may prove fruitful.

Thymopoietin pentapeptide can increase suppressor T-lymphocytes in atopic patients but has no demonstrable effect on the serum IgE levels or on the course of the disease [42].

Levamisole, an immune-enhancing agent, has caused dramatic improvement in some patients with atopic dermatitis.

Interferon can induce suppression of in vitro IgE biosynthesis in asthmatic children and is being tested as treatment for atopic diseases [43].

Immunotherapy has been widely used to treat patients with allergic disease. It is effective when the patient is exposed to a low dose of the offending allergen. For example, immunotherapy for ragweed allergy is highly successful in Missouri, much less so in New York. Unfortunately, patients with allergies to pets (domestic cats and dogs) rarely respond to immunotherapy. A series of inoculations is required. Minute doses of extracts of the specific allergens the inhalation of which is causing the trouble are given weekly or biweekly and are followed by gradually increasing doses as tolerated by the patient. The dosage end point is usually determined either by the appearance of local or systemic allergic reactions to the injections or by the patient's satisfaction with the relief of symptoms. The efficacy of this form of treatment has been confirmed by many observers [44–46].

The development of nonreaginic (IgG) antibodies as a result of immunotherapy was first noted by Cooke and associates [47]. These blocking antibodies can neutralize an allergen, preventing it from reacting with reagins (IgE antibodies) in a Prausnitz-Küstner reaction [48]. The test for blocking antibodies is based solely on their ability to neutralize allergens.

Allergic symptoms develop in persons exposed to a particular allergen because they possess IgE antibodies directed against that allergen. Allergic persons also have small amounts of blocking (IgG) antibodies against the same allergens [49]. Immunization by the transmucosal route (which includes the conjunctiva) seems to lead to a relative preponderance of IgE antibodies [50]. Parenteral immunization, on the other hand, produces a striking increase in IgG antibodies [51, 52]. It may well be advantageous (by immunotherapy) to change the relative IgE-IgG antiallergen–antibody ratio in favor of the latter. Because the IgG can bind the allergen, yet not induce an allergic biologic response, it should be protective. However, although an increase in blocking antibody is often associated with a major reduction in clinical symptoms [53–55], causality is not proved. Some studies show no correlation between the patient's symptoms and the titers of either the blocking or the IgE antibodies (or both) [56, 57].

In addition to changing the titers of circulating IgG antibodies, immunotherapy may reduce the basic reactivity of the target cells to the allergen [58, 59]. Although there continues to be an unchanging level of

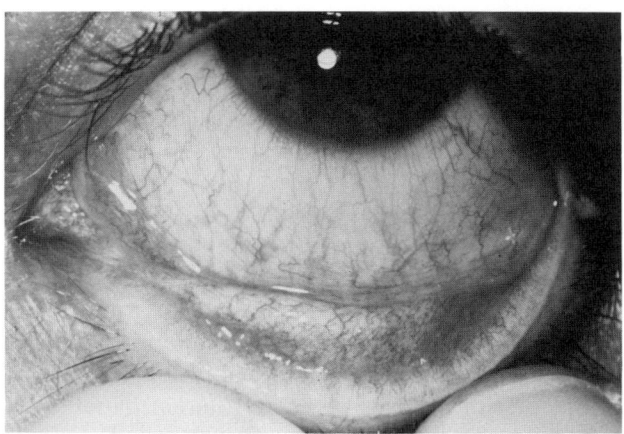

FIG. 3-3 Pale conjunctiva and watery discharge in a patient with mild hay fever conjunctivitis.

IgE that can sensitize cells, cell reactivity seems to diminish specifically. This reduced cell reactivity and the level of blocking IgG antibodies may be related to each other in a manner not yet apparent.

SPECIAL OCULAR CONSIDERATIONS

Allergic ocular disease comprises a group of conditions caused by exposure to allergenic materials and mediated by specific immunologic mechanisms that bring about the type I hypersensitivity response and possibly the type IV hypersensitivity responses such as the cutaneous basophilic type. The characteristic symptoms vary according to the tissue affected. In the acute phase the usual symptoms are tearing, itching, and burning, and the usual signs are swelling of the eyelids, chemosis and hyperemia of the conjunctiva, and a teary discharge (Fig. 3-3). In the chronic stages there may also be papillary hypertrophy, pallor of the conjunctiva (owing to chemosis), and a mucoid or stringy discharge.

Allergen Exposure

An extensive discussion of inhaled and ingested allergens is presented in general considerations of atopy. Particulate allergens (pollens, dander), which can be readily introduced onto the ocular tissues and temporarily trapped in the inferior cul-de-sac, can set up an allergic response. Insect bites or stings can introduce allergens directly into the ocular tissue. Because we do not know the permeability of the conjunctival mucosa to small molecules the size of allergens (10–100 μm), their mode and rate of penetration are not known. But because the cells that participate in the allergic reaction (mast cells, basophils, eosinophils, and lymphocytes) are located in the submucosa, the allergenic proteins probably do penetrate the mucosal barrier.

It has been shown that antibody within the rabbit's oral and intestinal mucosa retards the penetration of intact antigen, but that immune reactions may enhance the penetration of unrelated macromolecules [60].

The presence of IgE in the tears and of elevated levels of IgE in patients with assumed allergic disorders [61] substantiates the concept that the immune reaction between allergen and IgE is occurring locally in the conjunctival mucous membranes. Recently histamine and major basic protein have also been found in the tears of patients with vernal keratoconjunctivitis [62].

Topical agents can produce acute allergic reactions, and although they have infrequently been recorded, there are a number of unreported cases. In some patients, an acute onset of edema of the eyelids and chemosis of the conjunctiva followed the topical administration of proparacaine hydrochloride. Chronic allergic reactions to medications are commonplace and are a special problem when frequent topical administration of drugs is necessary (i.e., in patients with keratoconjunctivitis sicca or contact lenses).

Contact lenses can trap allergens and present them to the conjunctival tissue, thus setting the stage for a chronic allergic response.

Sensitization

So far as is known, the ocular physiologic findings of allergic persons do not differ intrinsically from those of the general population. Nevertheless, when allergic patients are exposed to an appropriate allergen, they respond by developing the symptoms of allergic ocular disease.

Mast cells are found in abundance in the ocular tissues. Allansmith [63] reported on the distribution of mast cells in the rat. The lid contained 495,000 mast cells and the conjunctiva 108,000 [63]. In the normal human conjunctiva no mast cells were noted in the epithelium but between 5000 and 12,000 cells/mm^3 were present in the substantia propria. The interstitial mast cell seems to be the one present [64]. This type is of uncertain origin and differs in appearance and possibly function from the mucosal (T-cell derived) type of mast cell.

The location of mast cells close to small vessels and the presence of basophils, eosinophils, and neutrophils within these vessels (and occasionally in the extravascular spaces) pave the way for the appearance of allergic phenomena when allergen and antibody (principally IgE) interact.

Recently interleukin-3, a substance that can activate mast cells, was discovered in the corneal and conjunctival epithelium [65]. The exact role of this factor in ocular allergy has not been elucidated. In addition, the roles of the conjunctiva-associated lymphoid system and Langerhans' cells in ocular allergy have not been studied.

H_1 and H_2 receptors are present in the conjunctiva and may play an important role in the manifestations of ocular allergy [66, 67].

Graham and co-workers [68] found that basophils contained only half of the histamine in the blood vessels, and that eosinophils and neutrophils contained the rest. The process of sensitization is also influenced by the temperature of the allergen-IgE environment: The rate of passive sensitization increases twelvefold as the temperature rises from 4° to 37°C [69]. The concentration of nonantibody IgE also affects sensitization: By *competition*, high concentrations of purified nonantibody IgE can block the Prausnitz-Küstner reaction [70].

The mediators of allergic reactions are discussed in Chapter 1. Although in most instances no convincing evidence exists that all these mediators play a major role in human allergic reactions, a strong case can certainly be made for histamine. The hyperemia and edema that characterize allergic conjunctivitis can be produced by exogenous histamine, and antihistaminic drugs can alleviate the symptoms of allergic conjunctivitis. In addition, a correlation seems to exist between histamine release in vitro and the extent of clinical illness caused by ragweed hay fever [71]. Tear histamine levels are elevated in patients with vernal keratoconjunctivitis (VKC) [63].

Certain factors worsen the allergic reactions in a nonspecific manner. Noxious stimuli, infections, and emotions may aggravate allergic ocular disease, and both Wolfe and associates [72] and Holmes and associates [73] have performed experiments that demonstrate the aggravating effect of emotions on preexisting allergic disease.

Enhancement can also occur when one allergic stimulus is added to another. A hay fever patient with normal ocular tissue may respond to out-of-season pollen exposure with a modest but definite amount of chemosis and hyperemia. During hay fever season, when the ocular tissues are already chemotic and hyperemic, the same patient may respond to additional exposure to pollen with a more violent reaction than previously experienced.

A priming effect, nonspecific and local, was demonstrated by Corvell [74]. When, on successive days, he exposed ragweed-sensitive patients to inhalations of pollen in sufficient amounts to evoke symptoms, he found that the reaction was elicited with less pollen each day. Under these circumstances, the threshold may be lowered fiftyfold.

Repeated exposure to one pollen can induce overreactivity to another, immunologically unrelated pollen. Priming may result from increased permeability of the mucous membrane, which allows the allergen to reach target cells more readily. In this way a one-time exposure to an allergen may cause an acute ocular response followed by rapid improvement, but repeated exposures may cause an intense, immediate response that lasts longer. In allergic rhinitis, if only one nostril is exposed, the unexposed nostril does not become primed. An analogous situation may exist in the ocular tissues, accounting for unilateral or asymmetric allergic ocular responses.

Specific Ocular Diseases

The specific ocular diseases in which atopy plays a role include hay fever, vernal keratonconjunctivitis (VKC), atopic keratoconjunctivitis (AKC), giant papillary conjunctivitis, and insect stings and bites.

HAY FEVER. Hay fever is probably the most common atopic condition involving ocular tissue.

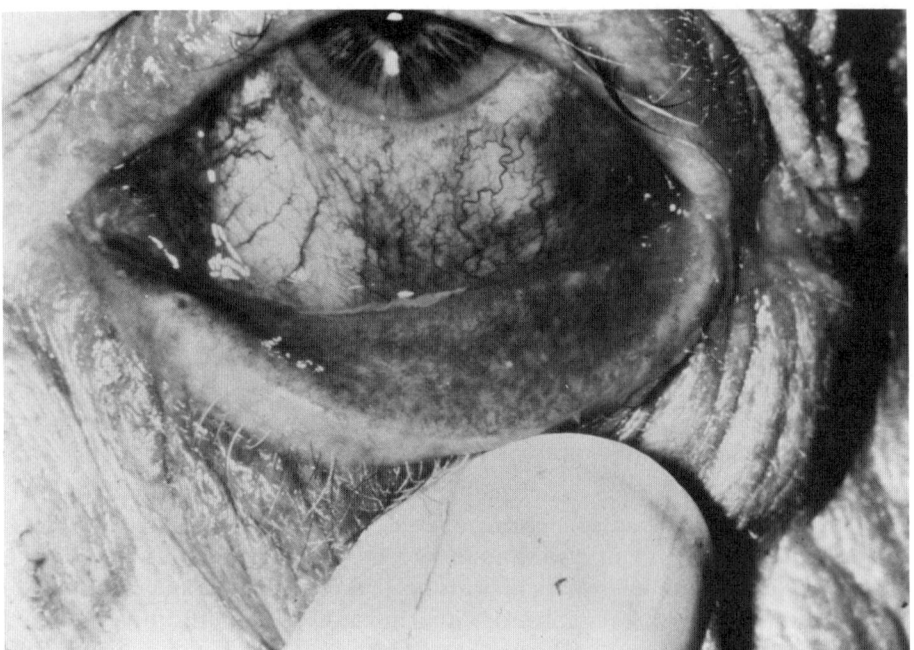

FIG. 3-4 Conjunctival hyperemia and white stringy exudate in inferior cul-de-sac in patient with severe and chronic hay fever conjunctivitis.

History and Cause. One of the first descriptions of hay fever was approximately 1683 as an ocular reaction to roses. Since then many substances have been found to act as allergens and to trigger this type of reaction (i.e., a localized form of anaphylaxis or type I hypersensitivity). Airborn allergens (i.e., pollens, dust, molds, dander) are mainly associated with hay fever reactions.

Clinical Features

SYMPTOMS. Hay fever may be seasonal or perennial. When the conjunctiva alone is affected, the symptoms are itching (often severe), tearing, and burning. If the cornea is affected, there may also be blurred vision and slight photophobia; if there are delle, there may be pain, photophobia, and blurred vision.

SIGNS. Rarely this entity may present with no discernible signs. The commonest ocular manifestations are rapid vascular congestion and conjunctival chemosis. The conjunctiva looks milky or pale pink. The exudative material is clear or whitish if the ocular reaction is acute, and whitish, thick, and even stringy if the reaction is chronic. A mild papillary hypertrophy may occur (Fig. 3-4).

Clinically visible edema of the conjunctiva and eyelids, often severe, usually occurs within hours after exposure to the allergen. If the allergic insult is to one eye only (e.g., if a particular allergen enters the cul-de-sac of only one eye), the changes may be unilateral. The conjunctival

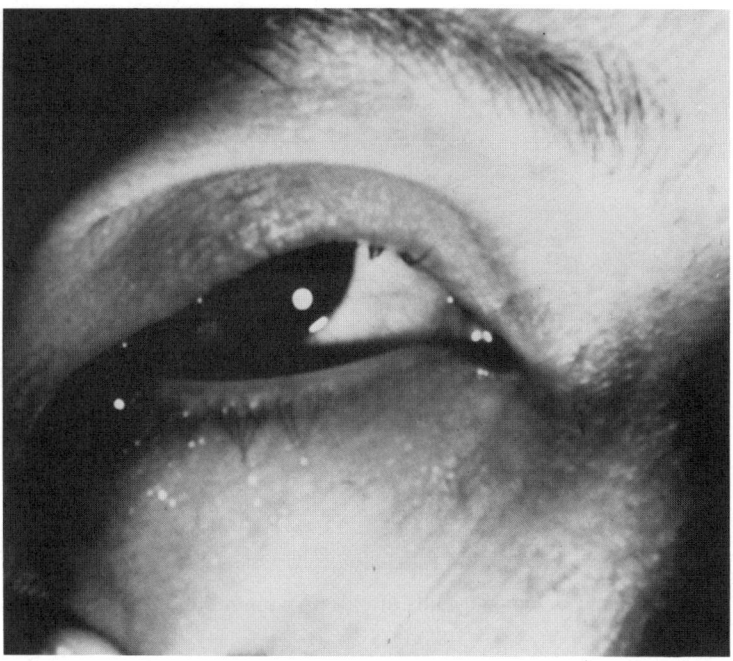

FIG. 3-5   Acute swelling of eyelid of child: allergic urticarial response to animal dander.

chemosis may be very intense and may produce a breakup of tear film. In eyes with severe conjunctival chemosis, we have seen corneal delle that disappeared when the chemosis subsided (after treatment with epinephrine). The conjunctival changes are usually accompanied by chemosis of the eyelids.

Urticaria (localized patches of edema in the epidermis) differs from angioedema, which affects principally the dermis. Both conditions can occur in the eyelids, and both may be either immunologic in origin (type I and other hypersensitivity reactions) or nonimmunologic (Figs. 3-5, 3-6). Physical urticarias may have an allergic component. The histopathologic changes of urticaria and angioedema are the same except for the difference in their tissue predilections (i.e., urticaria occurs in the epidermis, angioedema occurs in the dermis). These changes are edema, dilatation of venules and capillaries, and infiltration by lymphocytes and neutrophils. Eosinophilic infiltrations appear in the type I IgE–mediated reaction.

Urticaria is typically a circumscribed plaque of edema with an erythematous margin and a blanched center. Angioedema has localized dermal edema and an essentially normal epidermis.

A limitless number of drugs can produce allergic skin reaction [75], and it is fallacious to assign a particular type of skin reaction to a particular drug. It is more accurate, in fact, to say that any antigenic agent can occasionally cause urticaria. Some agents that commonly do so are pen-

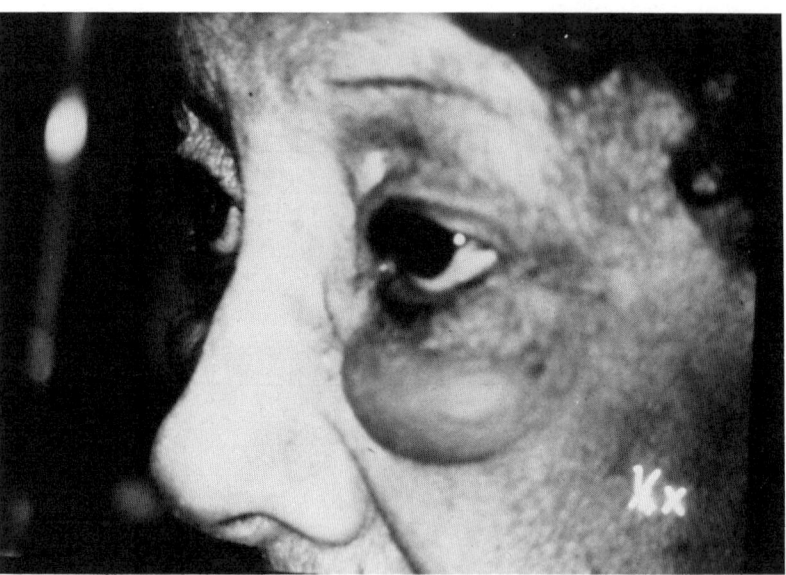

FIG. 3-6   Edema of eyelids of elderly woman: allergic response to pollen.

icillin, sulfonamides, salicylates, radiopaque dyes, vaccines [76–78], and topically applied proparacaine hydrochloride [79].

A variety of foods, infections, bites and stings, inhalants, and systemic diseases can cause allergic reactions.

Foods: seafoods, nuts, eggs, berries, milk products, and some additives
Infections: hepatitis [80], *Candida albicans* [81], infectious mononucleosis [82], coxsackie virus [83], and severe chronic bacterial infections
Inhalants: pollens, dander, and epidermal hairs
Systemic diseases: malignancies, collagen-vascular diseases [84], endocrine disorders [85], dermatitis herpetiformis, dysproteinemias, and pemphigoid (in these systemic diseases the pathogenic mechanisms are not always understood)

Urticaria can also be caused, triggered, or worsened by mechanical, thermal, solar, cholinergic, and psychological factors [86].

Corneal edema occurs rarely and is a transient condition that may accompany the attacks of urticaria or angioedema [87]. It may also follow the introduction of an allergen (e.g., bee sting) into the cornea and is then a complex reaction that is discussed in more detail later in the section Atopic Reactions to Insect Bites and Stings. A transient epithelial keratitis may also develop.

Neuroretinal edema is also a rare condition and may appear in association with generalized urticaria and angioneurotic edema [88].

Anterior uveitis is a condition that is related to allergy (a transient, exudative iridocyclitis) [89, 90]; hay fever [91] and animal dander [92] are implicated as its causes.

Diagnosis. The diagnosis of hay fever allergic ocular disease can be made on the basis of history, clinical appearance, special tests, and response to the appropriate treatment. There is usually a family history of atopic disease and sometimes a personal history of previous or current allergic responses (i.e., of allergic rhinitis or bronchial asthma). Although the signs and symptoms may be nonspecific, the clinically typical picture is a pale, boggy conjunctiva, a mild papillary response, lid edema, and a watery or white discharge. The classic symptom is itching (Fig. 3-5, 3-6).

The standard clinical test for the diagnosis of type I hypersensitivity reactions is the intradermal skin test. A small amount of the suspected allergen (usually diluted) is applied to a cutaneous scratch or injected intradermally. The rapid appearance, within seconds or minutes, of a wheal and flare indicates a positive reaction. Topical instillations of allergenic substances into the conjunctival sac have also been used diagnostically. A positive response is the nearly immediate onset of swelling of the eyelids, chemosis, hyperemia of the conjunctiva, and itching. Such tests are not innocuous and may indeed be fatal [93].

In an experimental study, Silverstein [88], injected allergen into the vitreous of sensitized animals and produced hyperemia of the iris, serous exudation, and aqueous flare.

The Prausnitz-Küstner test, which can be used to show the allergic nature of ocular disease, is described in the section Definition of Atopy.

In any chronic conjunctivitis that causes itching, one should look for eosinophils and the rare basophil. Because there should be no eosinophils in the nonallergic conjunctiva, the presence of one is important (unless bleeding occurs). Biopsy of ocular tissue is usually not warranted as a diagnostic procedure.

Because it requires time for the eosinophils to enter the tear film, they are usually not present in the acute allergic states [94]. When the allergic condition becomes chronic, eosinophils are more plentiful.

A rapid response to appropriate therapy may be useful in making a correct diagnosis. Epinephrine locally, corticosteroids locally, or systemic or local antihistamines often rapidly ameliorate the signs and symptoms of ocular allergic disease.

Levels of serum IgE, tear IgE, and tear histamine can all be determined. Most atopic persons have notably higher IgE levels than nonatopic persons. The levels are usually moderately elevated in patients with allergic rhinitis, bronchial asthma, and hay fever, and are markedly elevated in atopic dermatitis and chronic ocular allergic conditions. Not all atopic persons have elevated serum IgE levels, and elevated levels also occur in patients with a variety of diseases such as intestinal nematode infestations, cutaneous larva migrans, visceral larva migrans, celiac disease, cirrhosis, multiple myeloma, pulmonary hemosiderosis, cystic fibrosis, thymic hypoplasia, and pulmonary aspergillosis.

Brauninger and Centifanto [61] reported that in two of four hay fever patients studied, the tear IgE levels were increased. McClellan and associates [95, 96] reported that in three patients with hay fever conjunctivitis and three patients with perennial allergic rhinitis, tear IgG or IgA levels were normal. Unfortunately, tear IgE levels were not reported. Tear histamine levels, on the other hand, are known to be elevated in most allergic conditions [62, 97], but are normal in hay fever conjunctivitis [63].

Persons with hay fever conjunctivitis may have normal eosinophil counts and then show a definite increase in the pollen season. Eosinophil counts of more than 500 cells/ml seem to be associated with elevated IgE levels, but eosinophilia is also seen in nonatopic diseases such as parasitic infestations, serum sickness, multiple myeloma, polyarteritis nodosa, glomerulonephritis, and rheumatic fever [98].

The amount of histamine released from sensitized basophils may be determined spectrophotometrically by observing degranulation and by its biologic effect on guinea pig ileum. This test may be used as an assay of specific allergens and as an index of the number of molecules of IgE bound to basophils or mast cells.

The radioallergosorbent test [99] may be used for the assay of allergens and to determine the amount of IgE antibody present that is specific for that allergen. The technique in brief is as follows: The allergens are coupled to insoluble particles on a paper-disk carrier. The IgE in the sera of allergic patients then attaches itself to the allergens. I-labeled anti-IgE interacts with the IgE molecules, and the amount of bound IgE-^{125}I may be determined with a gamma counter.

Of the many ocular inflammations with which hay fever reactions may be confused, the following are important:

1. *Epidemic keratoconjunctivitis* (EKC) can arise suddenly with lid and conjunctival edema, hyperemia, and a watery discharge. If a pseudomembrane forms early, and necrosis and a polymorphonuclear leukocyte infiltrate results, then the discharge may be mucoid and yellowish-white. EKC can be differentiated from hay fever–type reactions by the absence of itching, a mononuclear response in the conjunctiva (unless a pseudomembrane or membrane forms), a follicular conjunctival reaction (Fig. 3-7), and a more prolonged course sometimes complicated by characteristic corneal infiltrates.
2. *Acute inflammation caused by toxic or irritating substances.* Miotics, insecticides, chemical ammonia, and other similar substances can cause an acute ocular response. Conjunctival and lid edema and hyperemia, a watery discharge, and an occasional burning sensation and photophobia may be present. There is no itching, however. The conjunctival response is follicular. The serum and tear IgE levels and the serum eosinophil level are normal because the pathogenesis of the condition is unrelated to the type I hypersensitivity response.
3. *Contact dermatitis* of the lids may show some lid edema, hyperemia, and itching. Because it is one of the CMI types of responses, however, no alterations in the IgE or eosinophil levels are to be expected.
4. *VKC* is characterized by a papillary conjunctival reaction, some conjunctival chemosis and hyperemia, and a pale conjunctiva, and a thick, ropy exudate. The eyes may be photophobic and may itch and burn.

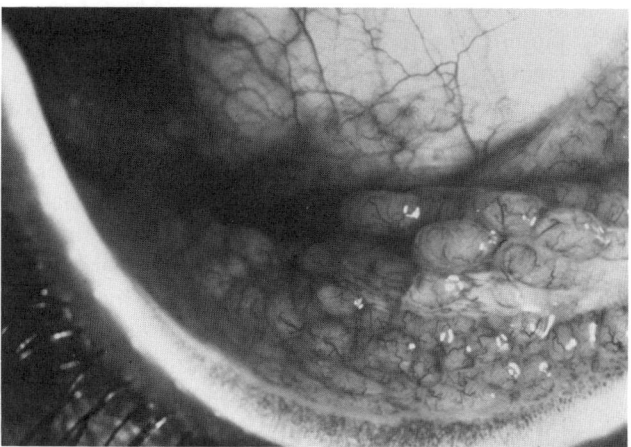

FIG. 3-7   Follicles in inferior palpebral conjunctivitis indicate viral or chlamydial disease or toxic reaction; papillae indicate allergic reaction.

Because the disease is partially the result of type I hypersensitivity, the IgE and eosinophil levels locally and systemically are usually elevated. Conjunctival eosinophils abound. There are seasonal exacerbations, and the disease runs a chronic course. The papillary conjunctivitis usually progresses to giant papillae or "cobblestones," which are located principally in the palpebral conjunctiva of the upper tarsal area. The cornea may develop a whitish syncytium or may ulcerate. Cysts or gelatinous masses may be present at the limbus, and the exudate often becomes thick, white, and stringy.

AKC and VKC are not chronic forms of the hay fever type of ocular responses (see Fig. 3-7). The pathogenetic mechanisms are not the same. Mononuclear-cell infiltration of the ocular tissues, which is never seen in hay fever conjunctivitis, is characteristic of both AKC and VKC, and the presence of these lymphocytes and macrophages suggests that both diseases have a more complex pathogenesis than hay fever.

The hay fever type of reaction is due to type I hypersensitivity. The allergen, the mast cell or basophil, and IgE all play a role in the release of the pharmacologic mediators (e.g., histamine, platelet-activating factor, eosinophil-chemotactic factor), and this release brings about the clinical and histopathologic changes of allergy. But the AKC and VKC types of reactions vary in that the type I hypersensitivity response certainly occurs but other pathogenetic mechanisms are also in operation. There are T-cell alterations, changes due to cell-mediated immunity, and large numbers of lymphocytes and macrophages at the affected sites. It is believed that the CMI response (type IV hypersensitivity) plays a particularly important role, and that both the cutaneous basophilic responses and the tuberculin type of CMI response may participate.

5. *Hypothyroidism* may be accompanied by lid edema, especially when the patient rises from sleep: but aside from a loss of brow hairs and some changes in the skin of the lids, there are no other ocular signs or symptoms that should confuse this condition with the hay fever type of disease.
6. In *hereditary angioedema* (HAE), the C1 esterase inhibitor is lacking. The disease is characterized by recurrent, circumscribed, subepithelial edema of the skin, mucosa, gastrointestinal and upper respiratory tracts, and eyelids. A faint macular or serpiginous erythema occasionally precedes the cutaneous lesion, which may develop at one site or another over a period of several hours. It does not pit, and it is not pruritic. In some patients, local trauma has clearly precipitated an attack. This process differs histologically from urticaria in that it affects the submucosa and deeper skin layers. The subcutaneous administration of epinephrine seems to reduce localized HAE as it would reduce the hay fever type of reaction, but the hay fever symptoms of itching, burning, photophobia, conjunctival eosinophilia, and alteration in IgE or serum-eosinophil levels are not present.

    The diagnosis of HAE must be considered in any patient with a history of recurring attacks of diffuse, circumscribed, nonpruritic edema. Association of edema with trauma, abdominal pain, hoarseness, and a choking sensation may be present. Treatment may include intubation or tracheostomy in severe cases along with the infusion of fresh plasma. Antibiotics, ε-aminocaproic acid, and epinephrine may be of great therapeutic value.

    The long-term treatment of HAE is prophylactic. Androgens (danazol) have been reported to be of great value.
7. A *foreign body* under the upper lid may cause acute chemosis and hyperemia of the bulbar conjunctiva, lid edema, a watery discharge, keratitis, and a burning sensation, and photophobia. Itching is absent, however. The eye hurts, there is a foreign-body sensation, there may be linear vertical scratches in the cornea, and a foreign body may be seen in the upper palpebral conjunctiva. No alteration occurs in the IgE or eosinophil levels unless the foreign body is allergenic as well as traumatizing. A chalazion can act as a foreign body.

TREATMENT. When feasible, an effort should be made to remove the patient from the offending allergen, and if this is a logistic impossibility, it may be possible to limit his or her exposure to it. Wearing a mask to prevent the inhalation of animal dander and wearing goggles to prevent ocular exposure to various allergens may be effective if the exposure time is short. For example, several of our technicians can work with rabbits or guinea pigs only when they wear goggles, masks, and gowns to protect them from the dander. Their symptoms are tolerable when exposure to the allergen is limited by these means.

Lid edema and hyperemia and symptoms of itching and burning can all be lessened by vasoconstriction induced by the use of cold compresses. These can be applied for 20 to 30 minutes several times a day.

Epinephrine, either topically or subcutaneously, gives dramatic symptomatic relief. The acute conjunctival chemosis and hyperemia respond rapidly to topical applications, and the eyelid edema often improves after repeated subcutaneous 0.2- or 0.3-ml doses of epinephrine 1 : 1,000 [100].

If a corneal delle complicates the conjunctival chemosis, the use of epinephrine topically (1 or 2 drops of the 1 : 1,000 aqueous solution) may reduce the chemosis enough to clear the delle. A bland ointment and patching can also diminish the size of the delle or eliminate them.

Sunglasses can relieve photophobia secondary to keratitis or uveitis.

Vasoconstricting agents such as naphazoline 0.05% or 0.10% may reduce the loss of both fluid and immune cells (eosinophils and basophils) from the blood vessels in mild cases of allergic conjunctivitis. No rebound vasodilation has been noted after discontinuance of usage [101].

The use of systemic antihistamines is discussed earlier in this chapter in the section Specific Drug Therapy. Topical antihistamine solutions are effective in mild ocular disease of the hay fever type. Anesthesia of the external ocular tissues has not been a problem. Because histamine is the only pharmacologic mediator released from mast cells or basophils that has been shown definitely to play a notable role in human allergic type I hypersensitivity reactions, antihistamines, either local or systemic, would be expected to be beneficial. Occasionally, however, topical antihistamines can be irritating and even allergenic [102].

Antazoline phosphate 0.5% has been shown to be effective topically as an antihistamine. Combined therapy using an antihistamine and vasoconstrictor topically is frequently more effective than using either drug alone [103]. Many such products are currently available and are essentially equally effective [104]. The preparation with a lower concentration of naphazoline (Naphcon-A) seems most comfortable.

Recently DSCG has been used in a 2%, 3%, or 4% solution topically for certain allergic ocular disease. In acute ocular allergies, the results have been conflicting, but a 4% solution has so far been consistently helpful in VKC and mild chronic hay fever conjunctivitis [105]. The drops are applied topically four times a day. DSCG has resulted in a diminution of symptoms and fewer eosinophils in the conjunctival scrapings of the VKC patients [106]. Several patients who had been on long-term topical corticosteroid therapy were able to reduce the dose or discontinue the drug when they started using DSCG.

The therapeutic benefit derived from the use of topical DSCG in two patients with ligneous conjunctivitis [107] suggests that this bizarre disease may sometimes be allergic in origin.

The tricyclic antidepressants have been demonstrated to have both H_1 and H_2 histamine receptor-blocking activity [108]. Treatment of hay fever conjunctivitis with imipramine, one such agent, resulted in measurable improvement in signs and symptoms [109].

Mucolytic agents are usually unnecessary for treating this disease.

Indomethacin has been used both systemically and topically to reduce inflammation in a variety of conditions in which prostaglandins play an important role. Its role in allergic eye disease is limited by its effects on cAMP [110].

Desensitization is discussed earlier in this chapter.

The use of systemic and subconjunctival corticosteroids is usually not warranted in the hay fever type of ocular allergy, but topical corticosteroids may be indicated when more conservative forms of therapy (e.g., vasoconstrictors and antihistamines) are ineffective. Low doses (prednisolone 0.12% b.i.d. or t.i.d.) may be very effective in counteracting the inflammation, and because low doses are associated with fewer complications, they should be tried first. If adequately beneficial effects are not forthcoming, then the dosage can be increased. High doses (prednisolone 1.0% every 2 hours) are immunosuppressive as well as antiinflammatory and should be effective in acute allergic ocular disease states because of both actions.

In selecting the appropriate corticosteroid, several factors should be borne in mind. If a suspension is used (hydrocortisone acetate [Hydrocortone Acetate 2.5%], prednisolone acetate [Prednefrin 0.12% and 1.0%], or fluorometholone [FML 0.1%]), then the medication must be shaken well before ocular delivery. The particulate matter in suspensions can be trapped between giant papillae (e.g., in VKC) and cause irritation and corneal epithelial damage. In such a case it is better to use a solution than a suspension.

Drops are preferred during the day because they do not interfere with vision. Ointment is preferred at night when blurred vision is not a consideration and a prolonged effect is desirable.

Of the solutions, prednisolone acetate penetrates the intact corneal epithelium better than prednisolone sodium phosphate [Hydeltrasol 0.5%; Metreton 0.5%; Inflamase 0.12% and 1.0%]. This particular feature of the acetate is probably not important in acute allergic diseases in view of their superficial nature.

Medrysone [HMS 1.0%], a progesteronelike compound, probably has the least antiinflammatory effect; others with minimal effect are prednisolone acetate suspension 0.12%, prednisolone phosphate solution 0.12%, and fluorometholone suspension. Those with a more potent effect are hydrocortisone acetate 2.5% suspension, prednisolone phosphate 0.5% solution, and dexamethasone phosphate 1.0% solution (Decadron) or suspension (Maxidex), and those with the most potent effect are prednisolone acetate 1.0% suspension and prednisolone phosphate 1.0% solutions [111].

The advantages of using corticosteroids topically are the high local concentrations achieved (when needed), the few systemic side effects, and the ease with which they can be applied and monitored. The possible disadvantages are local irritation caused by the medication (especially the suspensions), the development of allergies to the medication [112] or vehicle, elevation of the intraocular pressure, the development of posterior subcapsular cataracts, less efficient wound healing [113], keratopathy from the vehicle, corneal thickening, ptosis, and mydriasis.

VERNAL KERATOCONJUNCTIVITIS. VKC can be a serious manifestation of ocular allergy.

History. VKC was first described by Arlt in 1846 on the basis of several patients with inflammation and limbal infiltrations that he had seen. In 1871 von Graefe described the characteristic proliferations that occur on the tarsal conjunctiva and referred to them as "pavement-like granulations"—the cobblestones that are a classic feature of the disease. A year later Saemisch introduced the term *vernal catarrh* or *spring catarrh* after recognizing the seasonal exacerbations of the disease, and in 1880 Horner described "white points" or elevated dots on the nasal and temporal sides of the limbus. Trantas confirmed this observation 9 years later, and the lesions can to be known as *Trantas' dots.* In 1886 Gradle pointed out the similarities between vernal catarrh and hay fever conjunctivitis, and in 1903 Herbert discovered eosinophils in conjunctival scrapings from patients with the disease. Since then its allergic nature has been confirmed in numerous studies.

In 1888, Emmert described three major types of VKC, which he classified as limbal, palpebral, and mixed. Despite the invention of other systems of classification since then, this original one seems best suited to the disease. The palpebral type affects mainly the conjunctiva overlying the upper tarsus. The limbal type arises at the lateral aspects of the limbus and in severe cases may spread circumlimbally to involve the entire limbus.

Cause. Although there is substantial evidence that VKC is a localized form of allergy (type I hypersensitivity response), it is clearly also a CMI response (type IV hypersensitivity response) [114]. Atopic dermatitis is seldom associated with it, but many patients with VKC (26%–82%) have personal and family histories of atopy [115, 116].

In 1961 Allansmith [117] found reaginic antibodies to grass in 69 percent of patients with VKC, and Neumann and colleagues [116] reported positive skin tests to bacteria and fungi in 50 percent and 42 percent, respectively, of the 400 patients with VKC he studied. He concluded that in VKC, the patient is in some way "hypersensitive." In patients with VKC, tear IgE is elevated. This finding has been demonstrated by both the Prausnitz-Küstner reaction [118] and radioimmunodiffusion. Tear histamine, major basic protein and Charcot-Leyden crystal levels are also elevated [119].

Tear IgG–specific antibodies to rye grass and ragweed pollen have been reported [120].

There is a high incidence of large numbers of eosinophils in conjunctival scrapings. Alimudden [121] reported that 90 percent of 1050 patients with VKC had local eosinophilia, and that 40 percent had systemic eosinophilia of between 4 and 12 percent. The number of eosinophils in the conjunctival scrapings is so high that there are also large numbers of eosinophilic granules. The presence of these numerous free granules can be used as a minor differentiating point between VKC and other atopic reactions in the eye such as AKC. In VKC, basophils and mast cells were found in both tissues and conjunctival scrapings [122–124].

The positive therapeutic effect of cortisone and DSCG on VKC further confirms the atopic nature of the disease.

Epidemiologic Findings. In most of the reported series of patients with VKC, males predominate 75 percent to 25 percent until puberty when the prevalence in females rises, and by age 20 the incidence of VKC is almost equal in each sex. With its onset between 6 years of age and puberty, VKC is essentially a disease of childhood and youth. The youngest patient on record was 1 month old and the oldest 75 years, with the greatest prevalence between 11 and 13 years. The disease starts to diminish in severity between the ages of 16 and 21, and the patient usually "outgrows" it by his or her early 20s. Approximately 60 percent are between 11 and 20 years of age, only 17 percent are between 21 and 30, and only 6 percent have active disease after age 30.

All races are affected but the limbal form of the disease may be more common in blacks and American Indians than in others. VKC in two or more members of the same family has often been reported. Neumann and co-workers [116] found the frequency of multiple cases in a single family to be 28 percent among their 400 cases. A family history of atopy in one form or another is common.

VKC varies greatly in prevalence and severity from area to area according to the climate. Because it occurs more often and is more severe in hot climates, its prevalence in the northern hemisphere is highest in the Middle East, the Mediterranean basin, the Balkans, North Africa, and Central America. In San Francisco, VKC is almost nonexistent in the fog belt and relatively prevalent in the sunnier, warmer part of the city a few miles away. The tarsal conjunctival form predominates in Central and Northern Europe, the limbal form in most Mediterranean countries [125].

Seasonal variation is a characteristic feature of VKC. In temperate climates, the usual onset of the disease is in the spring. (Horner called it "Easter's gift.") It continues throughout the summer and then gradually abates during the fall. Occasionally a second exacerbation occurs near the end of the summer. The symptoms diminish during the cool months, but the proliferative changes usually persist with only slight regression. The limbal form is the more likely to regress, and in patients with mild disease, often regresses completely.

VKC in countries below the equator shows the same seasonal pattern; exacerbations also occur during the spring and summer months, September through February. Seasonal changes are naturally less marked in tropical countries, and regression is rare.

During the first years of the disease, variation is a hallmark of VKC, but later the symptoms may persist throughout the winter as well [115]. Although the disease is bilateral, one eye may be more severely affected than the other.

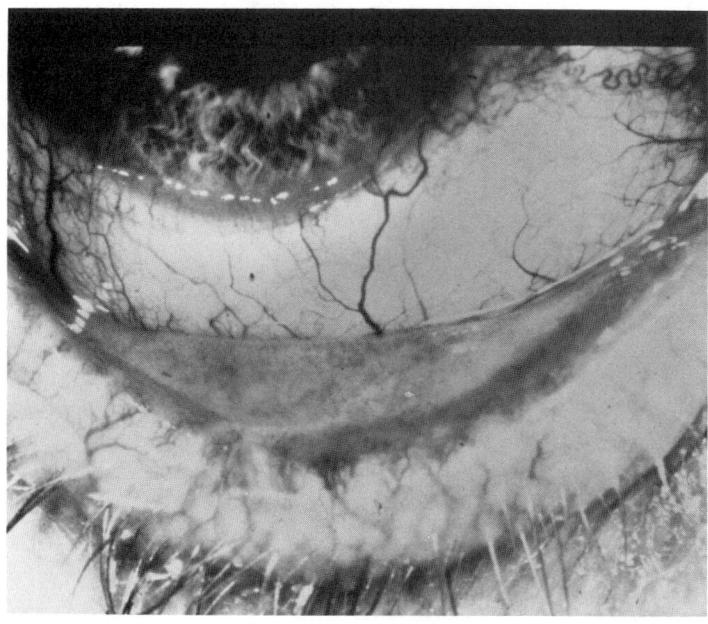

FIG. 3-8 Pale, inferior palpebral conjunctivitis and gelatinous infiltrate at inferior limbus in patient with palpebral and limbal (mixed) type of VKC.

Clinical Features

SYMPTOMS. The principal symptom is itching: If pruritus is absent, the clinician should strongly consider other diagnoses. It is usually the earliest symptom. It can be intense, persistent, and precede all tissue changes. It worsens toward evening and may be aggravated by exposure to dust, wind, bright light, or physical exertion associated with sweating. Rubbing the area that itches can increase the itching. Other less common symptoms are photophobia, foreign-body sensation, burning sensation, and lacrimation.

SIGNS. During the earliest stages of VKC, there may be a simple hyperemia that cannot be differentiated from the hyperemia of various other diseases that cause acute conjunctivitis. But in VKC, hyperemia is quickly followed by diffuse tissue hyperplasia. In the palpebral form of the disease, hyperemia is manifested by a dull, lusterless, pale pink conjunctiva in which the blood vessels and meibomian glands are obscured, often most markedly in the lateral areas with more or less early sparing of the central portion of the tarsal conjunctiva. In the limbal form of the disease, a flat, focal lesion, or a uniformly wide, opaque limbus, results (Fig. 3-8).

Papillary hypertrophy, predominantly on the upper tarsal conjunctiva, develops with a central capillary tuft in each papilla. The papillae may evolve slowly from minute elevations 0.1 mm in diameter up to the characteristic large, grayish pink, irregularly polygonal, vegetating excrescen-

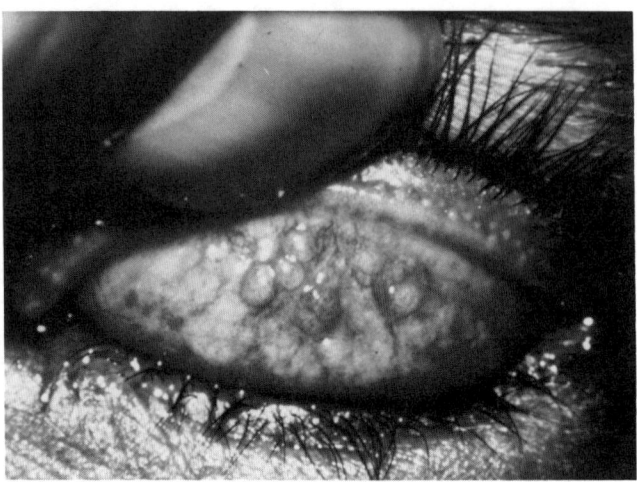

FIG. 3-9 Few large papillae in upper palpebral conjunctiva in patient with vernal keratoconjunctivitis.

ces that may reach 7 to 8 mm in diameter (Fig. 3-9). These papillae may appear on the entire strip along the free border of the eyelid. The largest of them have flattened tops and are separated from each other by intertwining crevices. When they are tightly packed, the tarsal conjunctiva may take on the classic cobblestone appearance (Fig. 3-10). The weight of these lesions may produce a mechanical ptosis (Fig. 3-11). They are the result of marked hyperplasia of connective tissue and of inflammatory infiltration (with eosinophils, mast cells, basophils, lymphocytes, and macrophages predominating) and do not represent the enlargement of just one papilla.

Limbal nodules (the counterpart of the tarsal papillae) may be single or multiple. They appear as small, semitransparent, smooth, gelatinous elevations, usually in the interpalpebral fissure. Their corneal edge is sharp but their conjunctival edge blends gradually with the normal tissue. Their color may vary from grayish white to pink depending on the degree of vascularization. These limbal masses may continue to grow and coalesce until they completely surround the cornea. Occasionally they extend centrally, with minimal to extensive corneal invasion.

The white points (Horner's points or Trantas' dots) in these circumlimbal vegetations were first described in 1880. They are small, grayish white to whitish yellow dots appearing singly or in large numbers, usually at the upper limbus (Fig. 3-12). They are sometimes seen on the bulbar conjunctiva and semilunar folds, however, and very rarely on the tarsal conjunctiva. A case of Trantas' dots atop a corneal plaque has been reported [125]. They are present in approximately 69 percent of patients with mixed VKC, in 41 percent with limbal VKC, and in 21 percent with palpebral VKC. They usually last for 2 to 3 days but may last as long as a week. Pathologically they are small cysts filled with eosinophils, gran-

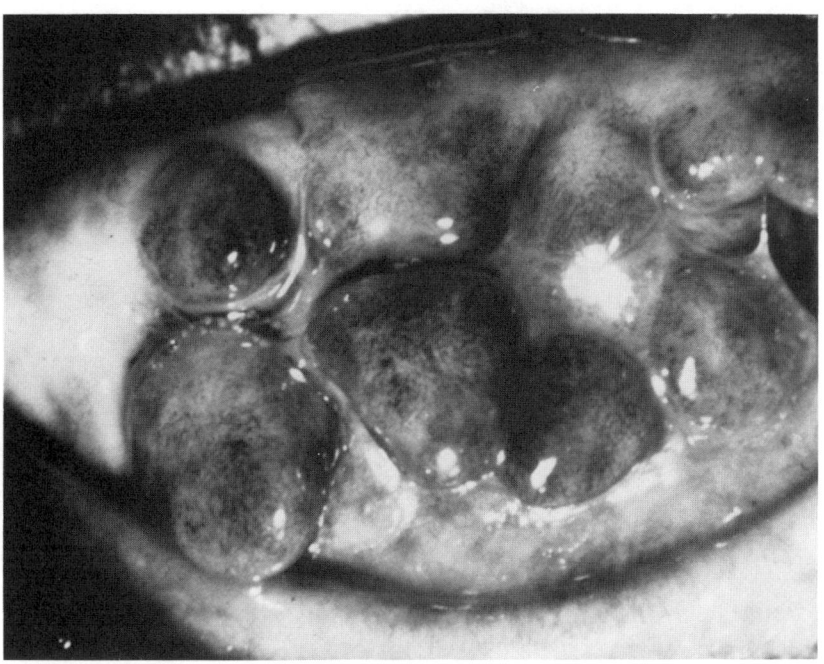

FIG. 3-10   Giant cobblestones in upper palpebral conjunctiva of patient with vernal keratoconjunctivitis. (Courtesy of Dr. P. Thygeson.)

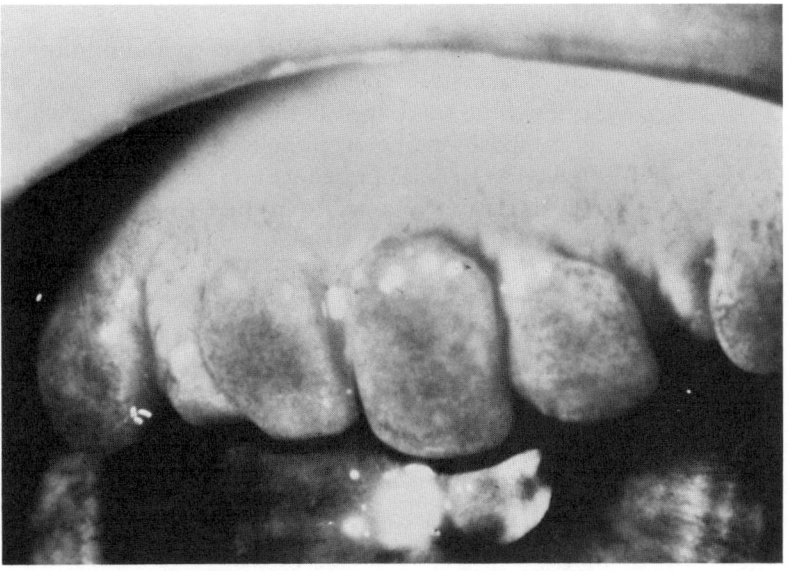

FIG. 3-11   Giant papillae in upper palpebral of patient with vernal keratoconjunctivitis. Note cataract. (Courtesy of Dr. P. Thygeson.)

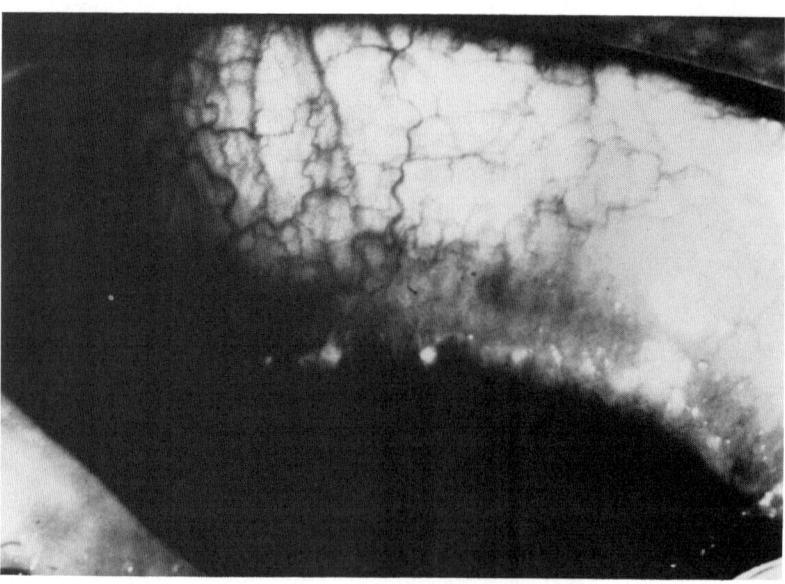

FIG. 3-12   Horner's points (Trantas' dots) at upper superior limbus in patient with vernal keratoconjunctivitis.

ules, and epithelial cells undergoing rapid degeneration. They are the tip of the iceberg the bulk of which lies in the deeper layers of the epithelium.

In the limbal form of VKC, cysts and minute marginal "pits" also occur. The cysts are ovoid, closely packed in some areas, contain clear, colorless fluid, and appear to be elevated. They are true cysts formed by the apposition of two epithelial layers between papillae, and they contain mucin as well as epithelial and inflammatory cells (Fig. 3-13). The marginal pits appear as transparent, round to oval, glassy spots in the opaque limbus, 1 to 5 mm in diameter. They are confined to the superior limbus. They are not depressed and represent areas in which the limbal infiltration has almost returned to normal. They are not to be confused with the Herbert's peripheral pits of trachoma, which are larger and permanent (Fig. 3-14).

The bulbar conjunctiva away from the limbus and on the plica may show hyperemia and mild chemosis and may develop reddish gray, colored elevations nasally or temporally and slightly above the interpalpebral area.

The fornices and plica are rarely affected. The lower tarsus is relatively free of giant papillae and usually shows only the gray discoloration and a slight degree of thickening.

The limbal lesions may extend into the cornea. Thickening, broadening, and opacification at the upper limbus may extend onto the cornea as a semitransparent hood. Peripheral vascularization of this area may extend into the cornea as a micropannus, rarely as a gross pannus. The

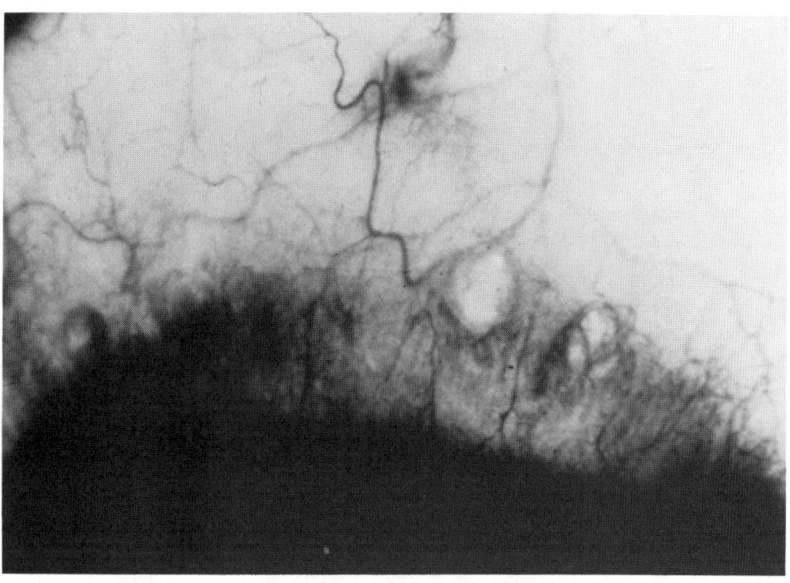

FIG. 3-13   Clear cysts and gross pannus in patient with vernal keratoconjunctivitis.

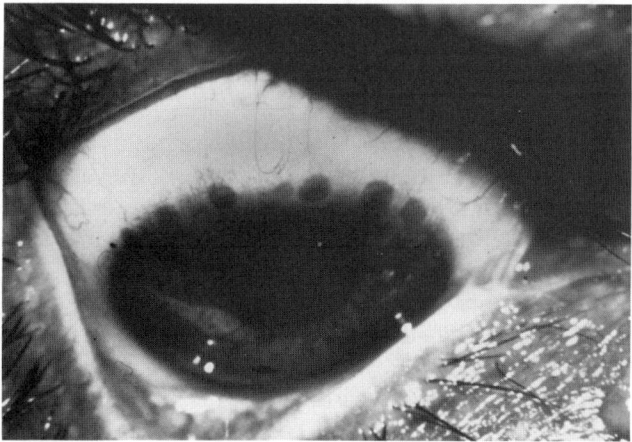

FIG. 3-14   Herbert's peripheral pits of trachoma and pannus at superior limbus of patient with trachoma.

pannus eventually clears, leaving ghost vessels and a few gray opacities. Occasionally the gelatinous limbal nodules extend centrally to cover the entire cornea, and in a few patients the corneal nodules have not been connected to the limbus.

The corneal epithelium may contain minute, dull, grayish points that look like flour dust. The upper part of the cornea is the part mainly

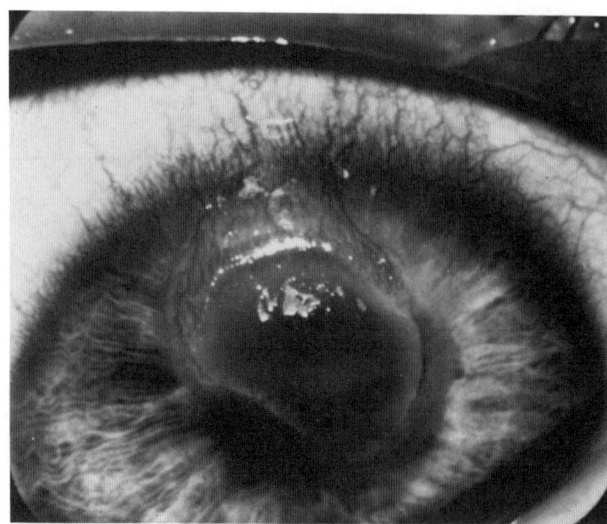

FIG. 3-15 Shallow corneal ulcer and superficial pannus in patient with vernal keratoconjunctivitis. Note gray opacification in ulcer bed and surrounding cornea.

affected, and there is relative sparing of the periphery. This syncytium-like lesion was well described in 1935 by Tobgy [126] and in 1961 by Jones [127]. The gray points remain discrete and stain irregularly. Fluorescein application shows many finely stained points on the cornea. Small intraepithelial cysts and areas of edema may be seen. If a punctate keratopathy affects principally the lower one-third of the cornea, then the clinician should rule out concomitant staphylococcal disease.

This syncytium like keratitis is most often associated with the palpebral type of VKC when the tarsal conjunctiva is covered with giant papillae. The limbus, in fact, may not be affected at all. The epithelium may eventually break down, forming a corneal ulcer, and this condition may happen in spite of therapy. The ulcer is very typical. It is transversely oval or shield shaped, smooth, affects the upper half of the cornea, is centrally located, and rarely vascularizes. It is shallow and shows a whitened roughening of the epithelium at its edges. The exposed Bowman's layer is slightly grayish, and the stroma may show varying degrees of cellular infiltration (Fig. 3-15). With time this area may develop a smaller, grayish plaque that heals slowly, leaving an oval, gray zone in Bowman's layer. The plaque is also transversely oval and located superiorly (Fig. 3-16). These corneal ulcerations and plaques seem to occur mainly in the very young.

A fascicular and deep keratitis has also been seen in patients with VKC. The most common degenerative change in the cornea is the pseudogerontoxon. It is an arclike or annular opacity, separated from the limbus by a narrow, lucid zone resembling arcus senilis. The opacity is focal and yellowish gray, and it occasionally ulcerates, leaving a gutterlike furrow covered with epithelium. A change in corneal curvature also oc-

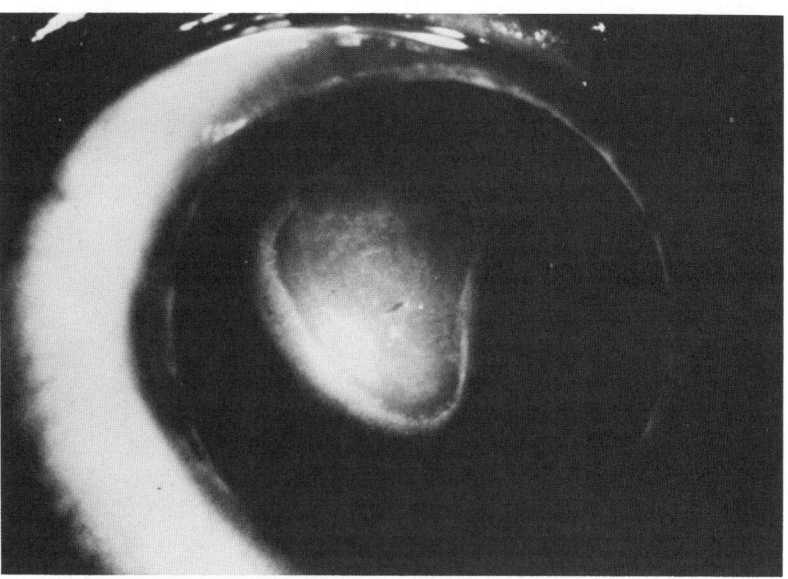

FIG. 3-16 Corneal ulcer and plaque in patient with vernal keratoconjunctivitis.

curs. There is a steepening of the cornea accompanied by myopic astigmatism, and late in the disease there may be ketatoconus [128] and keratoglobus.

The atopic type of cataract can occur in VKC; this is discussed later in the section on AKC. It occurs less frequently than keratoconus.

The conjunctival exudate in VKC is characteristic. It is a thin, ropy, milk-white, fibrinous secretion composed chiefly of fibrin and mucus (Fig. 3-17). Around the structureless core of this stringy matrix are epithelial cells, polymorphonuclear leukocytes, eosinophils, and free eosinophilic granules. The increased amount of hyaluronic acid [129] in VKC may be responsible for the stickiness of the discharge. Hyaluronidase also seems to be elevated, and the pH of the exudate is on the alkaline side—8.0 to 8.1.

Eversion of the upper lid and its exposure to heat may result in the formation of a thin, fibrinous pseudomembrane that can be readily peeled off without causing any bleeding. This peeling membrane is called Maxwell-Lyons' sign (Fig. 3-18). An extra lid fold may be present in VKC (Fig. 3-19), which is called Dennie's line.

PROGNOSIS. VKC is a self-limited disease lasting 4 to 6 years, with a few cases lasting longer. Eventually there is complete regression of all conjunctival signs. No conjunctival scarring has been recorded unless the tissues have been altered by treatment such as radiation or operation. The permanent corneal sequelae are micropannus, myopic astigmatism, keratoconus and keratoglobus, pseudogerontoxon, marginal furrows, and superficial opacities. If these alterations interfere with vision (and they usually do not), they can be corrected by spectacles or contact lenses.

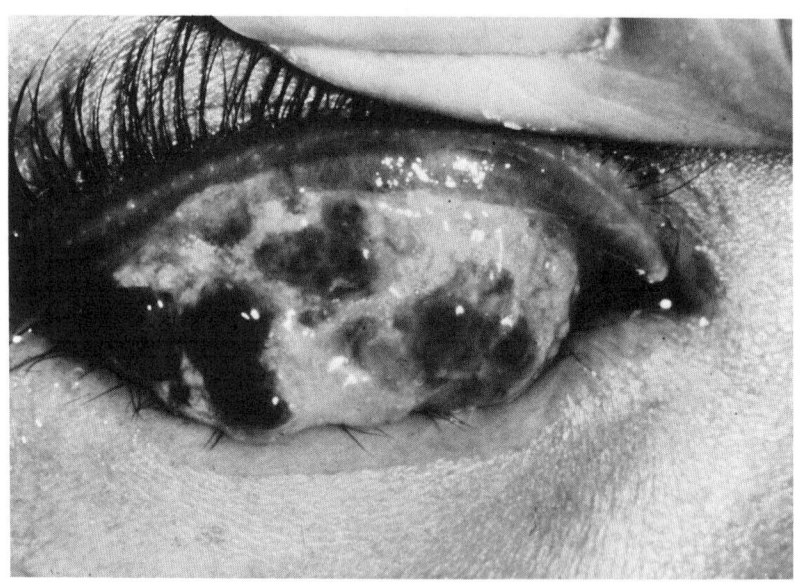

FIG. 3-17 Thick, ropy discharge on upper palpebral conjunctiva of patient with vernal keratoconjunctivitis.

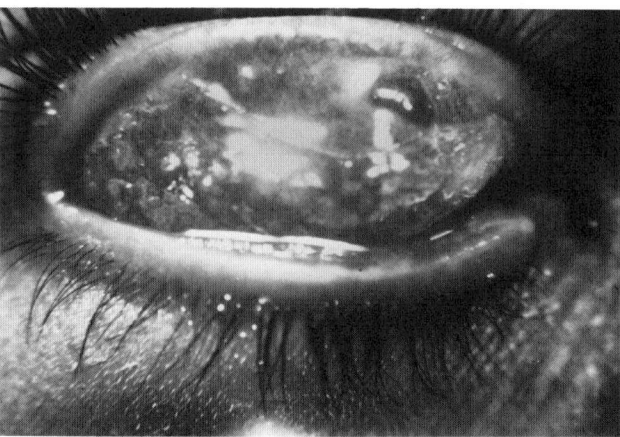

FIG. 3-18 Thin fibrin coagulum on upper palpebral conjunctiva of patient with vernal keratoconjunctivitis whose lid was everted under intense illumination for several minutes (Maxwell-Lyons sign).

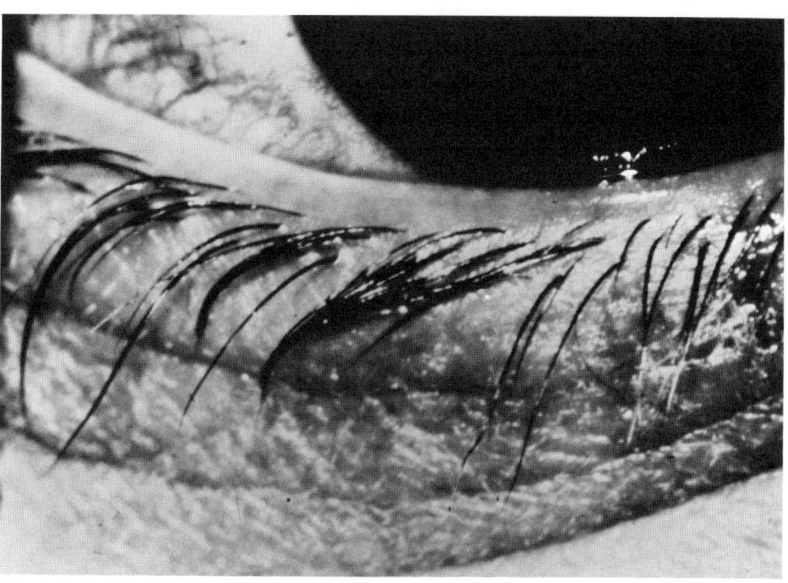

FIG. 3-19   Extra lid fold (Dennie's line) in patient with vernal keratoconjunctivitis.

The atopic type of cataract persists but may not alter the visual acuity materially.

Histopathologic Findings. The early stages of VKC are characterized by hyperemia, new-vessel formation, and the formation of papillae by the infiltration of polymorphonuclear leukocytes, eosinophils, basophils, and mast cells. The eosinophils are plentiful. Later in the course of the disease, mononuclear cells (lymphocytes and macrophages) appear. A marked percent of the mast cells appear degranulated [130].

Hyperplasia of the connective tissue extends upward to form large, sessile, giant papillae. The collagen and the walls of the blood vessels become hyalinized. The epithelium proliferates, and the normal two layers of the conjunctiva may increase to between five and ten layers of irregular, edematous, epithelial cells. As the papillae increase in size, the epithelial layers atrophy at the apex until only one layer remains, which may become keratinized. There is a columnar epithelial downgrowth and an increase in the number of goblet cells, especially in the crevices between the papillae. At the limbus the epithelial overgrowth is more extensive, and 30 to 40 cell layers may form (acanthosis).

Charcot-Leyden crystals have been seen in the corneal ulcer bed [131].

Diagnosis. In classic VKC, diagnosis is rarely a problem. If there is any confusion, it is most likely to be with chronic AKC. Both entities are probably IgE-mediated, chronic, type I hypersensitivity and CMI type IV reactions. Both are therefore associated with itching, local and systemic eosinophilia, more than the usual amount of tear IgE, and a family history of atopy. Both AKC and VKC may be exacerbated by warm weather, VKC regularly and AKC only rarely.

The characteristics of chronic AKC that help differentiate it from VKC are as follows: (1) conjunctival scarring and shrinkage of the fornix occur in AKC, rarely in VKC; (2) deep corneal vessels appear more commonly in AKC; (3) AKC affects principally the lower tarsal conjunctiva and causes small papillae, whereas VKC affects principally the upper tarsal conjunctiva and causes large papillae; (4) the exudate in AKC frequently is more watery than the thick, white, fibrinous exudate of VKC; (5) there are fewer eosinophils and minimal or no free eosinophilic granules in conjunctival scrapings from AKC; (6) AKC is not as seasonal (hot-weather related) as VKC and may be severe in winter; (7) AKC lasts longer than VKC and occurs more often in teenage and older patients (up to the early 40s) and less often in children than VKC; (8) unlike VKC patients, AKC patients rarely have limbal points or dots or corneal ulcerations; (9) AKC patients respond better to vasoconstrictors and antihistamines than VKC patients; (10) AKC patients may have atopic dermatitis of the lids; and (11) AKC patients may have sequelae of atopic dermatitis elsewhere on the body.

Some patients have the signs and symptoms of both diseases. Because the two entities are probably different manifestations of the same basic disease process, this is not surprising. In the spectrum of clinical disease, pure VKC can be readily differentiated from pure AKC. These pure forms can perhaps be considered the extremes of the spectrum; however, a large number of patients exhibiting atopic disease have manifestations of both entities.

Because trachoma affects predominantly the upper tarsal conjunctiva and may produce superior pannus and superior limbal pits, it too is a possible source of confusion with VKC. But unlike VKC, trachoma produces follicular conjunctivitis, conjunctival scarring, and limbal follicles, and scrapings from the trachomatous conjunctiva may contain neutrophils, plasma cells, lymphocytes, Leber cells, and epithelial-cell inclusion bodies but no eosinophils (Fig. 3-20). Again, VKC and trachoma may coexist, and in that event the VKC seems to be more severe and intractable than when it occurs alone.

TREATMENT. Treatment of VKC consists of general measures and the use of drugs. First the parents and the patient must be educated to the chronic, self-limited nature of the disease. The advantages and complications of the medications available should be discussed as well. For example, a family favoring corticosteroid therapy may be eager to consider alternatives when the complications of long-lasting corticosteroid therapy are explained.

General Measures. Climatotherapy (exposing the patient to a cooler climate) is the treatment of choice when it can be arranged, and for many patients it may be the only effective therapy. It can be particularly valuable in California: Moving short distances from the inland valleys to the fog-enshrouded coastal area always results in dramatic relief.

When moving is not feasible, air conditioning offices and especially bedrooms may be of value in reducing symptoms. If the disease is not

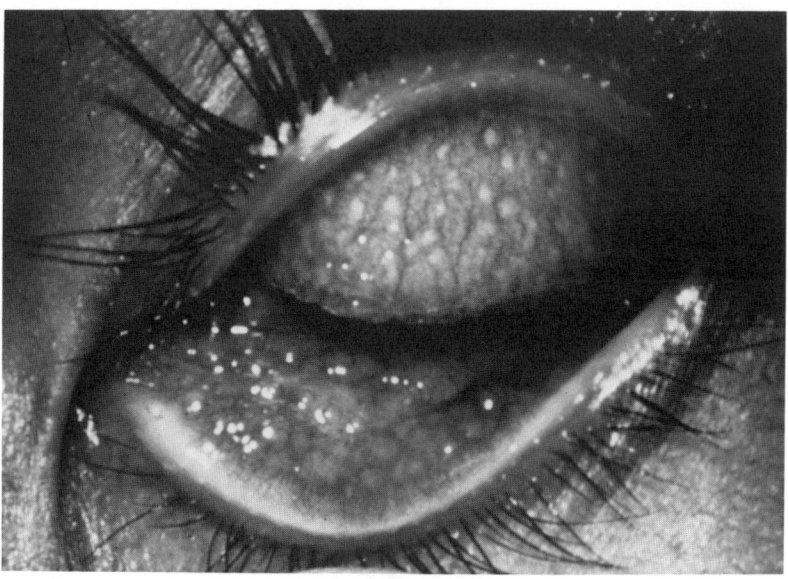

FIG. 3-20 Follicles in upper and lower conjunctivae of patient with active trachoma.

too severe, using cold compresses frequently may alleviate some of the symptoms. Removing such irritative factors as dusts and molds by vacuuming and oil mopping floors may also have a limited effect.

Patching has a dramatic effect on both symptoms and signs and is useful as a temporary measure in very severe limbal VKC complicated by ulcerative keratitis. The beneficial effect is transient, however, and lasts only as long as the eyes are fully covered.

Desensitization does not seem to be an effective form of therapy. Psychotherapy may be helpful, but because of the time and expense, it is unlikely to have more than limited value to a small segment of the population with severe disease. Hospitalization may bring about rapid improvement for a variety of reasons. Removing patients from their home environment may remove them from some of the allergens causing the problem, it may be a form of psychotherapy, and it certainly makes it possible to administer medication frequently and adequately.

Drug Therapy. The thick, ropy, sticky exudate characteristic of VKC is a sensitive indicator of disease activity and plays an important role in the production of symptoms. The irritation caused by it is responsible for the formation of some of the corneal lesions [132]. To remove this mucous secretion, sterile saline irrigations and very dilute acid solutions have been used with limited success. Mucolytic agents (e.g., 10–20% acetylcysteine drops) have also been useful, both in removing the exudate and in alleviating the symptoms caused by it. The dosage depends on the amount of exudate and the severity of the symptoms. The 10% solution is better tolerated than the 20% solution. Physical removal of the secretion is also possible but of limited, transient value.

Vasoconstrictors, which temporarily reduce hyperemia and edema, may offer some symptomatic relief. In severe VKC, however, the relief is insignificant.

The use of antihistamines, both topically with vasoconstrictors and systemically, in atopic eye disease is discussed earlier in the chapter.

DSCG has been used at several centers abroad [133, 134] and at the University of California Medical School in San Francisco. The original dosage prescribed was a 2% solution four times a day for 6 to 24 months. The result indicated that 18 percent of the patients with VKC could be controlled by DSCG alone, the remaining 72 percent also required topical corticosteroid therapy for a limited time. Ostler and associates [135] have found that a 4% solution of DSCG is the most effective concentration. This solution is now commercially available. Many patients who require corticosteroids are able to stop them or to reduce the dosage when the 4% DSCG solution is added to the therapeutic regimen. The discomfort that some patients experience after instilling DSCG may be due to the vehicle preservatives in which it is placed for delivery. It requires several weeks before beneficial results are seen. In no instance has the topical use of DSCG caused serious complications, although a local allergic reaction has been reported [136].

The topical use of corticosteroids has the most dramatic and beneficial effect of all of the medications used to treat VKC. Their systemic use for a short 1- to 2-week course (usually 2 to 3 tablets q.i.d.) may be necessary when the disease is severe, or when blepharospasm and photophobia make topical instillation extremely difficult or impossible. When administered topically, solutions are preferable to suspensions because the particles in the suspensions may lodge between the papillae and cause corneal damage.

The corticosteroid ophthalmic preparations should be used in as low doses and for as short a time as possible. Long-term corticosteroid therapy carries with it the danger of too many complications to be acceptable.

Aspirin orally has been reported to be effective in treating VKC [137]. Conflicting reports [36] and lack of confirmation make these results questionable at present.

Because atopic patients are more susceptible to infection than nonatopic patients, and because corticosteroids may aggravate this susceptibility, the practitioner must be careful to watch for secondary infections, especially with *Staphylococcus aureus* and herpes simplex virus. The other complications of the use of corticosteroids are discussed in Chapter 1.

Soft contact lenses may be of value in treating VKC by protecting the cornea from the irritative effect of the palpebral excrescences. The patient's increased susceptibility to infection makes their use more dangerous than usual, however, and fitting them may be more difficult than usual if there are limbal excrescences. The lenses may also irritate the patient.

Radiation should not be used to treat VKC, and although operation has been recommended for the removal of the corneal plaques [98], many believe it is not warranted as a form of treatment for this disease.

Recently mucous membrane grafting has been recommended for severe palpebral VKC [138]. A cryoprobe has also been used for severe palpebral VKC [139].

ATOPIC DERMATITIS AND ITS OCULAR MANIFESTATIONS

History. Atopic dermatitis, perhaps the best-defined atopic disease, is a common disorder and a source of some confusion. The nomenclature is confusing: The disease is often called eczema, allergic eczema, allergic dermatitis, and even neurodermatitis. The diagnostic features can be misleading. Typically the disease is a chronic hereditary dermatitis that usually starts in childhood and is characterized by severe pruritus and a persistent superficial inflammation. Although it tends to subside spontaneously by age 2, a number of patients have remissions and exacerbations into adult life, and the skin lesions in the child may differ vastly from the lesions in the same patient 15 to 20 years later. Unfortunately, moreover, histologic examination may provide little assistance in making the diagnosis.

Carr and colleagues [140] found a 3 percent incidence of atopic dermatitis in the general population. Approximately 70 percent of all patients have a family history of atopy. Roth and Kierland [141] found that when both parents are affected, the dermatitis is likely to be more severe in the offspring, to occur in more than one sibling, and in 55 percent of patients to be associated with asthma, hay fever urticaria, migraine headaches, rhinitis, or conjunctivitis.

Cause. The physiologic and immunologic causes of atopic dermatitis are complex, interrelated, and still not fully understood. That there are physiologic defects is obvious. The skin is extremely dry and pruritic [142], and the vasoreactions of the skin are abnormal; (1) the temperature of the skin of the fingers is diminished [143], (2) white dermatographism occurs, and (3) the blanch response to cholinergic agents is delayed [144]. It has been suggested that a blockade of β-adrenergic receptors in the tissues is the underlying cause of the disease (Szentivanyi's hypothesis) [145].

Concerning the immunologic associations of atopic dermatitis, there are associations with other allergic entities, abnormalities of both humoral and cell-mediated immunity, associations with immunodeficient states, and alterations of the cAMP system.

A transient deficiency of IgA at age 3 months has been associated with increased risk of developing atopy within the first year. Taylor and coworkers [146] suggested that this transient letdown of a mucosal IgA barrier against antigens could lead to an inappropriate stimulation of IgE-producing lymphocytes and the consequent development of atopy. Some recent work has shown a prevalence of HLA antigens in patients with atopic dermatitis, which suggests that the tendency to become atopic may be HLA-related [147]. (This subject is discussed in detail in Chapter 1.)

Increased levels of serum IgG and IgM and decreased levels of IgD have been observed in patients with atopic dermatitis [148, 149]. Complement and immunoglobulin, mainly IgG, were found in the skin of these patients. The all-important question of the role of IgE is still a puzzle. Many observers have noted elevated levels of IgE in patients with pure atopic dermatitis [150–152]. Others, however, have failed to do so. The interpretation of these results is clouded because IgE is a tissue-fixing antibody, and hence serum levels do not necessarily indicate total body levels. Skin and ocular IgE levels may be elevated while serum levels are not [153]. It can be stated unequivocally, however, that B-lymphocytes carrying IgE are measurably increased in patients with atopic dermatitis [154] (T-lymphocytes bearing fragment, crystallizable [Fc] receptors of IgE also exist in human beings), and that increased level of tear and serum IgE is one of the features of the disease, however uncertain its role.

Several lines of evidence attest to the dysfunction of the CMI response in atopic dermatitis patients. The most obvious is the susceptibility of these atopic patients to unusually severe cutaneous and ocular infections, especially viral infections such as vaccinia, herpes simplex, and molluscum contagiosum. The high carriage rate of S. aureus on the skin in atopic dermatitis patients has been recently reaffirmed [155]. The higher than average risk of patients with atopic dermatitis acquiring herpes simplex keratitis and S. aureus ocular infections is well known.

Cutaneous anergy has also been noted among patients with atopy. Some fail to respond to a battery of naturally occurring antigens such as tuberculin, candidin, and streptokinase-streptodornase [156]. All atopic patients, moreover, are less sensitized to dinitrochlorobenzene (DNCB) than normal persons [157].

In atopic dermatitis patients, the number of T cells [148] (rosette-forming cells) is reduced [158]. When their number was plotted against serum IgE levels, a roughly inverse correlation was found. The possibility that IgE may directly affect T cells is intriguing.

Lymphocyte transformation to phytohemagglutinin and concanavalin A is reduced in atopic patients, and the chemotaxis of both polymorphonuclear cells and monocytes is depressed [159–161]. Ascorbic acid may correct monocyte defect in vitro and in vivo.

Interferon production is decreased and natural killer cells are increasingly active [162].

Skin lesions resembling those of atopic dermatitis are manifestations of diseases associated with depressed immune responses (e.g., the lesions of the Wiskott-Aldrich syndrome [163], ataxia telangiectasia [164], X-linked agammaglobulinemia [165], and the hyperimmunoglobulin E syndrome of Buckley [166].

The increased sensitivity of atopic patients to histamine and cholinergic agents has been appreciated for many years and could be the result of an inadequate β-adrenergic counterbalance [167]. Serum factors that could act as β-adrenergic blockers play an as yet undefined role in the pathogenesis of atopic dermatitis. (See Chapter 1 for a complete discussion.)

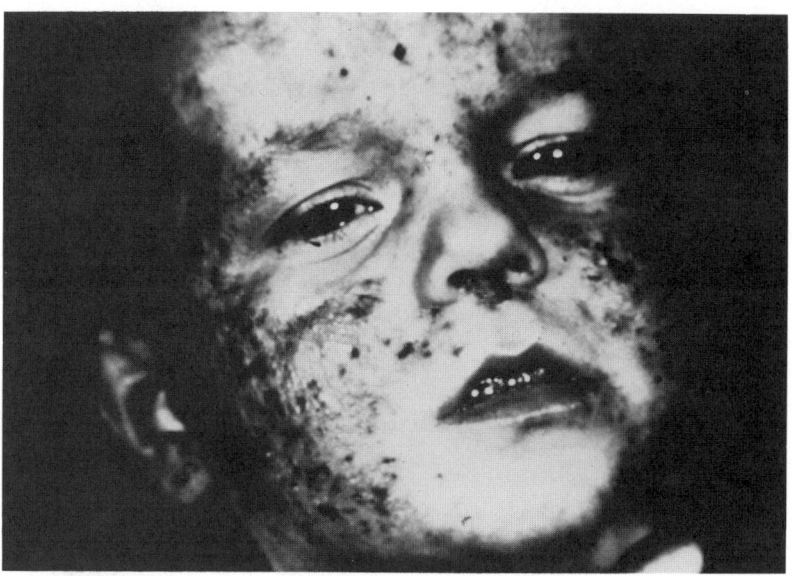

FIG. 3-21   Severe atopic dermatitis on face of young child.

Clinical Features

SKIN. Atopic dermatitis evolves through three age-related stages: infantile, childhood, and adult. Approximately 80 percent of patients onset is within the first year of life. But although the dermatitis usually develops in the first few months of life, it may also start at any later age, even over the age of 50.

In the infant the patches of dermatitis are usually poorly defined and are located on the cheeks, on the flexor surfaces of the forearms and legs, and less commonly on the trunk and in the diaper area. The eruption is usually symmetric, often begins with a slightly rough, gritty feeling to the touch, and has a light or dark reddish orange color. The surface develops scattered, fine scales but often looks glossy. Frank weeping, with the development of crusts, is quite common (Fig. 3-21).

In some patients the scalp and postauricular areas are affected, and in a few weeks the whole body becomes involved. The areas first affected seem to be those than can be rubbed against bed clothing, but as the baby matures and starts to crawl and walk, lesions appear on the exposed surfaces, especially the extensor surfaces.

From 18 months on, the sites most frequently affected are the elbow and knee flexures and the sides of the neck, wrist, and ankles. Lichenification replaces the erythematous, edematous papules. The skin becomes dry and thickened with excoriations. Pruritus is intense. By 2 years of age, 50 percent of the children have clear skins, and 50 percent may have recurrences between ages 5 and 9 and again at puberty. Those who continue to have dermatitis past the age of 2 are more likely to have

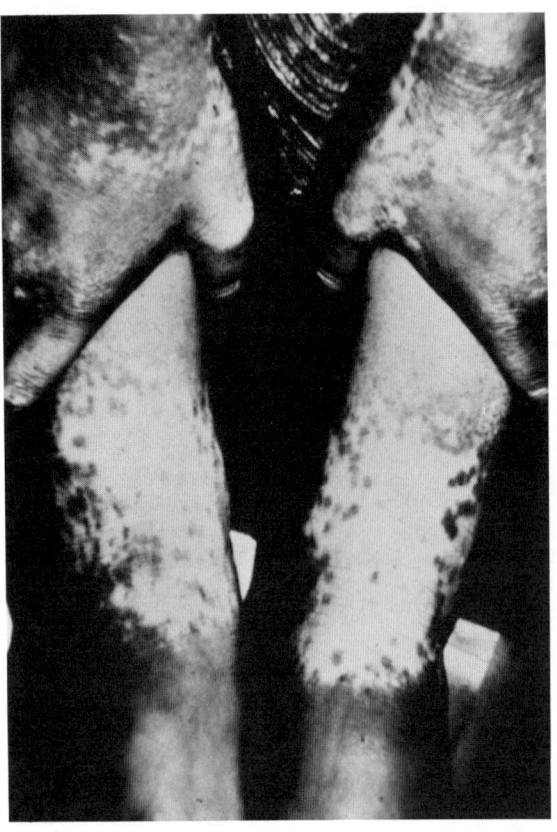

FIG. 3-22 Depigmented areas on flexure surfaces of forearms of child with atopic dermatitis. Areas on mother's hands also depigmented, indicating history of atopic dermatitis.

it on into adult life. At that time the lesions tend to localize on the hands, feet, and genitalia (Figs. 3-22, 3-23).

Hanifin's [168] diagnostic criteria for atopic dermatitis are listed in Table 3-1.

ATOPIC KERATOCONJUNCTIVITIS. Although it was generally realized that patients with atopic dermatitis occasionally develop the hay fever or VKC type of ocular disease, no specific keratoconjunctivitis was associated with the skin disease until 1953 when Hogan [169] described five patients with what he called "atopic keratoconjunctivitis."

All of Hogan's patients (and most of those we have seen since his original series) were men between the ages of 29 and 47. Most of his patients had had atopic dermatitis as children (which cleared by age 2), and some had had recurrences thereafter. This now well-established ocular disease usually appears in the late teens and lasts for many years. It most often improves or subsides when the patient approaches 30 years of age, but occasionally continues into the fourth or fifth decades of life.

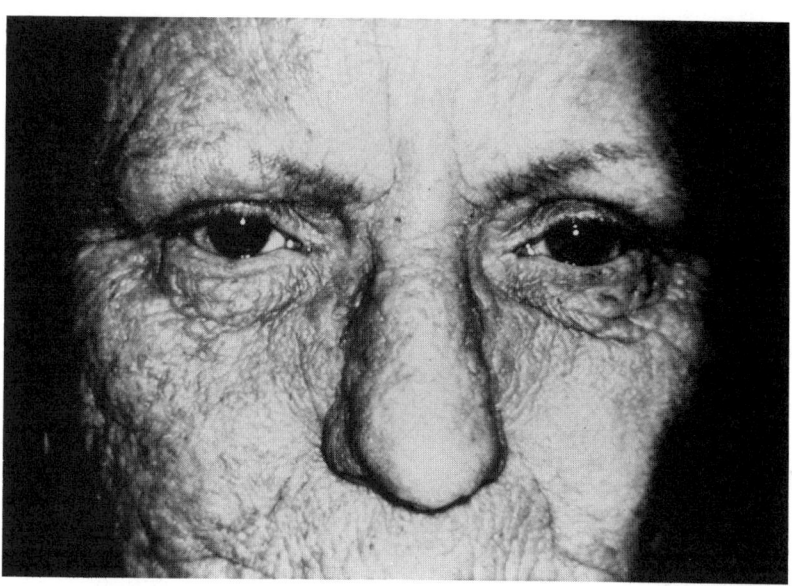

FIG. 3-23   Atopic dermatitis in an elderly patient.

The ocular disease occurs in the winter as well as in the spring and fall; the seasonal variation and association with hot weather are much less noticeable in AKC than in VKC. AKC is invariably bilateral, and the symptoms are itching, burning, tearing, and a watery to mucopurulent, white discharge. The signs, which include changes discussed in the section on VKC, are as follows: a pale conjunctiva; limbal infiltration; Horner's points (Trantas' dots); corneal pannus, ulceration, and scarring; keratoconus; keratoglobus; pseudogeronotoxon; punctate epithelial keratitis; thick, broad opacification of the limbus (Fig. 3-24); and cataract formation.

AKC can cause scarring of the conjunctiva (principally of the inferior palpebral portion), shrinkage of the fornix, and deep corneal vascularization (Fig. 3-25). In more than one-half of the patients in whom atopic cataract develops (8%), the opacity is the polygonal, ganglionlike, white, anterior, subcapsular (shieldlike) type. When the shield becomes visible, the rest of the lens is usually slightly opaque. The overlying capsule may appear wrinkled (Fig. 3-26).

A typical posterior polar, complicated cataract has also been reported. The earliest change is a microscopic, polychromatic, subcapsular vacuolation or opacification, usually axial. Soon there are several opacities, and if no cutaneous flare-ups occur, they push into the substance of the lens, being separated from the capsule by newly laid down, healthy lens fibers. In the course of this process, intensification zones form that coincide with exacerbations of the dermatitis and look like the rings of a tree trunk [170].

The lens opacities, 89 percent of which are bilateral, first appear be-

TABLE 3-1 Diagnostic critera for atopic dermatitis

Absolute features:

Patients must have each of the following:
  Pruritis
  Typical morphologic findings and distribution:
    Flexural lichenification in adults
    Facial and extensor involvement in infancy
  Tendency toward chronic or chronically relapsing dermatitis

   plus

Two or more of the following features:
  Personal or family history of atopic disease (asthma, allergic rhinitis, atopic dermatitis)
  Immediate skin test reactivity
  White dermatographism, delayed blanch to cholinergic agents, or both
  Anterior subcapsular cataracts

   or

Four or more of the following features:
  Xerosis, ichthyosis, hyperlinear palms
  Pityriasis alba
  Keratosis pilaris
  Facial pallor, infraorbital darkening
  Dennie-Morgan infraorbital fold
  Elevated serum IgE
  Keratoconus
  Tendency toward nonspecific hand dermatitis
  Tendency toward repeated cutaneous infections

Source: J. M. Hanifin, Newer concepts of atopic dermatitis. *Arch. Dermatol.* 113:663, 1977.

tween the ages of 16 to 18 years and either progress slowly or mature in a few months. The role of corticosteroid therapy in the pathogenesis of the posterior subcapsular cataract must be appreciated. This type of cataract developed in atopic dermatitis patients before the introduction of the corticosteroids, but there is small doubt that the steroids increase its incidence or severity or both.

The typical clinical picture, a family and personal history of atopy, and the appropriate laboratory test responses all assist the clinician in diagnosing AKC. Persons with atopy usually show a positive intradermal wheal-and-flare reaction to a number of common antigens. The amount of histamine released from sensitized mast cells and basophils is usually elevated. Conjunctival scrapings contain eosinophils and some mononuclear cells; basophils and mast cells are rarely seen. Serum and tear

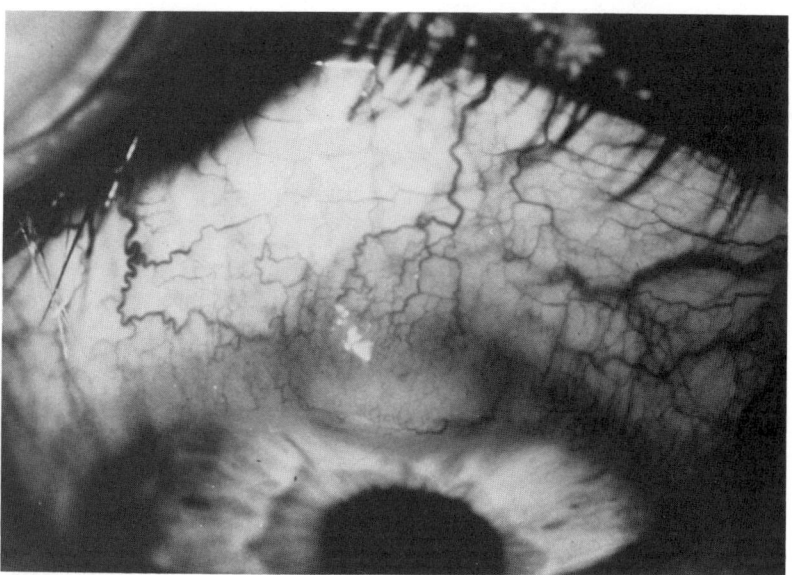

FIG. 3-24 Limbal gelatinous mass in patient with atopic keratoconjunctivitis.

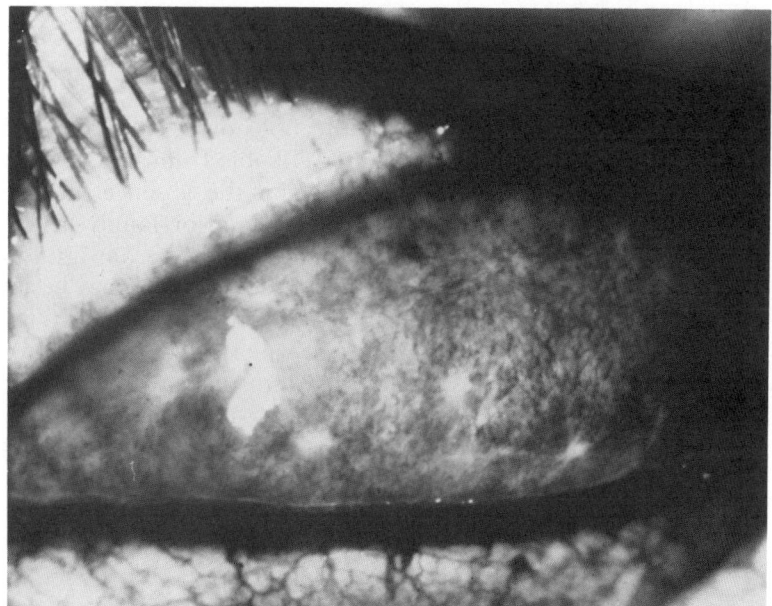

FIG. 3-25 Scarring of palpebral conjunctiva of patient with atopic keratoconjunctivitis.

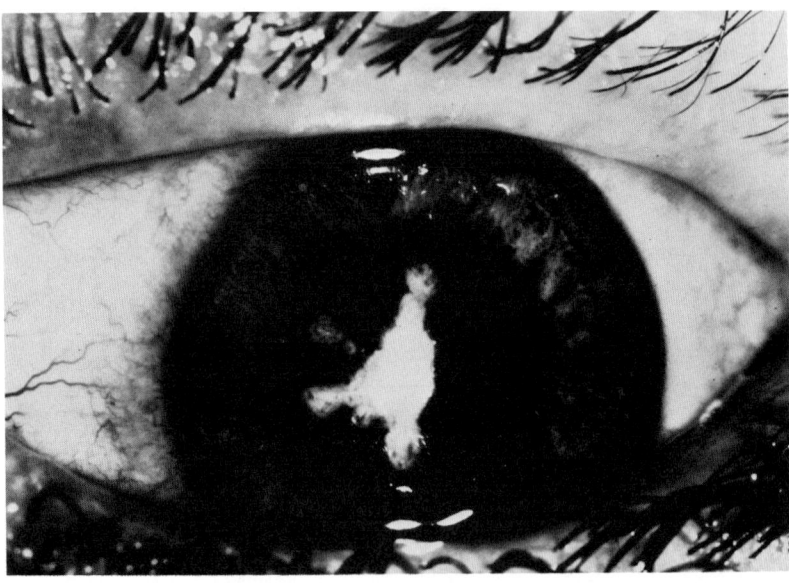

FIG. 3-26 Anterior cataract in the form of a shieldlike plaque in patient with atopic keratoconjunctivitis.

IgE levels are usually elevated, and serum eosinophils are sometimes elevated.

The conjunctival infections owing to viruses, chlamydiae, or toxic irritants are readily differentiable from AKC by virtue of their characteristic follicular reactions and the absence of conjunctival eosinophilia, atopic lid dermatitis, a personal or family history of atopy (except by coincidence), and elevated tear and serum IgE levels.

In contact dermatitis of the lids there may be severe itching associated with an erythematous, thickened skin lesion (Fig. 3-27). However, contact dermatitis is due to a type IV hypersensitivity response to an antigen, and for this reason there is usually a history of local exposure to an antigen (e.g., atropine, poison oak) and a positive delayed skin reaction to the antigen (Fig. 3-28). A detailed discussion of contact dermatitis is presented in Chapter 1.

The methods used to treat hay fever type conditions and the more chronic VKC can also be used to alleviate the symptoms of AKC. The chronicity of AKC, the susceptibility of the atopic patient to certain infectious processes, and the tendency for atopic cataracts to develop demand that the use of corticosteroids, which can be tolerated for brief periods when necessary, be kept to an irreducible minimum.

Retinal Detachment. Coles and Laval [171] found an incidence of 22 percent of retinal detachments associated with atopic cataracts. Possible causal mechanisms may be the frequent rubbing of the eyes and the headbanging and face slapping performed by a child who is attempting to alleviate the pruritus caused by the atopic condition.

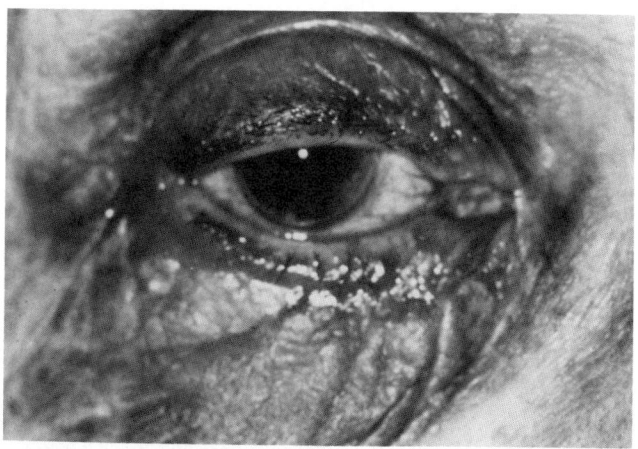

FIG. 3-27 Contact dermatitis of lids secondary to ophthalmic medication.

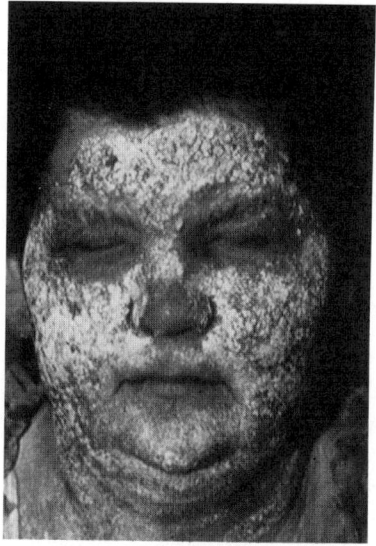
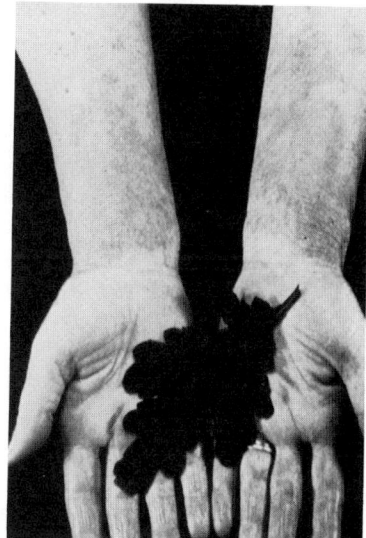

FIG. 3-28 Severe contact dermatitis on face and hands of patient exposed to poison oak.

Atopic Uveitis. Drug sensitivity of the uveal tract is rare but can be caused by atropine or physostigmine irritation of the external eye in atopic patients. The iritis presumably is due to absorption of the medication from the conjunctival sac. More frequently this type of uveitis is due to the inhalation or injection of an allergen [172].

GIANT PAPILLARY HYPERTROPHY. Loss of tolerance to contact lenses and the formation of giant papillae in the tarsal conjunctiva of the upper eyelids has been described in contact lens wearers [173]. It was first reported in 1974 [174] (Fig. 3-29). In our experience giant papillary hy-

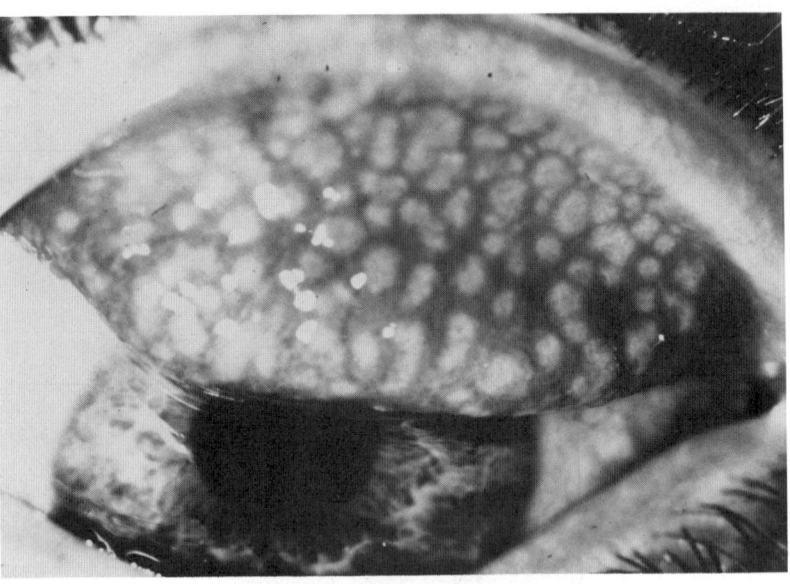

FIG. 3-29   Giant papillary conjunctivitis in a patient wearing soft contact lenses.

pertrophy (GPC) has occurred in approximately 3 to 4 percent of the patients wearing cosmetic hard contact lenses and in 5 to 10 percent of those wearing cosmetic soft contact lenses. It has been reported in patients after cataract extraction [175] and keratoplasty [176], and in patients with prostheses [177] and retained contact lenses (focal GPC) [178].

Although no association between this reaction and atopic disease has been reported [173], our own experience to date seems to indicate that there is such an association with a personal or family history of atopy or both. A substantiating fact is that atopic patients with GPC note an increase in the intensity of GPC symptoms during the spring pollen season.

The underlying cause of GPC is probably immunologic and traumatic. The presence of basophils, eosinophils, plasma cells, and lymphocytes points to its close relationship to VKC. VKC, AKC, and GPC may in fact be a mixed type I IgE and type IV CMI response.

Antigenic substances adhering to the foreign body on the eye (i.e., contact lens, prosthesis, suture) triggers the pathogenic process. Bacteria and other protein particles can provide a constant and marked dose of allergen to the upper tarsal conjunctiva. Trauma plus this immunologic exposure results in GPC.

The earliest symptoms are mild itching and a minimal white or clear exudate when the patient wakes. As the disease progresses, the itching and discharge increase and last all day, and more severe symptoms appear—increased awareness of the lens, pain on insertion of the lens, and blurring of vision. The lens no longer fits, and when the patient blinks completely, it may be pulled off the cornea and become fixed under the upper lid. The discomfort associated with wearing the lens may be so severe that it may have to be removed. The exudate usually becomes increasingly white and is quite thick and stringy.

Despite efforts to keep the lens clean, it becomes coated with fine, white deposits. The giant papillae form in the upper conjunctiva, enlarge, and then flatten. They often have the cobblestone appearance seen in patients with VKC. The surface of these papillae may stain with fluorescein during the active stages. There may be scarring of the upper palpebral conjunctiva, and in patients with severe disease a white syncytium may form in the upper half of the cornea. The bulbar conjunctiva becomes hyperemic and sometimes edematous. Trantas' dots and limbal inflammation may occur [179].

Histologic examination of the conjunctiva shows that the thickness of the epithelium overlying the giant papillae is irregular, and occasionally there is a tendency toward epidermalization and a reduction in the goblet-cell population. The epithelium contains mast cells, eosinophils, basophils, and polymorphonuclear leukocytes, and the stroma contain large numbers of lymphocytes and plasma cells [173].

Tear IgE, IgG, and IgM levels may be elevated in patients with GPC. These immunoglobulins are produced locally [180].

To treat this condition, the lens must be removed and cleaned of the deposits [181]. If the deposits cannot be cleaned, the lens must be replaced. When the same lens or a new lens of the same chemical composition is replaced in the eye, the syndrome may improve or disappear. From the improvement it can be inferred that the antigen initiating the disease is in the deposits on the lens and not in the lens itself. (The possibility exists that the lens may be defective and that monomers are present in the lens that cause the symptoms.) Sixty-five percent of patients who were treated by changing to a new lens of the same type were able to continue wearing their lenses satisfactorily [182]. Seventy-eight percent of patients whose symptoms returned after a new lens was replaced could be treated satisfactorily with a new lens and DSCG (1 drop 4 times a day). Seventy-seven percent of patients were able to be satisfactorily treated by initially changing to a different type of lens. Thus using all three modalities, 82 percent of patients were able to continue wearing contact lenses [182]. In severe cases, the patients may have to discontinue wearing the contact lens until the pathologic changes improve. The edema, hyperemia, and discharge improve rapidly whereas the giant papillae may persist for months. The use of vasoconstrictors, DSCG, or corticosteroids may speed the recovery of the ocular tissue.

In atopic patients with seasonal exacerbations of their symptoms, it may be best to remove the lens during the spring pollen season or, if this is not feasible, to institute DSCG therapy that may tide the patient over this difficult period.

ATOPIC REACTIONS TO INSECT BITES OR STINGS. The injection of foreign material into human beings by biting insects in the act of feeding is probably a universal experience, but the reactions to the foreign material differ from person to person. The commonest biting insects are the sand flies, black flies, fleas, mosquitos, and spiders.

Biting insect reactions that are severe enough to induce the victim to seek help of a physician are usually urticarial.

Hypersensitivity to stinging insects with serious or fatal anaphylactic reactions is confined almost entirely to the Hymenoptera, the most troublesome of which are honeybees, paper wasps, hornets, and yellow jackets. Fire ants are also a problem in the southern states [183].

Stinging insects inject venom into their victims, and the venom contains the sensitizing antigens. In venom there is histamine, serotonin, acetylcholine, kinin [184], hemolysin, neurotoxins, hyaluronidase, mellitin, apamine, and formic acid. Mellitin, the main toxin, can damage erythrocytes and leukocytes and can labilize lysosomal membranes. It also causes thrombocytes to release serotonin and mast cells to release their mediators [185]. Apamine acts exclusively at the neuromuscular junction. Formic acid presumably accounts for most of the pain that accompanies the stings of the Hymenoptera [186]. The major allergen in honeybee venom may be phospholipase A [187] or a combination of high-molecular-weight material and hyaluronidase [188].

Because the nonallergic inflammatory response that occurs after honeybee stings is primarily a toxic inflammatory response to mellitin or formic acid [189], it is clear that insect stings cause both immunologic and nonimmunologic responses. The allergens in the venom cause a type I IgE–mediated hypersensitivity response. There may be binding of complement as well as some of the components of the venom. Activation of the complement cascade results in inflammation of the affected tissue.

The immediate allergic reaction, ranging from simple urticaria to anaphylactic shock, makes up the majority (98%) of the hypersensitivity responses to venom. This event presupposes a previous, sensitizing sting. The much rarer delayed reaction, which appears from 24 hours to 14 days after the sting and resembles serum sickness with fever, joint symptoms, and urticaria, may accompany the patient's initial sting.

Most fatalities occur so quickly that there is no time to summon medical help. Parrish [190] reported that 92 percent of the fatalities whose records he collected from vital statistics occurred within 5 hours of the sting. Cerebral infarction may occur rapidly [191]. This finding suggests that the stinger may enter a capillary or venule. A fatality has also been associated with a corneal sting.

If the bite is on the conjunctiva, it is followed rapidly by conjunctival edema and hyperemia, and if the bite is on the cornea, there may be some corneal edema. Iritis and subsequent depigmentation of the iris may occur after wasp stings.

A patient in our care had a bee sting of the cornea. Almost immediately the patient had severe pain, which was accompanied in minutes by a reduction in visual acuity and photophobia. Four hours later there was central corneal edema around a small area of corneal staining, but no barb was found in the cornea. The bulbar conjunctiva was somewhat

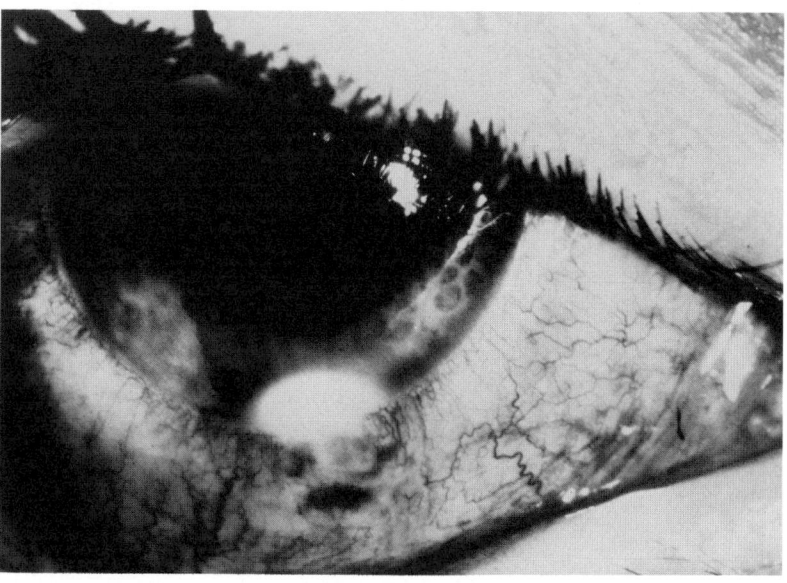

FIG. 3-30   Bee sting at corneal limbus. Sectoral infiltrate noted at site of sting. (Courtesy of Dr. Ira Wong.)

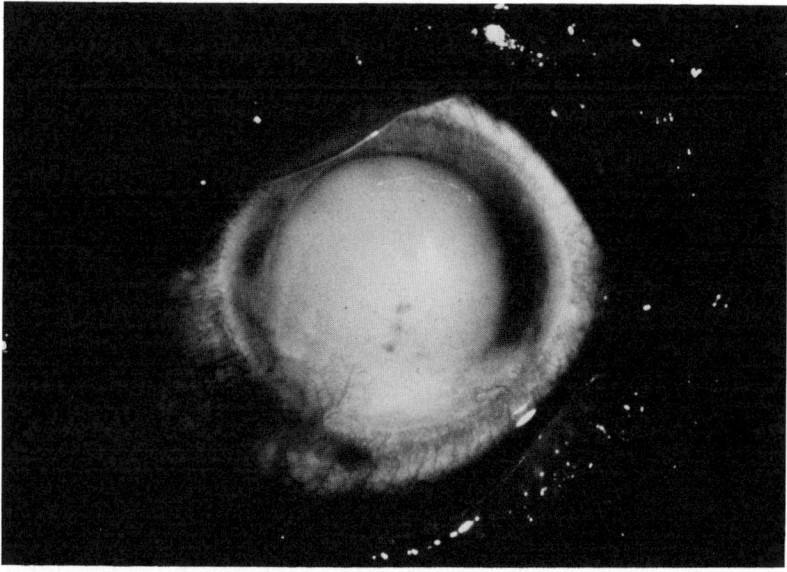

FIG. 3-31   Totally opaque cornea after wasp sting.

hyperemic, and the anterior chamber had a few cells and a trace of flare. The patient responded well to local treatment with one drop of 1 : 1,000 epinephrine and 1% prednisolone phosphate solution topically every 1 to 2 hours. Within 24 hours the reaction had subsided appreciably, and it soon disappeared without sequelae. Other cases of corneal bee stings have been associated with corneal infiltration (Figs. 3-30, 3-31). The barb itself seems to be inert [192].

Treatment consists of both emergency and preventive care. Emergency kits have been recommended for self-treatment of an acute attack [193]. Sublingual tablets of isoproterenol, 10 or 15 mg as indicated according to the age of the patient, provide protection until medical attention can be obtained. Epinephrine, 1 : 200 solution in a dispenser to use as an inhalant, should also be on hand in case of obstructive respiratory symptoms or shock. Transfusion of anti-bee venom antibody isolated from the blood of beekeepers (who are often stung) apparently neutralizes venom allergen before it can reach the patient's basophil- or mast-cell-bound IgE [194]. Desensitization [195] and hyposensitization [196] may also be effective ways to protect victims from insect stings.

General protective measures against stinging insects are (1) wearing light-colored clothes; (2) avoiding sweaty or objectionable odors, hair oils and perfumes; and (3) avoiding rapid, evasive tactics [197].

Miscellaneous allergic entities have been reported in the literature. These include an allergic periorbital mucopyocoele [198], an insect egg keratitis [199], and numerous skin reactions [200].

REFERENCES

1. Coca, A. F., and Cook, R. A. On the classification of the phenomena of hypersensitiveness. *J. Immunol.* 8:163, 1923.
2. Prausnitz, C., and Küstner, H. Studien uber die Ueberempfindlichkeit. *Zentralbl. Bakteriol. Mikrobiol. Hyg.* [A] 86:160, 1921.
3. Patterson, R. Investigation of spontaneous hypersensitivity of the dog. *J. Allergy Clin. Immunol.* 31:351, 1960.
4. Block, K. J. Immunoglobulin heterogeneity and anaphylactic sensitization. In K. F. Austen and E. L. Becker (Eds.), *Biochemistry of the Acute Allergic Reactions.* Oxford, Engl.: Blackwell, 1968.
5. Weiner, A. S., Zieve, J., and Fries, J. J. The inheritance of allergic disease. *Ann. Eugenics* 7:141, 1936.
6. Vaughan, W. T., and Black, J. H. *Practice of Allergy* (3rd ed.). St. Louis: Mosby, 1954.
7. Schwartz, M. *Heredity in Bronchial Asthma.* Copenhagen: Munksgaard, 1952.
8. Thommen, A. A. Hay fever. In A. F. Coca, M. Walzer, and A. A. Thommen (Eds.), *Asthma and Hay Fever in Theory and Practice.* Springfield, Ill.: Thomas, 1931.
9. Blanchard, G. C., and Gardner, R. The characterization of some of the antigens and allergens in ragweed pollen. *Ann. Allergy* 39:253, 1977.
10. Voorhorst, R. The human dander atopy. *Ann. Allergy* 39:295, 1977.
11. Voorhorst, R., et al. The house dust mite and the allergens it produces. *J. Allergy Clin. Immunol.* 39:325, 1976.

12. Hanson, L. A., Mausson, I. Immune electrophoresis studies of bovine milk products. *Acta Paediatr. Scand.* 50:484, 1961.
13. Fraser, C. M., Venter, J. C., and Kaliner, M. Autonomic abnormalities and autoantibodies to beta-adrenergic receptors. *N. Engl. J. Med.* 305:1165, 1981.
14. Venter, J. C., Fraser, C. M., and Harrison, L. C. Autoantibodies to beta$_2$ adrenergic receptors. *Science* 207:1361, 1980.
15. Fraser, C. M., and Venter, J. C. Autoantibodies to beta-adrenergic receptors and asthma. *J. Allergy Clin. Immunol.* 74:227, 1984.
16. Archer, C. B., Morley, J., and MacDonald, D. M. Impaired lymphocyte cyclic adenosine monophosphate responses in atopic eczema. *Br. J. Dermatol.* 109:559, 1983.
17. Kragballe, K., and Herlin, T. Antibody-dependent monocyte-mediated cytotoxicity in atopic dermatitis. *Allergy* 36:27, 1981.
18. Butrus, S. I., et al. Vernal conjunctivitis in the hyperimmunoglobulinemia E syndrome. *Ophthalmology (Rochester)* 91:1213, 1984.
19. Kjellman, N. M., Johansson, S. G. P., and Roth, A. Serum IgE levels in healthy children quantified by sandwich technique. *Clin. Allergy* 6:51, 1976.
20. Kjellman, N. M. Predictive value of high IgE levels in children. *Acta Paediatr. Scand.* 65:465, 1976.
21. Lenoir, M., Miller, J. R., and Wallace, W. Development of IgE and allergy in infancy. *J. Allergy Clin. Immunol.* 56:296, 1975.
22. Brasher, G. W. Clinical aspects of infantile asthma. *Ann. Allergy* 35:216, 1975.
23. Orgel, H. A., et al. Atopy and IgE in a pediatric allergic practice. *Ann. Allergy* 39:161, 1977.
24. Songsiridej, V., and Busse, W. W. Exercise-induced anaphylaxis. *Clin. Allergy.* 13:317, 1983.
25. Spiegelman, J., Blumstein, G. I., and Friedman, H. Effects of air purifying apparatus on ragweed pollen, mold and bacterial counts. *Ann. Allergy* 19:613, 1961.
26. Galant, S. P. β Adrenergic agonists 1984. *West. J. Med.* 141:513, 1984.
27. Taylor, W. A., et al. Anti-allergic actions of disodium cromoglycate and other drugs. *Int. Arch. Allergy Appl. Immunol.* 47:175, 1974.
28. Adachi, K., and Numano, F. Phosphodiesterase inhibitors. *Jpn. J. Pharmacol.* 27:97, 1971.
29. Falliers, C. J. Cromolyn sodium prophylaxis. *Pediatr. Clin. North Am.* 22:141, 1975.
30. Douglas, W. W. Histamine and antihistamines. In L. S. Goodman and A. Gilman (Eds.), *The Pharmacological Basis of Therapeutics* (3rd ed.). New York: Macmillan, 1965.
31. Halperin, M., Thorig, L., and Van Haeringen, N. J. Ocular side effects of antihistamine-decongestant combinations. *Am. J. Ophthalmol.* 95:563, 1983.
32. Rhoades, R. B., et al. Suppression of histamine-induced pruritus by 3 antihistaminic drugs. *J. Allergy Clin. Immunol.* 55:180, 1975.
33. Loew, E. R. Pharmacological properties of antihistamines in relation to allergic and nonallergic diseases. *Boston Med. Q.* 3:1, 1952.
34. Hui, H., Zeleznick, L., and Robinson, J. R. Ocular disposition of topically applied histamine cimetidine and pyrilamine in the albino rabbit. *Curr. Eye Res.* 3:321, 1984.
35. Rajka, G. Recent therapeutic events: Cimetidine and PUVA. *Acta Dermatov.* [Suppl.] 92:117, 1980.

36. Cummings, N. P., Morris, H. G., and Strunk, R. C. Failure of children with asthma to respond to daily aspirin therapy. *J. Allergy Clin. Immunol.* 71:245, 1983.
37. Rand, T. H., Clanton, J. A., and Colley, D. G. Arachidonic acid metabolism in the murine eosinophil. *J. Immunol.* 130:1356, 1983.
38. Flint, G. R., Morton, D. J. Effects of derivatization of the bioavailability of ophthalmic steroids. *Arch. Ophthalmol.* 102:1808, 1984.
39. Alvarez, O. M., et al. Effect of topically applied steroidal and nonsteroidal antiinflammatory agents on skin repair and regeneration. *Fed. Proc.* 43:2793, 1984.
40. Strannegard, I. L., et al. Transfer factor in severe atopic disease. *Lancet* II:702, Oct., 1975.
41. Dahl, B., et al. Lymphocyte transformation, IgE and T cells in eczema vaccinatum treated with transfer factor. *Acta Derm. Venereol. (Stockh.)* 55:187, 1975.
42. Strannegard, O., et al. FcIgG receptor-bearing lymphocytes and monoclonal antibody-defined T cell subsets in atopic dermatitis. *Int. Arch. Allergy Appl. Immunol.* 69:238, 1982.
43. Hsieh, K. Interferon-induced suppression of in vitro IgE biosynthesis in asthmatic children. *Ann. Allergy* 48:302, 1982.
44. Frankland, A. W. Seasonal hayfever and asthma treated with pollen extracts. *Int. Arch. Allergy Appl. Immunol.* 6:45, 1955.
45. Lowell, F. C., and Franklin, W. A double-blind study of treatment with aqueous allergenic extracts in cases of allergic rhinitis. *J. Allergy Clin. Immunol.* 34:165, 1963.
46. Lowell, F. C., and Franklin, W. A double-blind study of the effectiveness and specificity of injection therapy in ragweed hayfever. *N. Engl. J. Med.* 273:675, 1965.
47. Cooke, R. A., et al. Serological evidence of immunity with coexisting sensitization in a type of human allergy. *J. Exp. Med.* 62:733, 1935.
48. Loveless, M. H. Immunologic studies in pollinosis. *J. Immunol.* 47:165, 1943.
49. Lichtenstein, L. M., et al. In vitro studies of human ragweed allergy. *J. Clin. Invest.* 45:1126, 1966.
50. Salvaggio, J. E., et al. A comparison of the immunologic response of normal and atopic individuals to intranasally administered antigen. *J. Allergy Appl. Immunol.* 35:62, 1964.
51. Lichtenstein, L. M., Holtzman, A., and Burnett, L. S. A quantitative in vitro study of the chromatographic distribution and immunoglobulin characteristics of human blocking antibody. *J. Immunol.* 101:317, 1968.
52. Loveless, M. H. Immunologic studies of pollinosis. *J. Immunol.* 38:25, 1940.
53. Connell, J. T., and Sherman, W. B. The effects of treatment with emulsions of ragweed extract in antibody titers. *J. Immunol.* 91:197, 1963.
54. Feinberg, S. M., and Feinberg, A. R. Desensitization therapy with emulsified extracts. In M. Holub and J. Jarovkova (Eds.), *Mechanisms of Antibody Formation*. Prague, Czechoslovakia Academy of Sciences. New York: Grune & Stratton, 1960, p. 161.
55. Loveless, M. H. Humoral antibody and tissue tolerance induced in pollen sensitive individuals by specific therapy. *South. Med. J.* 33:869, 1940.
56. Arbesman, C. E., and Reisman, R. E. Repository pollen therapy. In E. A. Brown (Ed.), *Allergology*. London: Pergamon, 1962, p. 187.

57. Delorme, P. J., et al. Immunologic studies of ragweed-sensitive patients treated by a single repository antigen injection. *J. Allergy Clin. Immunol.* 32:409, 1961.
58. Van Arsdel, P. P., and Middleton, D. The effect of hyposensitization on the in vitro histamine release by specific antigen. *J. Allergy Clin. Immunol.* 32:348, 1961.
59. Sadon, N., et al. Immunotherapy of pollinoses in children. *N. Engl. J. Med.* 280:623, 1969.
60. Tolo, K., Brandtzaeg, P., and Jonsen, J. Mucosal penetration of antigen in the presence or absence of serum-derived antibody. *Immunology* 33:733, 1977.
61. Brauninger, C. E., and Centifanto, Y. M. Immunoglobulin E in human tears. *Am. J. Ophthalmol.* 72:558, 1971.
62. Abelson, M. B., et al. Histamine in human tears. *Am. J. Ophthalmol.* 84:417, 1977.
63. Allansmith, M. R. *The Eye and Immunology.* St. Louis: Mosby, 1982.
64. Allansmith, M. R. Personal communication, 1985.
65. Grabner, G., et al. Human cornea epithelial cells and a human conjunctival cell line producing an interleukin 3–like factor. *Invest. Ophthalmol. Vis. Sci.* 26:317, 1985.
66. Kirkegaard, J., Secher, C., and Mygind, N. Effect of the H_1 antihistamine chlorpheniramine maleate on histamine-induced symptoms in the human conjunctiva. *Allergy* 37:203, 1982.
67. Spada, C. S., et al. Histamine H_1 and H_2 receptors involved in eosinophil migration into the conjunctiva. *Invest. Ophthalmol. Vis. Sci.* 26:236, 1985.
68. Graham, H. T., et al. Distribution of histamine among the blood elements. *Blood* 10:467, 1955.
69. Levy, D. A., and Osler, A. G. Studies on the mechanisms of hypersensitivity phenomena. *J. Immunol.* 97:203, 1966.
70. Ishizaka, K., Ishizaka, T., and Terry, W. D. Antigenic structure of γ E globulin and reagenic antibody. *J. Immunol.* 99:489, 1967.
71. Lichtenstein, L. M., Norman, P. S., Osler, A. G., and Winkenwerder, W. In vitro studies of human ragweed allergy. *J. Clin. Invest.* 45:1126, 1966.
72. Wolfe, S., et al. An experimental approach to psychosomatic phenomena in rhinitis and asthma. *J. Allergy Clin. Immunol.* 21:1, 1950.
73. Holmes, T. H., Treuting, T., and Wolff, H. G. Life situations, emotions and nasal disease. *Psychosom. Med.* 13:71, 1951.
74. Corvell, J. T. Quantitative intranasal pollen challenge. *J. Allergy Clin. Immunol.* 41:123, 1968.
75. Warin, R. P., and Champion, R. H. *Urticaria.* London: Saunders, 1974.
76. Mathews, K. P. A current view of urticaria. *Med. Clin. North Am.* 58:185, 1974.
77. Shelly, W. B. Case report: An analysis of a case of chronic urticaria. *Ann. Allergy Clin. Immunol.* 24:421, 1966.
78. Zwemer, R., et al. Persistent toxic erythema and chronic urticaria. *Arch. Dermatol.* 104:390, 1971.
79. Wilson, F. M., II. Personal communication, 1985.
80. Lockshin, N. A., and Hurley, H. Urticaria as a sign of viral hepatitis. *Arch. Dermatol.* 105:570, 1972.
81. James, J., and Warin, R. P. An assessment of the role of *Candida albicans* and food yeasts in chronic urticaria. *Br. J. Dermatol.* 84:277, 1971.

82. Africk, J. A., and Halprin, K. M. Infectious mononucleosis presenting as urticaria. *J.A.M.A.* 290:1524, 1969.
83. Cherry, J. D., et al. *Coxsackie* A9 infections with exanthema. *Pediatrics* 31:819, 1963.
84. Cream, J. J., and Turk, J. L. A review of the evidence for immune-complex depositions as a cause of skin disease in man. *Clin. Allergy* 1:225, 1971.
85. Isaacs, N. J., and Ertel, N. H. Urticaria and pruritus. *J. Allergy Clin. Immunol.* 48:73, 1971.
86. Hanifin, J. M. Type 1 hypersensitivity diseases of the skin. *Ann. Allergy* 39:153, 1977.
87. Theodore, F. H., and Schlossman, A. *Ocular Allergy.* Baltimore: Williams & Wilkins, 1958.
88. Silverstein, A. M. Uveal hypersensitivity reactions to protein antigens. In A. E. Maumenee and A. M. Silverstein (Eds.), *Immunopathology of Uveitis.* Baltimore: Williams & Wilkins, 1964, p. 83.
89. Potvin, A., and Bossu, A. L'allergie en ophtalmologie. *Bull. Soc. Belge. Ophtalmol.* 106:1, 1954.
90. Leopold, I., and Leopold, H. Uveitis. In *Modern Trends in Ophthalmology* (3rd series). London: Butterworth, 1955.
91. Coles, R. S. Uveitis. In F. H. Theodore and A. Schlossman (Eds.), *Ocular Allergy.* London: Balliere, Tindall and Cox, 1958.
92. Walker, V. G. Iritis of allergic origin. *S. Afr. Med. J.* 30:132, 1956.
93. Rahi, A. H. S., and Garner, A. Immunopathology of the Eye. London: Blackwell, 1976.
94. Abelson, M. B. Conjunctival eosinophils in allergic ocular disease. *Arch. Ophthalmol.* 101:555, 1983.
95. McClellan, B. H., et al. Immunoglobulins in tears. *Am. J. Ophthalmol.* 76:89, 1973.
96. Allansmith, M. R., and McClellan, B. Immunoglobulin levels in human tears. *Invest. Ophthalmol.* 8:240, 1969.
97. Chodirker, W. B., and Tomasi, T. B., Jr. Gamma globulins. *Science* 142:1080, 1963.
98. Honsinger, R. W., Jr., Silverstein, D., and Van Arsdel, P. P., Jr. The eosinophil and allergy. *J. Allergy Clin. Immunol.* 49:142, 1972.
99. Ceska, M., Erickson, R., and Varga, J. M. Radio-immunosorbent assay of allergens. *J. Allergy Clin. Immunol.* 49:1, 1972.
100. Gordon, D. M. *Medical Management of Ocular Disease.* New York: Harper & Row, 1964, p. 104.
101. Abelson, M. D., Butrus, S. I., Weston, J. H., and Rosner, B. Tolerance and absence of rebound vasodilation following topical ocular decongestant usage. *Ophthalmology (Rochester).* 91:1364, 1984.
102. Wyngaarden, V. B., and Seevers, M. H. Toxic effects of antihistamine drugs. *J.A.M.A.* 145:277, 1951.
103. Abelson, M. B., Allansmith, M. R., and Friedlaender, M. H. Effects of topically applied ocular decongestant and antihistamine. *Am. J. Ophthalmol.* 90:254, 1980.
104. Smith, J. P., et al. Treatment of allergic conjunctivitis with ocular decongestants. *Curr. Eye Res.* 2:141, 1983.
105. Friday, G. A., et al. Treatment of ragweed allergic conjunctivitis with cromolyn sodium 4% ophthalmic solution. *Am. J. Ophthalmol.* 95:169, 1983.
106. Greenbaum, J., et al. Sodium cromoglycate in ragweed-allergic conjunctivitis. *J. Allergy Clin. Immunol.* 59:437, 1977.

107. Friedlaender, M. Personal communication, 1983.
108. Richelson, E. Tricyclic antidepressants and histamine H_1-receptors. *Mayo Clin. Proc.* 54:669, 1979.
109. Sugar, J., et al. Imipramine inhibition of ragweed allergic conjunctivitis. *Invest. Ophthalmol. Vis. Sci.* 25:217, 1984.
110. Belfort, R., Jr., et al. Indomethacin and the corneal immune response. *Am. J. Ophthalmol.* 81:650, 1976.
111. Hyndiuk, R. A., and Chin, G. N. Corticosteroid therapy in corneal disease. *Int. Ophthalmol. Clin.* 13:103, 1973.
112. Smolin, G. Medrysone hypersensitivity. *Arch. Ophthalmol.* 85:478, 1971.
113. Aquavella, J. V., Gasset, A. R., and Dohlman, C. H. Corticosteroids in corneal wound healing. *Am. J. Ophthalmol.* 58:621, 1971.
114. Meisler, D. M., et al. Late-phase hypersensitivity in vernal patients. *Invest. Ophthalmol. Vis. Sci.* [Suppl.] 20:187, 1981.
115. Frankland, A. W., and Easty, D. Vernal keratoconjunctivitis. *Trans. Ophthalmol. Soc. U.K.* 91:479, 1971.
116. Neumann, E., Blumenkrantz, N., and Michaelson, L. C. A review of 400 cases of vernal conjunctivitis. *Am. J. Ophthalmol.* 47:166, 1959.
117. Allansmith, M. R. Vernal conjunctivitis as an atopic disease. *Calif. Med.* 95:163, 1961.
118. Settipane, G. A., Connell, J. T., and Sherman, W. B. Reagin in tears. *J. Allergy Clin. Immunol.* 36:92, 1965.
119. Udell, I. J., et al. Eosinophil granule major basic protein and Charcot-Leyden crystal protein in human tears. *Am. J. Ophthalmol.* 92:824, 1981.
120. Ballow, M., et al. IgG specific antibodies to rye grass and ragweed pollen antigens in the tear secretions of patients with vernal conjunctivitis. *Am. J. Ophthalmol.* 95:161, 1983.
121. Alimuddin, M. Vernal conjunctivitis. *Br. J. Ophthalmol.* 39:160, 1955.
122. Morgan, G. The pathology of vernal conjunctivitis. *Trans. Ophthalmol. Soc. U.K.* 91:467, 1971.
123. Takakusaki, I. Fine structure of the human palpebral conjunctiva with special reference to the pathologic changes in vernal conjunctivitis. *Arch. Histol. Jpn.* 30:247, 1969.
124. Collin, H. B., and Allansmith, M. R. Basophils in vernal conjunctivitis in humans. *Invest. Ophthalmol.* 16:858, 1977.
125. Tabbara, K. F. Extralimbal Trantas' dots. *Ann. Ophthalmol.* 14:458, 1982.
126. Tobgy, A. F. Keratitis epithelialis vernalis. *Bull. Ophthalmol. Soc. Egypt* 28:104, 1935.
127. Jones, B. R. Vernal keratitis. *Trans. Ophthalmol. Soc. U.K.* 81:215, 1961.
128. Tabbara, K. F., and Butrus, S. I. Vernal keratoconjunctivitis and keratoconus. *Am. J. Ophthalmol.* 95:704, 1983.
129. Neumann, E., and Blumenkrantz, N. Mucopolysaccharide in the secretion of vernal conjunctivitis. *Br. J. Ophthalmol.* 43:46, 1959.
130. Henriquez, A. S., Kenyon, K. R., and Allansmith, M. R. Mast cell ultrastructure. *Arch. Ophthalmol.* 99:1266, 1981.
131. Rahi, A. H. S., and Buckley, R. J. Pathology of the Corneal Plaque in Vernal Keratoconjunctivitis. In G. R. O'Connor and J. W. Chandler (Eds.), Third International Symposium on the Immunology and Immunopathology of the Eye. New York: Masson Publ. U.S.A. Inc. In press, 1985.
132. Rice, N. S. C., et al. Vernal keratoconjunctivitis and its management. *Trans. Ophthalmol. Soc. U.K.* 91:483, 1971.
133. Easty, D. L., Rice, N. S. C., and Jones, B. R. Clinical trial of topical disodium

cromoglycate in vernal keratoconjunctivitis. *Clin. Allergy* 2:99, 1972.
134. Easty, D. L., Rice, N. S. C., and Jones, B. R. Disodium cromoglycate in the treatment of vernal keratoconjunctivitis. *Trans. Ophthalmol. Soc. U.K.* 91:491, 1971.
135. Ostler, H. B., Martin, R. G., and Dawson, C. R. The use of disodium cromoglycate in the treatment of atopic ocular disease. *Symp. Ocular Ther.* 10:99, 1977.
136. Ostler, H. B. Acute chemotic reaction to cromolyn. *Arch. Ophthalmol.* 100:412, 1982.
137. Abelson, M. B., Butrus, S. I., and Weston, J. H. Aspirin therapy in vernal conjunctivitis. *Am. J. Ophthalmol.* 95:502, 1983.
138. Tse, D. T., et al. Mucous membrane grafting for severe palpebral vernal conjunctivitis. *Arch. Ophthalmol.* 101:1879, 1983.
139. Singh, G. Cryoprobe for palpebral vernal catarrh. *J. Ocular Ther. Surg.* 1:273, 1982.
140. Carr, R. D., Berke, M., and Becker, S. W. Incidence of atopy in the general population. *Arch. Dermatol.* 89:27, 1964.
141. Roth, H., and Kierland, R. The natural history of atopic dermatitis. *Arch. Dermatol.* 89:209, 1964.
142. Arthur, R. P., and Shelley, W. B. The nature of itching in dermatitic skin. *Ann. Intern. Med.* 49:900, 1958.
143. Eyster, W. H., Jr., Roth, G. M., and Kierland, R. R. Studies of the peripheral vascular physiology of patients with atopic dermatitis. *J. Invest. Dermatol.* 18:37, 1952.
144. Lobitz, W. C., Jr., and Campbell, C. J. Physiologic studies in atopic dermatitis. *Arch. Dermatol.* 67:575, 1953.
145. Szentivanyi, A. The beta adrenergic theory of the atopic abnormality in bronchial asthma. *J. Allergy Clin. Immunol.* 42:203, 1968.
146. Taylor, B., et al. Transient IgA deficiency and pathogenesis of infantile atopy. *Lancet* 2:111, 1973.
147. Krain, L., and Terasaki, P. HLA types in atopic dermatitis. *Lancet* 2:1059, 1973.
148. Ohman, S., and Johansson, S. G. O. Immunoglobulins in atopic dermatitis. *Acta Derm. Venereol.* 54:1974.
149. Shakib, F., et al. Elevated serum IgE and IgG4 in patients with atopic dermatitis. *Br. J. Dermatol.* 97:59, 1977.
150. Johansson, S. G. O. Raised levels of a new immunoglobulin class (IgND) in asthma. *Lancet* 2:951, 1967.
151. Juhlin, L., et al. Immunoglobulin E in dermatoses. *Arch. Dermatol.* 100:12, 1969.
152. Jones, H. E., et al. Atopic disease and serum immunoglobulin E. *Br. J. Dermatol.* 92:17, 1975.
153. Jansen, C. T., Haapalahi, J., and Hopsu-Havu, V. K. Immunoglobulin E in the human atopic skin. *Arch. Dermatol. Forsch.* 246:299, 1973.
154. Carapeto, F. J., Winkelmann, R. K., and Jordon, R. E. T and B lymphocytes in contact and atopic dermatitis. *Arch. Dermatol.* 112:1095, 1976.
155. Raza, A., Maibach, H. K., and Shinefield, H. R. Microbial flora of atopic dermatitis. *Arch. Dermatol.* 113:780, 1977.
156. Rogge, J. L., and Hanifin, J. M. Immunodeficiencies in severe atopic dermatitis. *Arch. Dermatol.* 112:1391, 1976.
157. Palacios, J., Fuller, E. W., and Blaylock, W. K. Immunological capabilities of patients with atopic dermatitis. *J. Invest. Dermatol.* 47:484, 1966.

158. Gottlieb, B. R., and Hanifin, J. M. Circulating T cell deficiency in atopic dermatitis. *Clin. Res.* 22:159, 1974.
159. Clark, R. A., et al. Defective neutrophil chemotaxis and cellular immunity in a child with recurrent infections. *Ann. Intern. Med.* 78:515, 1973.
160. Hanifin, J. M., Bauman, R., and Rogge, J. L. Chemotaxis inhibition by plasma from patients with atopic dermatitis. *Clin. Res.* 25:198A, 1977.
161. Snyderman, R., Rogers, E., and Buckley, R. H. Abnormalities of leukotaxis in atopic dermatitis. *J. Allergy Clin. Immunol.* 60:121, 1977.
162. Strannegard, I., and Strannegard, O. Natural killer cells and interferon production in atopic dermatitis. *Acta Dermatov.* 92:48, 1980.
163. Rostenberg, A., Jr., and Solomon, L. J. Infantile eczema in systemic disease. *Arch. Dermatol.* 98:41, 1968.
164. Reed, W. B., et al. Cutaneous manifestations of ataxia-telangiectasia. *J.A.M.A.* 195:746, 1966.
165. Peterson, R. D. A., Page, A. R., and Good, R. A. Wheal and erythema allergy in patients with agammaglobulinemia. *J. Allergy Clin. Immunol.* 33:406, 1962.
166. Buckley, R. H., Ray, B. B., and Belmaker, E. Z. Extreme hyperimmunoglobulinemia E and undue susceptibility to infection. *Pediatrics* 49:59, 1972.
167. Busse, W. W., and Tee-Ping, L. Decreased adrenergic responses in lymphocytes and granulocytes in atopic eczema. *J. Allergy Clin. Immunol.* 58:585, 1976.
168. Hanifin, M. J. Newer concepts of atopic dermatitis. *Arch. Dermatol.* 113:663, 1953.
169. Hogan, M. J. Atopic keratoconjunctivitis. *Am. J. Ophthalmol.* 36:937, 1953.
170. Beetham, W. P. Atopic cataracts. *Arch. Ophthalmol.* 24:21, 1940.
171. Coles, R. S., and Laval, J. Retinal detachments occurring with cataracts associated with neurodermatitis. *Arch. Ophthalmol.* 48:30, 1952.
172. Fein, R., and Swinny, S. Atopic uveitis. *Ann. Allergy* 10:599, 1952.
173. Allansmith, M. R., et al. Giant papillary conjunctivitis in contact lens wearers. *Am. J. Ophthalmol.* 83:697, 1977.
174. Spring, T. F. Reaction to hydrophilic lenses. *Med. J. Aust.* 1:499, 1974.
175. Friedman, T. Giant papillary conjunctivitis following cataract extraction. *Ann. Ophthalmol.* 16:50, 1984.
176. Sugar, A., Meyer, R. F. Giant papillary conjunctivitis after keratoplasty. *Am. J. Ophthalmol.* 91:239, 1981.
177. Meisler, D. M., Krachmer, J. H., and Goeken, J. A. An immunopathologic study of giant papillary conjunctivitis associated with an ocular prosthesis. *Am. J. Ophthalmol.* 92:368, 1981.
178. Stenson, S. Focal giant papillary conjunctivitis from retained contact lenses. *Ann. Ophthalmol.* 14:881, 1982.
179. Meisler, D. M., Zaret, C. R., and Stock, E. L. Trantas' dots and limbal inflammation associated with soft contact lens wear. *Am. J. Ophthalmol.* 89:66, 1980.
180. Donshik, P. C., and Ballow, M. Tear immunoglobulins in giant papillary conjunctivitis induced by contact lenses. *Am. J. Ophthalmol.* 96:460, 1983.
181. Mondino, B. J., Salamon, S. M., and Zaidman, G. W. Allergic and toxic reactions in soft contact lens wearers. *Surv. Ophthalmol.* 26:337, 1982.
182. Donshik, P. C., Ballow, M., Luistro, A., and Samartino, L. Treatment of contact lens–induced giant papillary conjunctivitis. *C.L.A.O.* 10:346, 1984.
183. Carol, M. R., Derbes, V. J., and Jung, R. Skin response to the sting of the imported fire ant. *Arch. Dermatol.* 75:475, 1957.

184. Jacques, R., and Schacter, M. The presence of histamine, 5 hydroxytryptamine and a potent slow contracting substance in wasp venom. *Br. J. Pharmacol.* 9:352, 1954.
185. Mackler, B. F., and Kreil, G. Honey bee venom mellitin. *Inflammation* 2:55, 1977.
186. Brock, T. Resume of insect allergy. *Ann. Allergy* 19:288, 1961.
187. Sobotka, A. K., et al. Allergy to insect stings. *J. Allergy Clin. Immunol.* 57:29, 1976.
188. Hoffman, D. R., and Shipman, W. H. Allergens in bee venom. *J. Allergy Clin. Immunol.* 58:551, 1976.
189. Mackler, B. F., and Kreil, G. Honey bee venom mellitin. *Inflammation* 2:55, 1977.
190. Parrish, H. M. Analysis of 460 fatalities from venomous animals in the United States. *Am. J. Med. Sci.* 245:35, 1963.
191. Starr, J. C., and Brasher, G. W. Wasp sting anaphylaxis with cerebral infarction. *Ann. Allergy* 39:431, 1977.
192. Smolin, G., and Wong, I. Bee sting of the cornea. *Ann. Ophthalmol.* 14:342, 1982.
193. Barnard, J. H. Allergic reaction to insect stings and bites. *N.Y. J. Med.* 261:374, 1959.
194. Beekeepers can donate immunity to stings. *Clinical Trends* 15:8, 1976.
195. Mueller, H. L. Insect Allergy. In D. P. Brennemann (Ed.), *Practice of Pediatrics,* Vol. II. New York: Harper & Row, 1968.
196. Barr, S. E. Prolonged interval immunotherapy of hymenoptera sting allergy. *Ann. Allergy* 36:308, 1976.
197. Morse, R. A., and Ghent, R. L. Protective measures against stinging insects. *N.Y. J. Med.* 59: 1546, 1959.
198. De Juan, E., Jr., Green, W. R., and Iliff, N. T. Allergic periorbital mucopyocele in children. *Am. J. Ophthalmol.* 96:299, 1983.
199. Bullock, J. D., Albert, D. M., and Richman, S. J. Insect egg keratitis. *Am. J. Ophthalmol.* 78:339, 1974.
200. Schulz, K. H. Cutaneous Manifestations of Drug Allergy. In A. L. deWeck and P. Bundgaard (Eds.), *Handbook of Experimental Pharmacology.* Berlin: Springer-Verlag, 1983, p. 135.

4   IMMUNOLOGIC REACTIONS LIMITED TO THE EXTERNAL EYE

A large number of local, nonatopic immunologic diseases affect the external ocular tissue. For the purposes of this chapter diseases are divided into the type of hypersensitivity response they evoke.

CYTOTOXIC (TYPE II HYPERSEN-SITIVITY) REACTIONS

The immunoglobulins (antibodies) concerned with cytotoxic reactions are usually IgG and IgM. When they bind to antigens on the cell surfaces, they cause (1) phagocytosis of the cell by opsonic or immune adherence with complement factor 3b (C3b), (2) nonphagocytic extracellular cytotoxicity by the killer (K) lymphocytes, or (3) cell lysis through the operation of the full complement system up to C8,9. These mechanisms are discussed in detail in Chapter 1.

Corneal Allograft Reaction

A long-standing corneal allograft that has withstood the first onslaught of the cell-mediated immune (CMI) reaction can evoke antibodies in the host that are directed against the graft's surface-transplantation (histocompatibility; HLA) antigens. These antibodies can induce the three reactions listed in the preceding paragraph. A detailed discussion of the corneal graft reaction is presented in Chapter 6.

Drug-Related Reactions

In general, many drugs may elicit nonimmune or various types of immune reactions. For example, penicillin may elicit a type I, II, III, or IV hypersensitivity reaction, which can, respectively, manifest itself by (1) acute anaphylaxis or urticaria; (2) hemolytic anemia, thrombocytopenia, or interstitial nephritis; (3) serum sickness, drug fever, or cutaneous eruptions; or (4) contact dermatitis.

    When a drug acts as a hapten attached to a cell membrane, a cytotoxic type of reaction can occur. The hemolytic anemia that follows the systemic administration of a variety of medications is a cytotoxic reaction,

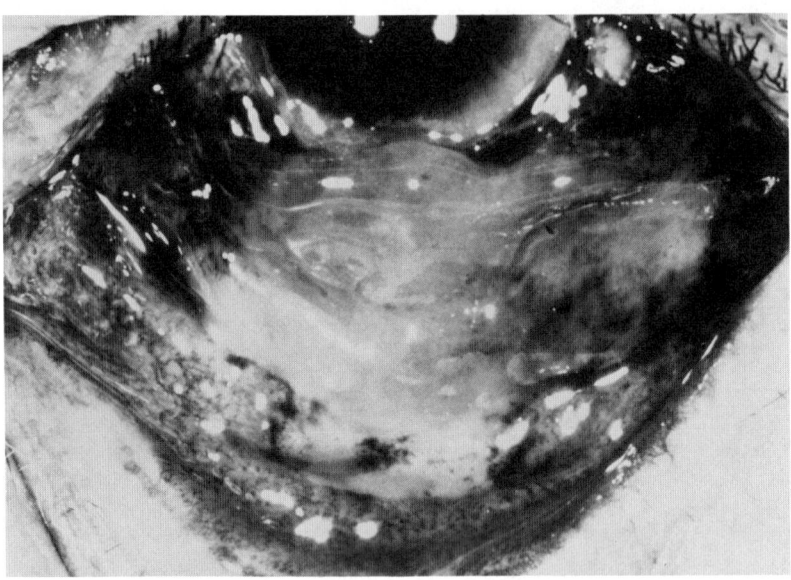

FIG. 4-1 Conjunctival slough and scarring after subconjunctival injection of gentamicin.

and certain locally applied drugs can cause a cytotoxic reaction in the ocular adnexal tissues. Although there are no proven examples of clearly cytotoxic drug reactions of the tissues of the external eye, several drugs—gentamicin, physostigmine (eserine), isoflurophate (diisopropyl fluorophospate; DFP), neostigmine, iododeoxyuridine (IDU), pilocarpine, phenylephrine (Neo-Synephrine), and furtrethonium iodide (furmethide)—can produce necrosis and subsequent scarring of the conjunctiva [1] in addition to nonimmune toxic effects (Figs. 4-1, 4-2). It may be that these drugs can act as haptens, attaching to external ocular tissue and ultimately causing an immune response to the tissue-drug complex.

Two cases of unilateral "ocular pseudopemphigoid" occurred after the long-term use of echothiophate iodide (Phospholine Iodide) [2] (Fig. 4-3). There was suggestive evidence that the reactions in these patients were type II hypersensitivity (cytotoxic) reactions, but the authors were unwilling to exclude the possibility that the clinical picture was produced by nonimmune toxic effects of the drug. In both patients the lesions were restricted to the eye in which the drug had been used.

The clinical signs in these two patients were conjunctival scarring and shrinkage, conjunctival epidermalization, symblepharon formation, foreshortening of the inferior conjunctival fornices, and punctal occlusion. The cornea was normal in one patient, but in the other there was an apparently sterile corneal ulcer with vascularization. Histopathologic examination showed subepithelial fibrosis, a reduced number of goblet cells, and stromal infiltration with plasma cells and lymphocytes. Immunofluorescent studies of the biopsy from one patient showed stromal plasma cells that stained for IgA, IgD, IgE, and C3, but there was no

4. REACTIONS LIMITED TO THE EXTERNAL EYE

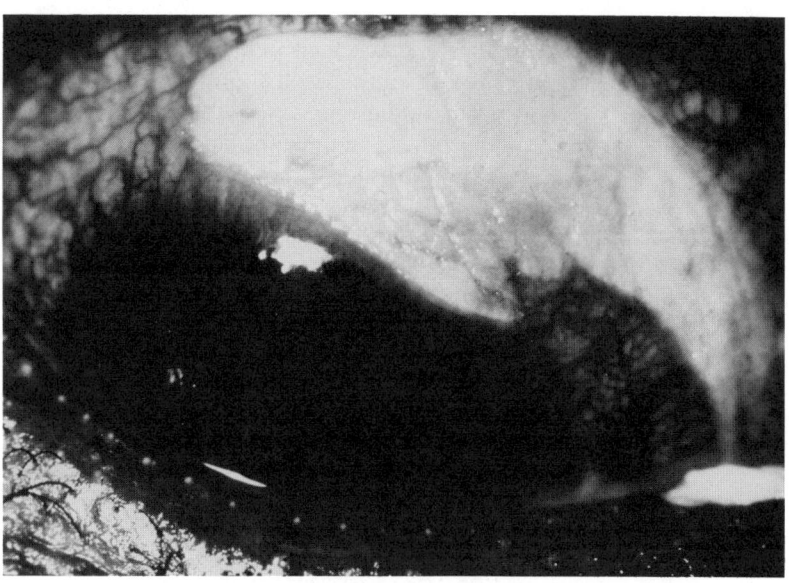

FIG. 4-2 Keratinization caused by toxic reaction to chronic use of pilocarpine.

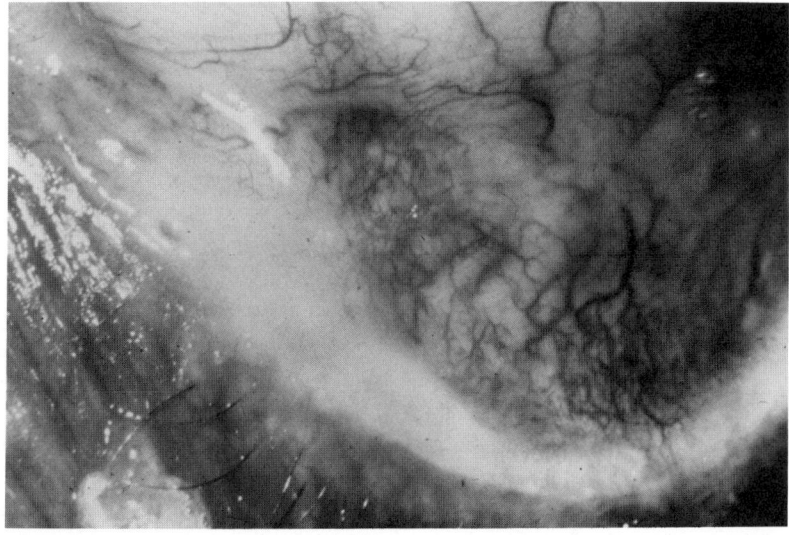

FIG. 4-3 Early symblepharon formation and scarring after long-term use of echothiophate iodide.

epithelial- or basement-membrane staining such as that seen in pemphigus vulgaris or cicatricial pemphigoid. The affected eye of the second patient showed plasma-cell staining for IgD, IgG, IgA, and IgE, and interepithelial and basement-membrane staining for IgG. The interepithelial and basement-membrane staining disappeared 3 weeks after the drug was discontinued.

Mooren's Ulcer Although Mooren's corneal ulcer, a clinical entity of uncertain origin, was first reported by Bowman in 1849 [3], Mooren is credited with being one of the first to recognize in 1867 the features of the disease that distinguish it from other types of corneal ulceration [4, 5].

PATHOGENESIS. Although strong evidence suggests that Mooren's ulcer is an autoimmune phenomenon, its precise cause remains something of a mystery. Because it is sometimes preceded by infection or trauma to the ocular tissue [5–7], it can be hypothesized that the corneal tissue is altered by this process so that it is no longer recognized as "self" and elicits an immune response. A number of investigators [8–10] have shown that the corneal epithelium possesses an organ-specific antigen. This antigen may diffuse into the anterior third of the stroma [8], and in its natural or altered form may play a role in initiating this immunologic response. This assumption would seem to be logical because the disease process is limited to the corneal epithelium and anterior third of the stroma, and because removal of this tissue can frequently bring about a remission of the disease process.

Patients with Mooren's ulcer may be more susceptible to responding to this self antigen because of an immune defect. Indeed, T-suppressor lymphocytes have been shown to be decreased in a Mooren's ulcer patient [11].

The abundance of plasma cells and eosinophils in the conjunctival and corneal tissue strongly suggests that patients with Mooren's ulcer have an immune disease. The plasma cells may be producing antibody that binds with the corneal antigen–binding complement, which then attracts polymorphonuclear leukocytes. (In several patients with Mooren's ulcer, complement has been found in the corneal epithelium in association with IgM and IgG [12].) In addition, IgG and C3 have been found in the conjunctiva. The large number of polymorphonuclear leukocytes in the overhanging edge may release the enzymes that degrade the collagen and corneal proteoglycans and produce the ulceration at the periphery of this edge and beyond. Collagenase may also be produced by the conjunctiva. In one patient with Mooren's ulcer, circulating antibodies to corneal tissue were found [13].

Some observers have concluded that the conjunctiva plays an important role in the immunopathologic process of Mooren's ulcer. Our belief is that the conjunctiva is no more important than the cornea in eliciting the immune response, but that for anatomic reasons it may later become laden with more effector cells and substances (e.g., plasma cells, lymphocytes, polymorphonuclear leukocytes, complement) than the cornea.

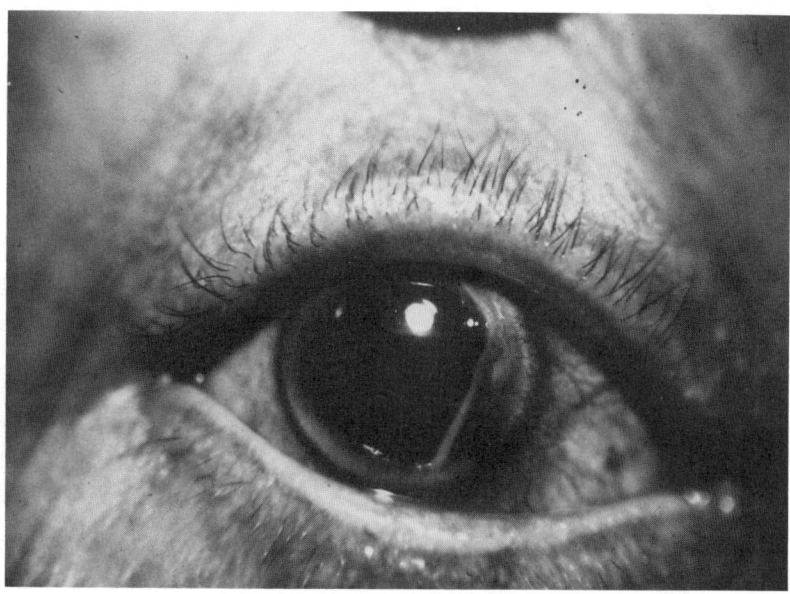

FIG. 4-4 Mooren's ulcer. Note gray overhanging edge.

The role of the CMI response in Mooren's ulcer is still being studied (several patients have demonstrated migration inhibition factor to corneal antigens in their serum) [14].

CLINICAL FEATURES. Mooren's ulcer is a chronic, progressive, marginal nonpurulent ulcer that begins as an infiltrate in the anterior stroma, destroys the epithelium overlying the stroma, and then spreads circumlimbally or centripetally. In approximately 35 percent or more of affected patients it is bilateral. Like the corneal ulcers that occur in Wegener's granulomatosis and polyarteritis nodosa, Mooren's ulcer shows no unaffected area between the corneal lesion and the limbus. (In this way it differs from the ulcers associated with rheumatoid arthritis or those that occur in Terrien's type of peripheral ulceration.)

Mooren's ulcer starts in the medial and lateral quadrants. Typically its gross features are a gray overhanging edge, involvement of the anterior one-third or one-half of the corneal layers, and minimal cicatrization (Fig. 4-4). Some of the ulcerated areas may be active while others seem to be healing. The ulcer normally runs a course of from 3 to 12 months and has been known to recur in scarred, healed corneas. The course is sometimes severe and leaves the patient with a badly damaged cornea and almost no vision (Fig. 4-5). Although the whole cornea may be covered with scar tissue, 2 or 3 years later the vision may improve to as much as 20/100. Corneal sensation remains normal or only slightly reduced, both hypopyon and perforation are rare, and the concomitant iritis is mild (Fig. 4-6).

Pain starts early in patients with Mooren's ulcer but only becomes se-

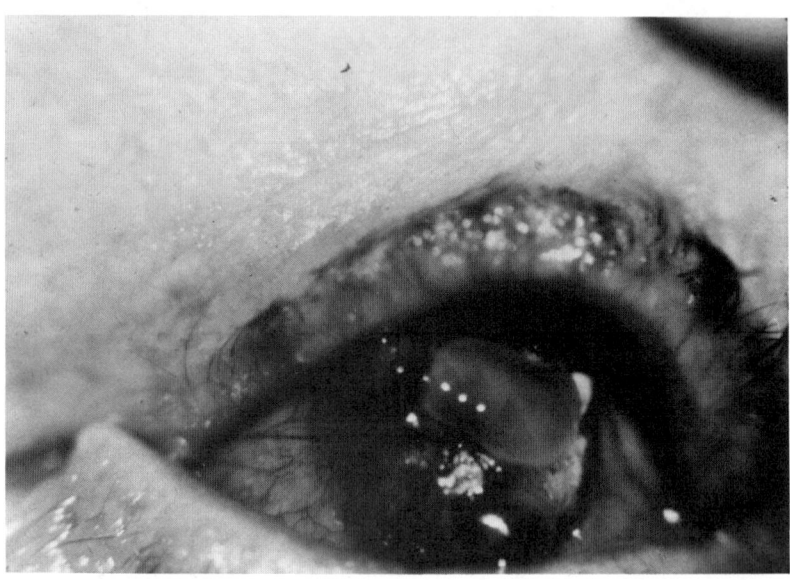

FIG. 4-5   Severely damaged cornea in Mooren's ulcer. Ectatic cornea present centrally.

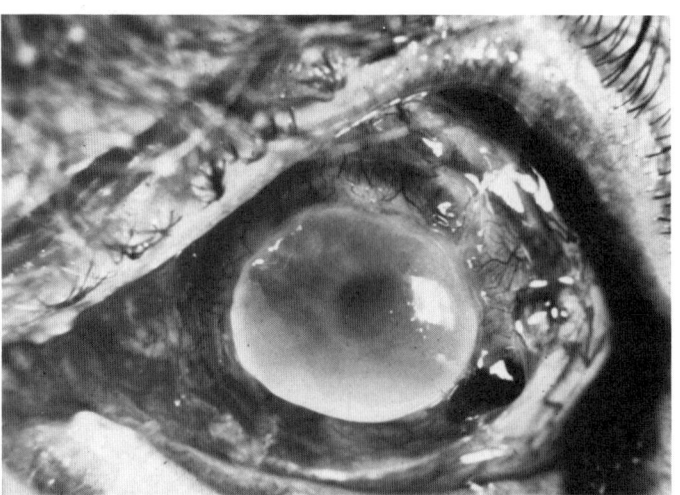

FIG. 4-6   Rare perforation in peripheral cornea in Mooren's ulcer.

vere as the lesion develops. The pain is often unresponsive to topical medication (anesthetics, antiinflammatory agents) and may be so severe that the patient wants the eye removed and sometimes, regrettably, is accommodated.

Mooren's ulcer seems to be more common in Africa than elsewhere and has been seen in persons of all ages. With reference to age, there appear to be two types. The type that occurs in young adults (third de-

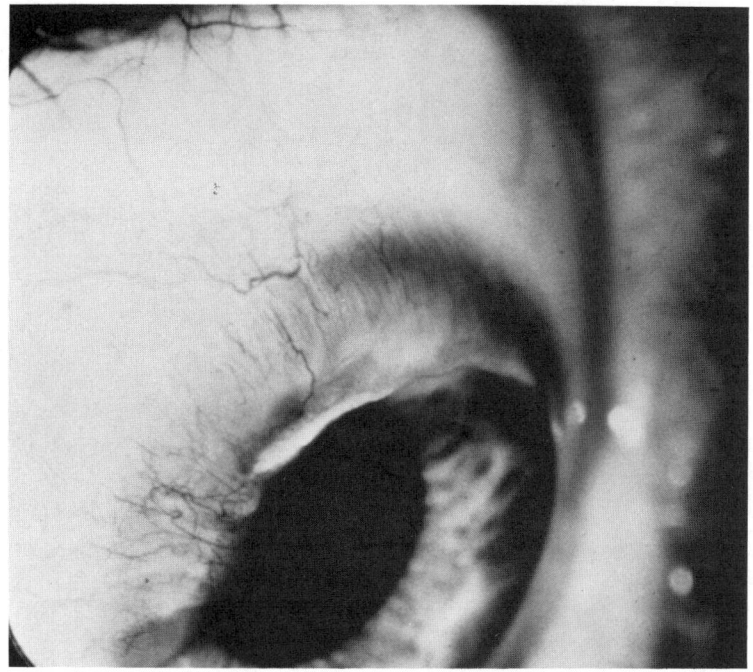

FIG. 4-7   Terrien's degeneration. Note vascularization and lipoidal deposits.

cade of life), occurs more frequently in men (3 : 1) and in blacks, is bilateral 75 percent of the time, and runs a rapidly progressive course [15]. The pain is severe, the prognosis poor, and fully one-third develop corneal perforation [16]. Frequently, there is an antecedent history of trauma or operation [6]. In the type that occurs in older persons, men are more frequently affected (3 : 2), there is no racial predilection, and it is bilateral 25 to 30 percent of the time. This type runs a slower, relentless course, perforations are rare, and the prognosis is fair [17].

DIAGNOSIS. In diagnosing this disease, a number of entities must be taken into consideration. In staphylococcal catarrhal ulceration an infiltrate near the limbus is followed by an epithelial breakdown. But the lesion usually does not progress; does not cause limbal ulceration; does not affect the sclera; does not develop the gray overhanging edge; and is not severely painful.

The marginal ulceration in Terrien's degeneration usually starts bilaterally in the superior nasal quadrant of each cornea. It may progress circumlimbally and become vascularized. In severe cases, inflammation and lipoidal deposits occur (Fig. 4-7). The sclera is usually not affected, the ulceration does not extend to the limbus or centrally, no overhanging edge develops, the pain is usually minor, and the disease runs a self-limited and more benign course than Mooren's ulcer. Perforation may

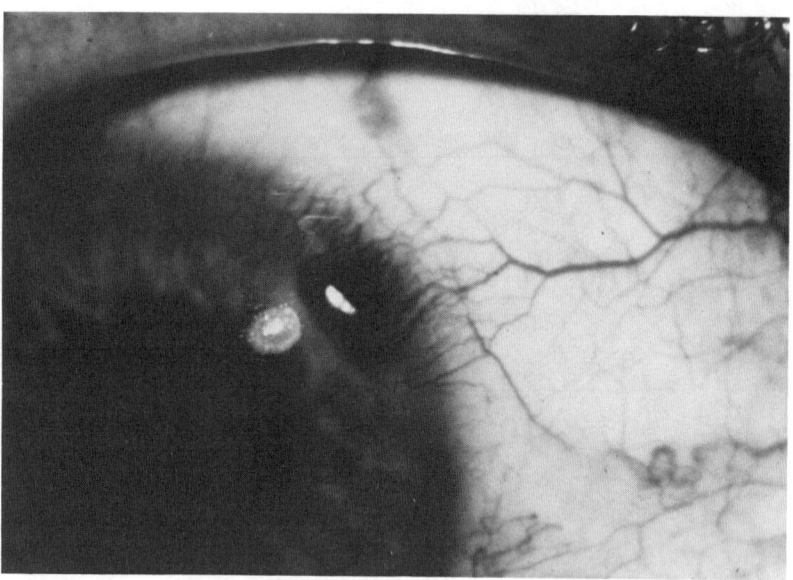

FIG. 4-8   Perforation in Terrien's degeneration.

occur (Fig. 4-8). The patient's visual acuity is often unaffected except for some astigmatic changes in refraction.

Infectious peripheral ulcers (e.g., pneumococcal, gonococcal) are more yellowish white than Mooren's ulcer, are often accompanied by a copious exudate (purulent on occasion), and show marked scleral hyperemia and corneal infiltration.

The corneal lesions that most clearly mimic Mooren's ulcer are those associated with Wegener's granulomatosis [18] and polyarteritis nodosa. Although both these conditions may start as infiltrates, later they ulcerate, and the ulceration may affect both limbus and sclera and progress circumlimbally. The ocular changes, although often concurrent with various systemic signs, may be the first indications of the two diseases with which they are associated.

Marginal ulcers owing to rheumatoid arthritis occur more frequently in females, are bilateral 50 percent of the time, and are associated with minimal or no pain; the ulcer has no gray overhanging edge. The limbus and sclera may not be involved in the process.

HISTOPATHOLOGIC FINDINGS. The pathologic examination of the corneal tissue from a Mooren's ulcer shows active inflammation in the anterior stroma, especially in the area of the overhanging edge. The cells are principally polymorphonuclear leukocytes, but there are also some lymphocytes and eosinophils. The posterior stroma is largely unaffected. There is necrosis in the anterior stroma, with loss of basement membrane, Bowman's layer, and epithelium. In the base of the ulcer, plasma cells abound [19, 20] and there are a number of lymphocytes and giant cells.

The conjunctival epithelium adjacent to the affected cornea is intact, and the subepithelial tissue is packed with plasma cells and an occasional polymorphonuclear leukocyte or monocyte. The metabolic products from a tissue culture of the conjunctiva in these eyes can degrade collagen and corneal proteoglycan.

TREATMENT. The treatment of Mooren's ulcer—medical and surgical—has had limited success.

Initial therapy is with topical corticosteroids, usually prednisolone acetate 1%. The medication is applied hourly, and application is increased to every 30 minutes around the clock if there is no evidence of epithelial healing within several days [21]. If the ulcer heals completely the medication is tapered and finally stopped. Topical antibiotics can be added (i.e., tobramycin or gentamicin t.i.d.) to prevent secondary bacterial infection.

If there is no response or an incomplete one, then conjunctival excision can be performed in the operating room. If both forms of therapy are ineffective then, in conjunction with an internist or oncologist, immunosuppressive therapy can be initiated systemically. The combination of cyclophosphamide, 100 mg/day, and prednisone, 60 mg/day, has been employed most frequently for the treatment of Mooren's ulcer. The drugs may have to be administered for months before a notable beneficial response is noted.

Older patients and those with unilateral Mooren's ulcer are more responsive to therapy. Bilateral, severe Mooren's ulcer may be unresponsive to any form of therapy.

Because Mooren's ulcer may be due to enzymes that degrade collagen and corneal proteoglycan, neutralizing this degradation with inhibitors of the enzymes has been attempted. Local applications of the patient's own serum seem to have some beneficial effect, and a new collagenase inhibitor (Provera) is now being used to alter the ulcer's unrelenting course. Patching the eye [22] and giving subconjunctival injections of heparin [23] have also been added to the therapeutic regimen, but without improved results.

Placing a hydrophilic contact lens over the ulcer may dramatically relieve the pain [24]. However, it in no way affects the course of the disease.

Both lamellar keratectomy and conjunctival flaps have been used without any apparent success. Gifford [25] recommended a delimiting keratectomy for the treatment of Mooren's ulcer. He reopened the wound daily so that the aqueous from the anterior chamber could pass through the diseased cornea. It was his conviction that this procedure lessened the severity of the disease materially, and some still advocate it when all other forms of therapy fail. Why this technique should work is obscure, however. It is thought that the secondary aqueous possesses factors (e.g., collagenase inhibitors or blocking antibodies) that alter the course of the disease.

Maumenee (personal communication, 1978) recommended removing the anterior third of the cornea, especially when a ring ulcer formed and the central cornea had a mushroom configuration. Brown and Mondino [21] found this form of therapy to be successful in a limited number of patients. It can perhaps safely be assumed that this procedure would remove the inciting antigen. In any event, the beneficial results of this therapy are consistent with our concept that the inciting antigen lies in the corneal epithelium and may possibly diffuse into the anterior third of the stroma.

IMMUNE-COMPLEX-MEDIATED (TYPE III) REACTIONS

Reactions Related to Infection

A comprehensive, general discussion of the immunology of infection is presented in Chapter 1. The immune-complex–mediated, cytotoxic, and CMI responses all play important roles in the development of ocular infectious disease, and all are discussed in this section for the convenience of covering infectious disease all in one place.

BACTERIAL INFECTIONS

Staphylococcal Infections. An important feature of staphylococcal infection is the organism's ability to produce extracellular substances that enhance its ability to multiply and spread widely in the tissues. These substances are exotoxins (extracellular bacterial toxins), leukocidins (bacterial toxins that destroy polymorphonuclear leukocytes), coagulases (enzymes that accelerate the formation of blood clots), and enterotoxins (toxins specific for the cells of the intestinal mucosa). *Staphylococcus aureus* is thought to be able to produce L-phase variants (viable bacteria without walls) in the presence of antibiotics, reemerging as fully virulent organisms when the antibiotic is withdrawn. The surface of the staphylococcus is covered with a substance called *protein A* that inhibits phagocytosis. Because phagocytosed staphylococci can remain viable for long periods, the organism is likely to produce chronic, latent, or smoldering infections of long duration.

Bacteria possess a large number of transmissible plasmids the genetic products of which induce bacterial resistance to a specific antibiotic when it is used to treat a host harboring a particular bacterium [26]. Staphylococci are particularly likely to develop resistant strains, but strains of *Pseudomonas* resistant to antibiotics such as gentamicin have also been reported [27].

When lymphocytes sensitized to *S. aureus* are reexposed to the organism, they can liberate lymphokines, including migration inhibition factor (MIF) [28]. Staphylococcal enterotoxins can stimulate both mitogenic activity and lymphokine production in lymphocytes [29]. The CMI response is clearly important in the body's defense against staphylococci and may play a major role in the pathogenesis of phlyctenulosis owing to staphylococci.

The rationale for using staphage lysate to treat recalcitrant staphylococcal ocular infections is to take advantage of the patient's previous exposure to the staphylococcus. The immune response induced by previous contact is a first step in the mobilization of cell-mediated immunity. The next requirement is for reticuloendothelial cells that are specially

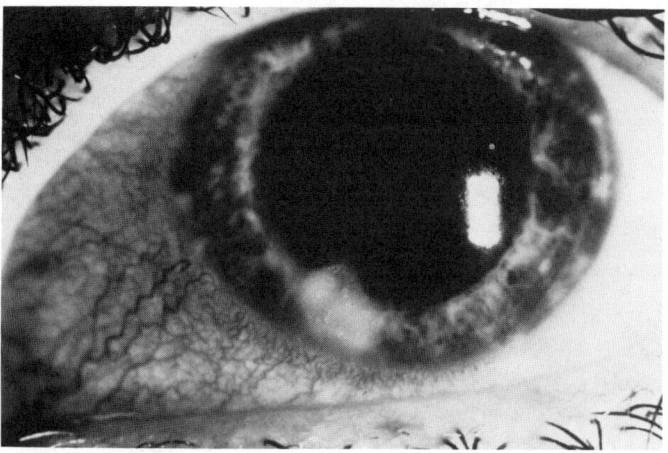

FIG. 4-9 Round catarrhal infiltrate with no overlying ulceration. Note lucid interval at limbus.

committed to action against *S. aureus* to come in contact with the antigen. When this intermediate step is completed properly, monocytes and macrophages become activated and symptoms improve [30].

In patients with neutrophil dysfunction, alteration of the normal bacterial flora probably occurs and marginal keratitis results [31].

The catarrhal marginal ulceration and infiltration seen with staphylococcal infections are probably antigen-antibody reactions to staphylococcal antigens and exotoxins. The immune complex binds complement, which then attracts the polymorphonuclear leukocytes that account for the clinical appearance of the lesion. The catarrhal infiltrates appear near the limbus and remain near or at the limbus, possibly because there is an appropriate concentration of antigen and antibody in this area (the zone of optimal proportions) (Figs. 4-9, 4-10).

This hypothesis would seem to be confirmed by the fact that if a limbal pannus exists, the catarrhal infiltrates do not occur at the limbus but centrally, some 1 to 2 mm from the pannus. No organisms are found in scrapings from the ulcerated area, which again suggests that the catarrhal ulceration is an immune phenomenon.

The marginal catarrhal ulcer begins as a marginal infiltrate that extends more deeply than the midstroma. There is a lucid interval between the infiltrate and the limbus, and the conjunctiva in the area is hyperemic. The infiltrate may be anywhere in the circumference of the cornea but is usually where the lid margin crosses the limbus (at the 10, 2, 4, and 8 o'clock positions). This location may be due to the concentration of the antigen or toxin at these sites.

The infiltrate may regress without scarring if no necrosis has occurred, or it may progress to an actual breakdown of the overlying epithelium, and finally to a peripheral ulcer. Necrosis may be followed by vasculari-

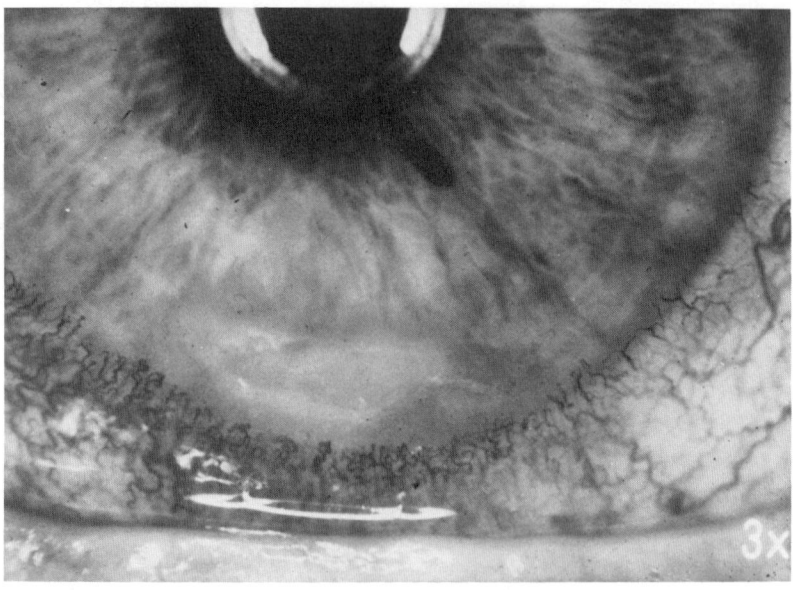

FIG. 4-10   Linear catarrhal infiltrate with overlying ulceration. This clinical pattern may be difficult to differentiate from marginal herpes simplex keratitis.

zation of the affected cornea. Untreated, the catarrhal infiltrate or ulcer usually clears in from 4 to 14 days after its onset.

Patients who wear contact lenses (especially soft lenses) sometimes develop peripheral catarrhal infiltrations and ulcerations of unknown cause, which may be clinically indistinguishable from the staphylococcal type of lesion described previously. Most of them also have mild to moderate staphylococcal blepharitis or keratitis. As in all staphylococcal blepharitis, the lids show (1) scales (hard, brittle, and fibrinous, or matted and crusted with underlying ulcers), (2) dilated blood vessels, (3) white lashes (poliosis), (4) lash loss (madarosis), (5) trichiasis, and (6) collarettes. Seborrhea, hordeolum (Figs. 4-11, 4-12), or angular blepharitis may be coexistent, and there is almost invariably a chronic papillary conjunctivitis. If there is also a toxic keratitis, it predominates in the inferior quadrants of the cornea as small, flat, punctate lesions that are regular in pattern and stain with fluorescein.

The peripheral catarrhal ulcerations owing to soft contact lens improve if the lenses are removed for a few days. If a more loosely fitting lens is used, the recurrence rate of the lesion is sharply reduced. It is the author's experience that treating any associated blepharitis with antibiotic therapy also lessens the likelihood of recurrence when the contact lenses are replaced. If rapid improvement of the catarrhal infiltrate is urgent then treating the eye with the medication usually used to treat staphylococcal catarrhal marginal infiltration will be effective. Taken together, these therapeutic results strongly suggest that the disease is related to anoxia or possibly staphylococcal blepharitis, or both.

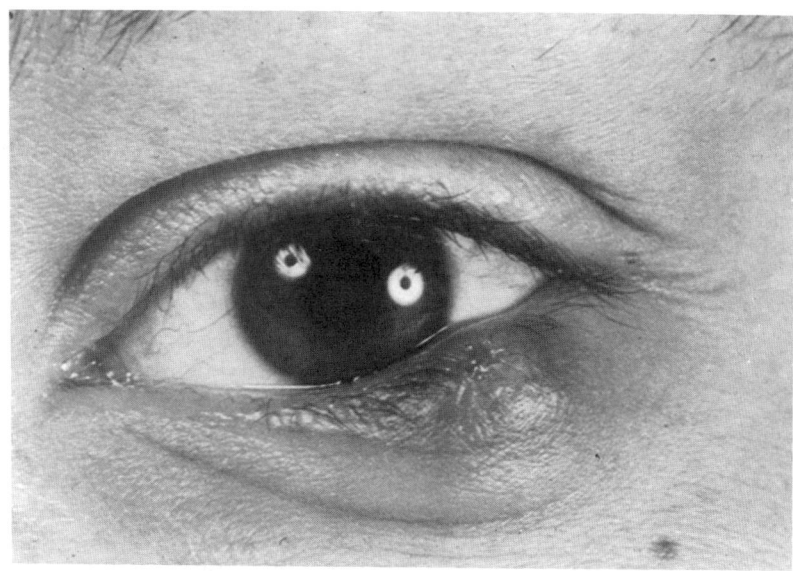

FIG. 4-11   Hordeolum.

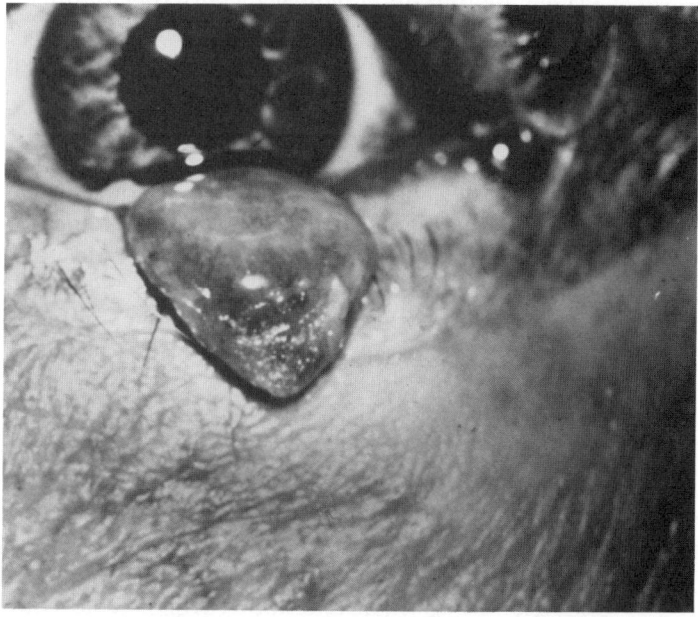

FIG. 4-12   Excessive granulation tissue produced in patient with chronic meibomian gland infection.

Catarrhal marginal ulcers are also seen occasionally in acute catarrhal conjunctivitis owing to *Hemophilus aegyptius* in adults, in chronic conjunctivitis owing to *Moraxella lacunata,* and in hemolytic streptococcal disease [31, 32]. In these infections the marginal lesions are presumed to be immune-complex-mediated reactions to the organisms.

It is important to differentiate the type of catarrhal infiltration described in the preceding paragraphs from marginal herpes simplex virus (HSV) infection. The first sign of marginal herpes is the epithelial defect. The infiltration arises later. This is the reverse of the catarrhal infiltration-ulceration sequence. The corneal sensation over the herpetic lesion is almost always greatly diminished or absent and only rarely normal; the corneal sensation over the catarrhal infiltrate is usually normal or slightly diminished.

Marginal herpetic keratitis causes fewer symptoms than the catarrhal ulcer. A history of a trigger or of previous herpetic ocular disease may also be helpful in differentiating the two types of lesions. The catarrhal ulcer responds rapidly (in days) to a therapeutic regimen that includes antibiotic and corticosteroid therapy, whereas the marginal herpetic lesion usually does not respond to such therapy or resolve spontaneously in so short a time.

Successful treatment of the staphylococcal catarrhal lesion depends on (1) eliminating the organisms where they originate (usually on the lids), and (2) altering the pathologic response of the peripheral cornea.

The appropriate antibiotic ointment is applied to the lids. In longstanding disease, the patient may have received many antibiotics, and running sensitivity tests on a culture of the organisms may be warranted. Because the applications of ointment may blur the vision for 10 to 15 minutes, they should be scheduled as conveniently as possible. The severity of the blepharitis dictates the frequency of application. A daily bedtime application may be successful in mild cases, but severe cases may require three or four daily applications. Sulfasoxazole (Gantrisin) [33], bacitracin, and erythromycin ophthalmic ointments are effective against most staphylococcal organisms and are excellent choices for the initial course of treatment. If necessary, gentamicin is an excellent alternative choice [34].

The catarrhal corneal ulcer can be treated by adding corticosteroid drops to this regimen. The dose ranges from 0.12% prednisolone two or three times a day to 1.0% four or more times a day. The low dose is principally antiinflammatory; the high dose may also be immunosuppressive [35] and therefore appropriate for the treatment of an immunologic reaction. An antibiotic-corticosteroid combination need not be used, however. The treatment of the lid-margin infection requires an antibiotic ointment, and the catarrhal ulcer is best treated by the addition of corticosteroid drops. If this regimen is followed, the catarrhal ulcer should heal within 24 to 48 hours [36].

In recalcitrant cases, especially those associated with acne rosacea, systemic antibiotics can be added to the treatment regimen. Tetracycline or erythromycin, 250 mg four times a day, is particularly effective.

In rare instances, multiple staphylococcal catarrhal infiltrates coalesce to form ring infiltrates; ring infiltrates are usually seen in association with gonococcal conjunctivitis or in cases of endophthalmitis or panophthalmitis [37]. In these latter conditions, the immunopathogenesis has yet to be worked out. Some investigators believe that the endotoxin from such gram-negative organisms as *Pseudomonas aeruginosa* and *Escherichia coli* can bind complement, attract polymorphonuclear leukocytes, and produce corneal rings [38].

OTHER BACTERIAL INFECTIONS. The following ocular responses that can be immunologically mediated can also be elicited by bacteria.

Membranous Conjunctivitis. Membranous conjunctivitis can be produced by severe infection with staphylococci, meningococci, gonococci, *Haemophilus* sp., and other microorganisms [39–41]. A true membrane is a massive exudation of fibrin and proteinacious fluid that permeates the conjunctival epithelium and superficial substantia propria and produces coagulative necrosis and cicatrization.

Ligneous Conjunctivitis. Ligneous conjunctivitis is a more severe but similar response [42, 43]. Its cause is uncertain, but β-hemolytic streptococcus has been implicated [44]. Whether only a certain type of β-hemolytic streptococcus can elicit this unusual response is unknown. One can hypothesize, however, that certain streptococci can do so (as they can in other tissues such as the heart, kidneys, and grafted tissue), and that the unusual response is a rare, bilateral, membranous conjunctivitis. Occurring in childhood, the disease is characterized by woodlike (hence "ligneous") induration of the palpebral conjunctiva. It runs a chronic and relentless course (Figs. 4-13, 4-14). Attempts to remove the membrane cause severe hemorrhages, and in a short time new membranes appear and are even thicker than the previous ones [45]. Rarely, extension of the membrane onto the bulbar conjunctiva occurs (Fig. 4-15).

Treatment with diathermy, sometimes combined with hyaluronidase and chymotrypsin, or with broad-spectrum antibiotics seems to have been somewhat successful [44, 45]. Several patients have been cured with cromolyn sodium (disodium cromoglycate; DSCG). The efficacy of DSCG may be the result of an alteration of the immune component of the disease; the drug reduces the release of pharmacologic mediators from mast cells and basophils.

If ligneous conjunctivitis is indeed caused by an unusual immune response to β-hemolytic streptococci in the ocular tissue, then appropriate antibiotic therapy (to eliminate the antigen), combined with an attempt to alter the tissue response with DSCG, α chymotrypsin, and hyaluronidase, seems like a reasonable approach to therapy.

Granulomatous Conjunctivitis. Granulomatous conjunctivitis was first described by Parinaud in 1889 [46]. The causative agents have since been determined, but the exact role of the immune response has yet to be elucidated. The disease is discussed here as an unusual immune response to a variety of infectious agents.

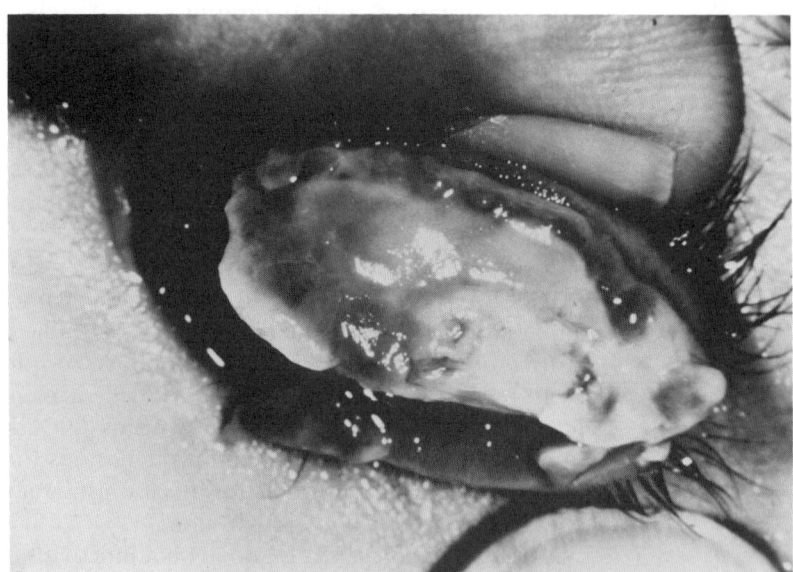

FIG. 4-13 Ligneous conjunctivitis.

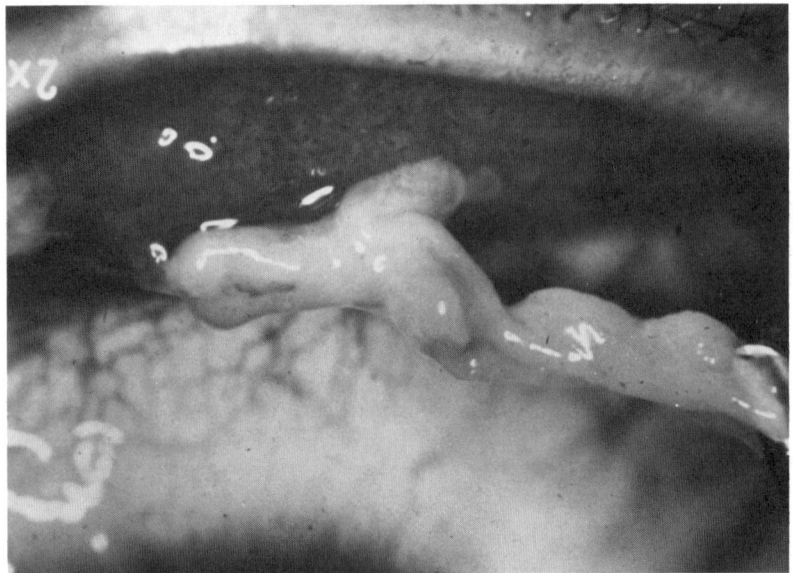

FIG. 4-14 Dissectable membrane formation in a patient with ligneous conjunctivitis.

4. REACTIONS LIMITED TO THE EXTERNAL EYE

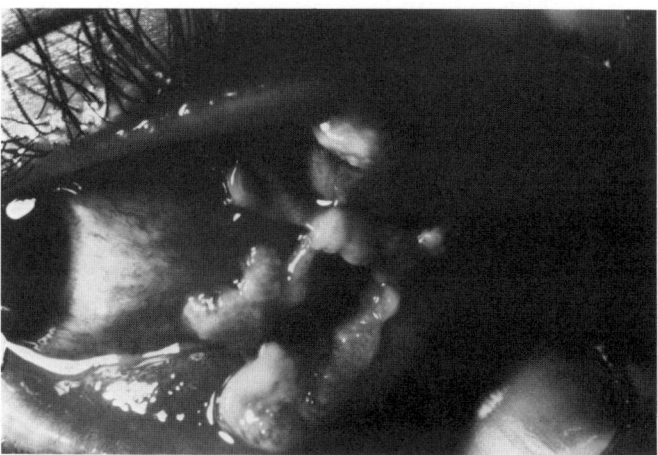

FIG. 4-15 Membrane in ligneous conjunctivitis extending onto bulbar conjunctiva.

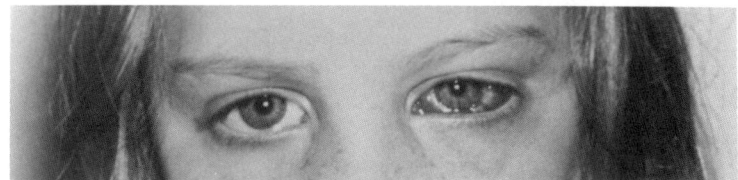

FIG. 4-16 Parinaud's oculoglandular syndrome (granulomatous conjunctivitis): unilateral conjunctivitis with enlarged regional lymphadenopathy.

Parinaud's patients had conjunctivitis with granulation and ulceration. There was regional lymphadenopathy that suppurated, and some patients had fever. The disease was self-limited, healing in 4 to 5 months (Fig. 4-16).

This now well-known conjunctivitis is usually unilateral and has granulomatous nodules or vegetations (with or without ulcerations or follicles) and regional lymphadenopathy (Figs. 4-17, 4-18). There may also be fever, malaise, diarrhea, and other systemic signs and symptoms. The diseases with which it is associated etiologically are most often cat-scratch disease [47–49], tularemia [50, 51], and tuberculosis [52]; less often syphilis, sarcoidosis, sporotrichosis [53], chalazion, and coccidioidomycosis [54]; rarely chancroid, yersinia, Hansen's disease (leprosy), glanders, listeriosis, lymphogranuloma venereum, actinomycosis, blastomycosis, infectious mononucleosis, and Mediterranean fever.

Pseudomonas species Ve-1 has been isolated from patients with cat-scratch disease. The criteria for diagnosing this disease is now: (1) a history of animal contact, (2) negative findings for other causes of lymphadenopathy, (3) a positive skin test for cat-scratch disease, and (4) pleomorphic gram-negative bacillus in the tissue.

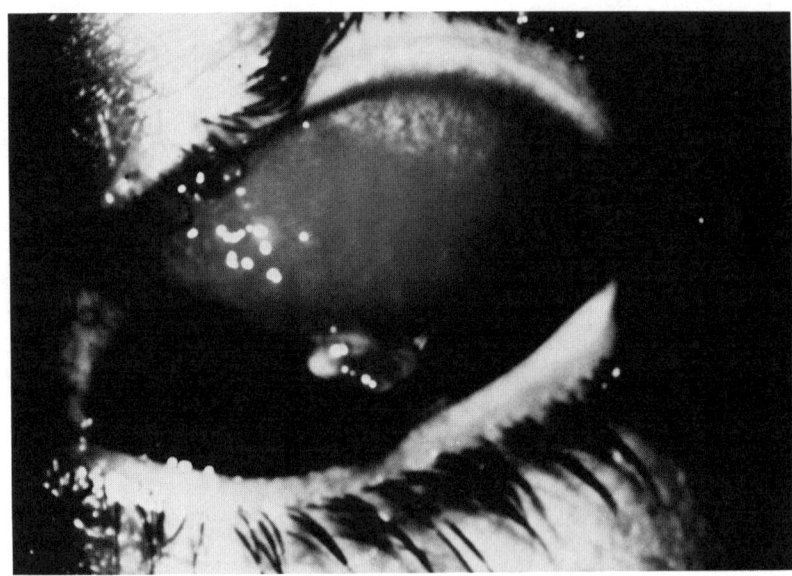

FIG. 4-17 Granuloma surrounded by papillary response in Parinaud's oculoglandular syndrome (granulomatous conjunctivitis).

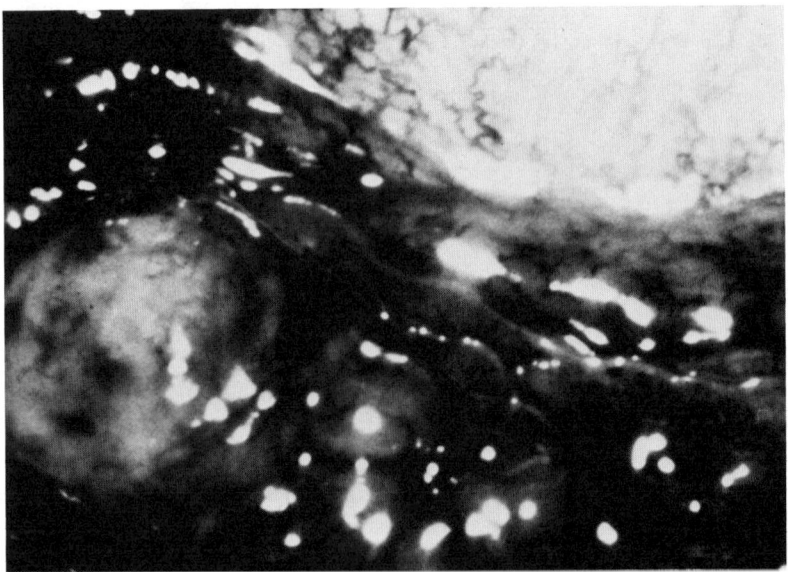

FIG. 4-18 Granuloma surrounded by follicular response in Parinaud's oculoglandular syndrome (granulomatous conjunctivitis).

CHLAMYDIAL INFECTIONS. With few exceptions (e.g., *Moraxella* infections in children), the response of the conjunctival tissues to bacterial infections is papillary. In contrast, chlamydial and viral agents usually evoke a follicular response in both the bulbar and palpebral conjunctiva. The pathophysiologic reason for this characteristic response has not been clearly established. When follicles heal, they sometimes leave scars that are pathognomonic of a specific disease (e.g., Herbert's pits at the limbus in trachoma).

Although IgG and IgM have been detected in the sera of animals infected experimentally with chlamydiae [55, 56], any antibody resistance to infection is apparently attributable to locally formed secretory IgA [57]. In human beings with chlamydial infections, elevated levels of IgA, IgG, and IgE have been found in the tears [58]. This alteration may be the result of an outpouring of the immunoglobulins from the dilated conjunctival blood vessels associated with the infectious process. There is no convincing evidence that these antichlamydial immunoglobulins exert any notable effect on the disease process, however [59]. Even after immunization, their protective effect is short-lived and of questionable value [60].

Studies of the trachoma organism have shown that trachoma-sensitive guinea-pig lymphocytes cultured in the presence of trachoma antigen release lymphokines (i.e., skin-reactive factors and lymphocytotoxic factor) [61], which is a clear indication that cell-mediated immunity [62] participates in the defense of the host against the chlamydial agent. It is also possible that the CMI response rather than any cytopathic quality of the chlamydial agent is responsible for the tissue necrosis [63]. Some investigators believe, in fact, that the immune response is totally responsible for the pathologic tissue findings in chlamydial disease [64].

VIRAL INFECTIONS. The herpetic antigen [65] and herpesviruslike particles [66] have been identified in the cornea, conjunctiva, tear film, iris, and trigeminal ganglion [67]. In stromal herpetic keratitis, herpetic antigenic determinants can be incorporated into the cell walls of infected cells. The cells are then permanent antigenic reservoirs and may stimulate subsequent immune reactions [68, 69]. Herpes simplex virus (HSV) may also possess collagenolytic activity [70], which would account for some of its virulence.

The sensory ganglion acts as a reservoir of HSV between attacks of overt disease [67]. When a trigger mechanism (e.g., fever, stress [71], or ultraviolet light) activates the HSV in the ganglion, the virus may be shed into the tear film and recurrence may follow. The trigger mechanisms themselves may so affect various components of the immune surveillance system that some control over the HSV is lost.

The role of antibodies in HSV keratoconjunctivitis is probably subsidiary to T-cell function. In patients subject to recurrent herpetic vesicles on the lips, there is evidence of impaired CMI [72] responsiveness and low levels of natural killer (NK) cells. NK cells may play an important role in the resistance to herpes in human beings [73]. A study of T-cell activity in patients with herpetic keratitis has shown that patients with impaired CMI responses are more likely to develop stromal lesions than patients with normal CMI response; those with intact T-cell function usually develop only epithelial lesions [74]. (There has been some difference of opinion on this point, however.)

Cells infected with HSV form a low-molecular-weight protein that can interfere with subsequent viral replication. The mechanism is complex, but it is probably that this protein (interferon) initiates the formation of a second protein that prevents the genetic information in the virus from being conveyed to the nucleic-acid replicating mechanism of the cell. The enzymes protein kinase and oligoadenylate may play a role. There is also evidence that T cells and activated macrophages can secrete "immune interferon" [75, 76]. Interferon appears in rabbit corneas soon after their injection with HSV and prior to the appearance of local antibody [77]. The early arrival of this lymphokine at the site of infection implies that it probably plays a role in the host's recovery from herpetic keratitis. By virtue of its minute size, the interferon particle is readily diffusible and can prevent adjacent cells from forming more virus. Interferon affects viral adherence and penetration of a cell and viral multiplication within the cell. It may stimulate NK cell activity.

In several studies [78], human interferon and interferon inducers have been used to treat herpetic keratitis. In one study [79] the inducers were somewhat helpful in treating the active corneal infection but had no effect on recurrences, and in other studies the topical application of interferon was effective in diminishing the recurrence rate [80] and viral shedding [81, 82].

Viral infections are associated, first with increased levels of IgM, then with increased levels of IgG in the circulating bloodstream, and finally with the appearance of IgA antibodies in the mucosal secretions. It is the CMI response that plays the major role in controlling intracellular virus or viral antigen in the cell walls. The local and systemic antibody produced by the initial infection may play a role in reinfection [78] or in the systemic spread of the infection.

Antibodies destroy the extracellular virus. Viruses that are combined with antibody, especially IgA, are prevented from adhering to cell membranes and thus infecting tissue cells. The opsonization and immune adherence (expressions of the type II cytotoxic hypersensitivity response) that are promoted by IgG antibodies facilitate the phagocytosis and neutralization of the virus. Complement fixation and subsequent lysis of the virus occur only when the outer antigenic mantle is derived from the membrane of the infected cell; otherwise the virus may continue to be viable despite its combination with antibody.

The HLA-B5 antigen was found to be notably more common in patients with corneal HSV infection than in a control population and HLA-B8/DRw3 was found more often in patients with herpes labialis, a difference which suggests a relationship between recurrences of HSV keratitis and a genetically abnormal immunoreactivity [83].

Different strains of HSV have different virulences, and the severity of

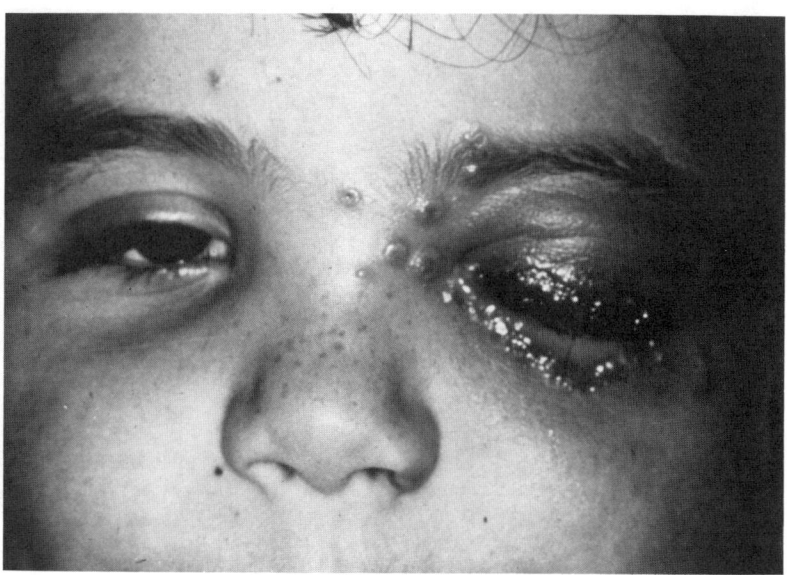

FIG. 4-19   Herpetic lid vesicles and ulcers. Concomitant conjunctivitis is present.

the clinical disease may depend not only on the host's immune response but the strain of HSV as well.

Clinical Features. In primary HSV ocular infection the lesions usually affect the lids and conjunctiva. Corneal lesions may occur later. The infection is usually acute and severe, and there may be pseudomembrane formation; subconjunctival hemorrhages; follicular hypertrophy of the conjunctiva; enlarged, tender preauricular nodes; and lid vesicles and ulcers (Fig. 4-19). There is an associated rising titer of serum antibody to HSV.

In recurrent HSV ocular infection, the typical corneal lesion (an exceedingly rare conjunctival lesion) is the epithelial dendrite, often marginal (Fig. 4-20). Follicular conjunctival hypertrophy predominates, and there are abundant mononuclear cells and a few multinucleated giant cells in corneal and conjunctival scrapings. HSV may affect both stromal corneal tissue and uveal tissue. Cases of recurrent attacks of presumed HSV infection have been reported in which an initial uveitis was followed by corneal disease later in the same attack or in a subsequent recurrence. The stromal or uveal HSV disease may be associated with some form of CMI depression [84–89] owing to medication (e.g., corticosteroids) or to the host's currently depressed state as a result of malnutrition, old age, or systemic disease.

The several types of stromal infiltration may be related to direct viral cytotoxicity (necrosis) or to the host's immune response; that is, to antigen-antibody complexes (ring infiltrate) or to the CMI response (disciform edema and infiltrate).

The partial or complete ring infiltrate appears to be identical to the

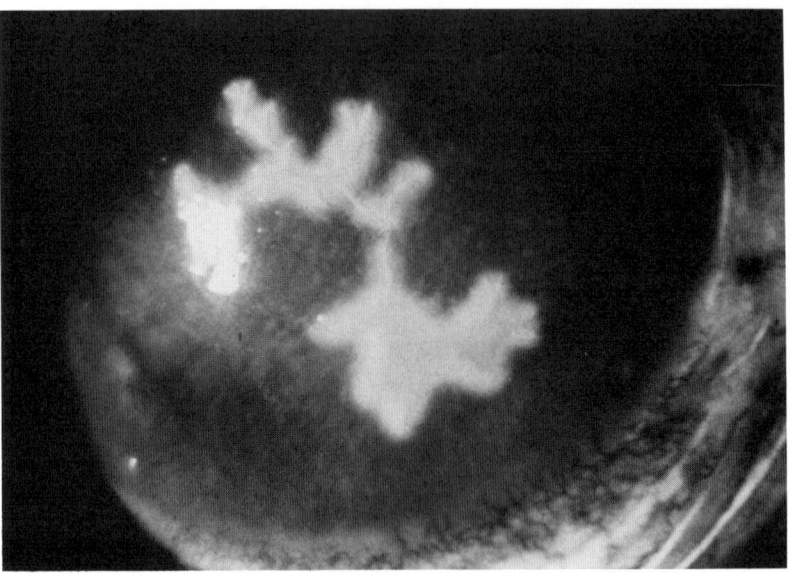

FIG. 4-20   Dendritic herpetic lesion.

Wessely ring produced in the corneas of experimental animals by the intracorneal injection of a foreign antigen. These ring infiltrates are clearly an immune phenomenon and have been produced in the rabbit cornea by the intrastromal injection of HSV antigen into animals previously systemically sensitized to HSV [88]. This experimentally produced ring represents the local accumulation of polymorphonuclear leukocytes brought to the area by HSV antigen, HSV antibody, and complement complexes. The formation of the ring can be blocked if the animals receive treatment to suppress their polymorphonuclear leukocyte response, or if the complement component C3 is inactivated by cobra venom.

In disciform keratitis, the disk-shaped area of clouding varies in size and shape, and its density depends on the amount of edema and infiltration with lymphocytes and polymorphonuclear leukocytes (Fig. 4-21). Histopathologic features include edema, minimal focal necrosis of the stromal lamellae, and swelling of the keratocytes. If the necrosis is extensive, vascularization may also take place [89]. Mild disciform keratitis usually heals with little or no scarring despite its persistence for weeks or months. Small amounts of corticosteroids may produce a partial or complete clearing of the edema and infiltrates [90]. The disciform lesions may be the CMI response to the viral antigens incorporated into the cell membrane [91–93].

The corneal subepithelial infiltrates noted in adenoviral infections may also be an immune response to the foreign viral antigen (Fig. 4-22). The initial disease affects the corneal epithelium, and then, some 1 or 2 weeks later, the subepithelial opacities arise. This interval may be the

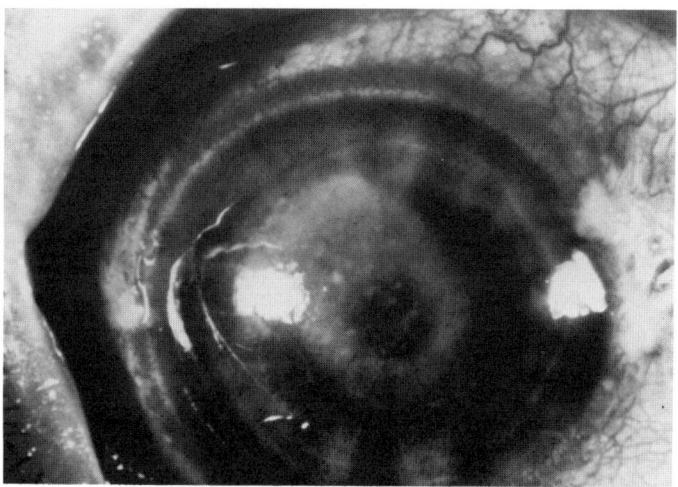

FIG. 4-21   Disciform edema in herpetic keratitis. Note underlying keratic precipitates.

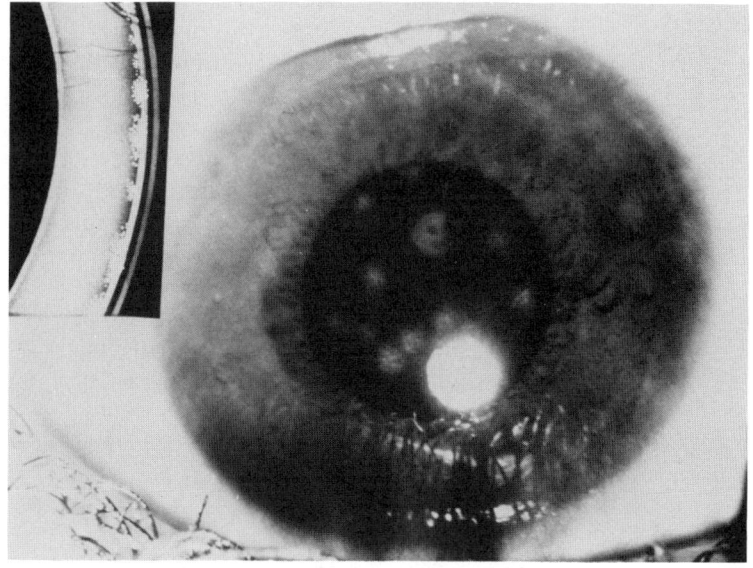

FIG. 4-22   Subepithelial infiltrates in patient with adenovirus infection.

time required for the initial viral antigenic challenge to evoke an immune response, which then sends sensitized effector cells into the cornea. Histologically the infiltrates consist of a minimal accumulation of lymphocytes and polymorphonuclear leukocytes. No viral particles can be identified in these subepithelial areas. It is also possible that they are a direct result of viral cytotoxicity (the virus residing in the epithelium). Corticosteroids can clear the subepithelial opacities rapidly, but as soon as the medication is withdrawn, they reappear [94]. There is an interesting report of a Stevens-Johnson syndrome occurring with an adenovirus conjunctivitis [95].

TREATMENT. To date treatment of acute corneal epithelial HSV keratitis, consisting of debridement or topical chemotherapy (or both) aimed at preventing viral synthesis and adherence, has been effective. But in chronic HSV keratitis (epithelial or stromal) and HSV uveitis, local treatment has been somewhat disappointing. Antiviral (especially acyclovir) and corticosteroid therapy has been used for stromal and anterior uveal herpetic inflammation. Cyclosporin and trifluorothymidine has also been employed for herpetic stromal disease [96] on the premise that the effector cells and virus are both directly or indirectly responsible for the inflammation.

Systemic antivirals (acyclovir) may be especially effective for herpes zoster infections affecting the eye [97] (Fig. 4-23). Topical acyclovir is also helpful [98].

Early reports of viral inactivation by topically applied dyes combined with exposure to ultraviolet light have prompted many clinical trials [99]. The results have been inconsistent. Recently the desirability of the method has been subject to considerable speculation because of reports that it has apparently produced in vitro malignant transformation of infected animal cells [100]. The potentiation of humoral immunity with such procedures as smallpox vaccination to induce a "bystander" response is of little or no benefit [101], and autoinoculation [102] and vaccines have been equally disappointing [103]. Immune globulin has been used to treat viral ocular infections (e.g., vaccinia, herpes zoster) [104], but in patients so treated there has been more disciform keratitis (probably a manifestation of an immune reaction).

The use of immunopotentiators for the treatment of ocular viral infections is still experimental and controversial [105], but it offers an exciting avenue for future research. The use of leukocyte interferon is discussed in Chapter 1. Some of the other agents that have been used successfully are levamisole [106–108], transfer factor [109, 110] and other lymphokines [111–113], *Mycobacterium bovis* (bacillus Calmette-Guerin; BCG) [114–116], *Corynebacterium parvum* [117–119], vitamin A [120, 121], thymosin [122, 123].

Levamisole acts by boosting the stimulating effect of an antigen on phagocytic and lymphocytic function rather than directly. Depressed hosts are most affected, and the cells that are stimulated are principally macrophages and T-lymphocytes. Levamisole has little or no effect on humoral immunity and little toxic effect. There have been a few reports of agranulocytosis associated with levamisole administration [124, 125]. When patients with recurrent corneal ulcers, recurrent herpes labialis, and recurrent herpes genitalis were treated with levamisole, the majority responded with a rapid and dramatic reduction in the duration and severity of the lesions and in the frequency of recurrences [107]; and after treatment was discontinued, many patients remained symptom-free for

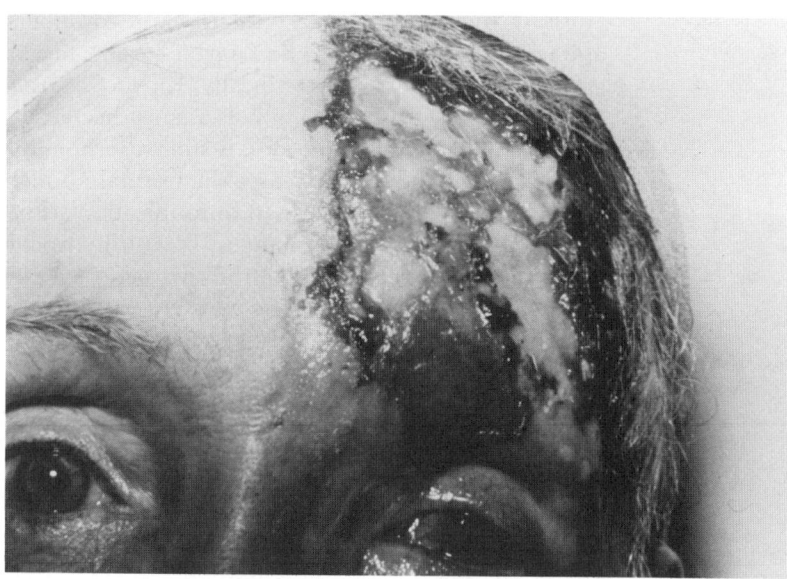

FIG. 4-23 Herpes zoster ophthalmicus in elderly patient. Note unilaterality.

extraordinarily long periods of time. In animal experiments, levamisole has shortened the course of chronic herpetic keratitis [126] and prevented or lessened the severity of reinfection of the animal's second eye [127].

Transfer factor is a dialysable extract of sensitized lymphocytes that can transfer delayed hypersensitivity from a skin-positive donor to a skin-negative recipient. It has a potent nonspecific influence on the CMI response and has apparently been effective in the treatment of cytomegalic retinitis [128], coccidioidomycosis [129], and chronic mucocutaneous candidiasis [130]. Other lymphokines have been effective against yeast cells [131] HSV [112, 113], *Listeria monocytogenes* [132], and staphylococci [133], for example. It has failed to affect HSV guinea pig keratitis [105], however, and a number of investigators have questioned its value in many infectious diseases. Neither of these two agents are presently being used.

In several diseases, *BCG* confers nonspecific resistance when the host has received an inoculation of attenuated live organisms [134]. The resistance is related to the host's CMI response and to his specific immunity to BCG itself. The intravenous and aerosol routes of administration are better than the dermal route. In the immunosuppressed patient, BCG can cause systemic disease, but this possibility can be avoided by the use of the methanol-extracted residue from BCG. To date, immunization of animals with BCG has not been effective in altering the course of experimentally induced HSV keratitis [135].

Killed *C. parvum* works by being taken up by cells of the reticuloendothelial system. This process is followed by prolonged hyperphagocytosis owing to the emergence of large numbers of activated macrophages. It is nontoxic when given locally but may depress the CMI response when given systemically. Killed *C. parvum* does not cause disease and in fact protects animals against bacterial and viral infection. Its use in established viral disease is still experimental.

Vitamin A markedly increases the normal number of antibody-forming cells generated in response to immunization with sheep red blood cells. If it is administered simultaneously with hydrocortisone, moreover, the immunosuppressive effect of the hydrocortisone can be prevented [120, 121]. In animals, nonspecific resistance to infection can be induced by vitamin A [122], and high doses of vitamin A can improve the course of chronic HSV keratitis [78].

On the basis of this series of experimental results, it can be conjectured that the future treatment of recalcitrant HSV corneal infection may depend, not on new and better chemotherapeutic agents, but on new and better means of stimulating the patient's reticuloendothelial system and CMI response.

MYCOTIC INFECTIONS. Early in the twentieth century, *Candida albicans* and *Aspergillus* sp. were almost the only mycotic organisms that had been found in ocular tissue infections in the urban population. This situation has recently changed radically. Altered host resistance has led to numerous mycotic infections that were never before a problem (Fig. 4-24).

The role of the CMI response in defending the host against mycotic infection has been clearly established [136–138]. For example, the CMI response of many patients with chronic mucocutaneous candidiasis has been shown to be defective both in vivo and in vitro. The sera of some of these patients inhibited the proliferation of normal control lymphocytes when stimulated by *Candida* antigens [139]. Other patients showed in their saliva a selective deficiency of IgA antibody directed against *C. albicans* [140]. The successful treatment of one patient with phlyctenular keratitis and superficial candidiasis consisted of reconstitution of the CMI response by means of allogeneic lymphocyte transfusion, supplemented by transfer factor and amphotericin B [141].

It is also possible that patients with disseminated candidiasis have blocking antibodies. In one study [142], the inhibition of candidacidal leukocyte activity appeared to be related to high titers of IgG antibodies against *C. albicans* in the sera of patients with disseminated candidiasis.

The pathogenesis of ocular mycotic disease seems to be related to (1) a break in the protective barriers (e.g., by the baring of the cornea in chronic herpetic infection) [143], (2) conjunctival or corneal trauma (especially with vegetable matter) [144], (3) intraveous drug inoculation, or (4) keratoplasty with stored grafted material. When one of these events is combined with an alteration in the host's immunologic response to disease [145, 146] or with immunosuppressive therapy, contamination with normally innocuous fungi is very likely to result in infection. Topically applied corticosteroids seem peculiarly disposed to actuate the growth of fungal opportunists [147, 148].

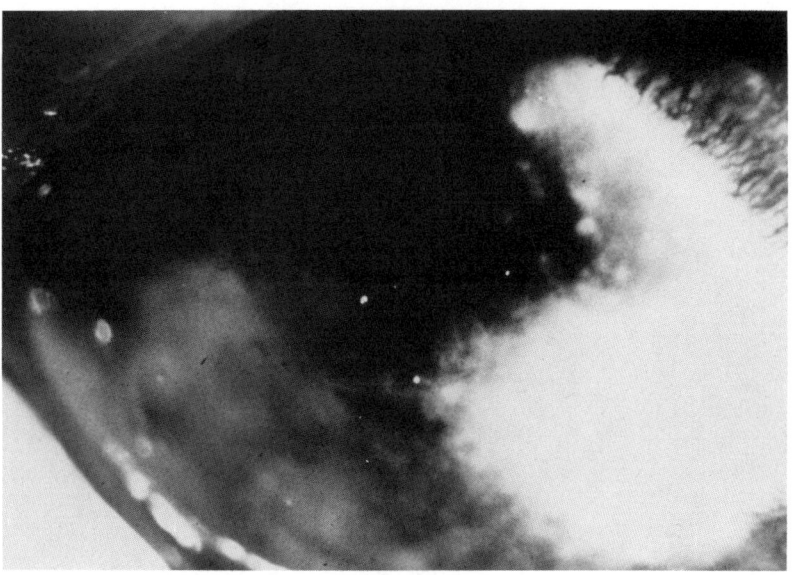

FIG. 4-24   Mycotic corneal infiltrate. Note satellite lesions and feathery edges.

Reactions Not Related to Infection

WESSELY RING. The classical reaction of Wessely (a white ring in the peripheral cornea) can occur from 10 to 12 days after the experimental introduction of a foreign antigen (e.g., bovine serum albumin, bovine gamma globulin) into the cornea. The ring, which consists largely of antigen-antibody complex, complement, and polymorphonuclear leukocytes, slowly migrates centripetally and diminishes in intensity until it disappears. (It is possible for aggregated immunoglobulin or a bacterial endotoxin to combine with complement to form a similar ring. Such a ring appears sooner than one caused by the introduction of an antigen that depends on an antigen-antibody complex to bind complement in the classical way.) Although a Wessely ring usually leaves no sequelae when it clears, pannus has occasionally been noted, indicating that some necrosis has occurred.

An immune ring has been seen in patients with severe corneal burns. It can be assumed that the heat altered the corneal protein so that it could evoke an immune response to itself. Antigenic foreign bodies (usually animal parts) can elicit immune rings (Fig. 4-25). Some animal parts can elicit anaphylaxis, some a toxic response, and others a granulomatous response possibly mediated by immune mechanisms.

Caterpillar hairs, burdock burrs, hop vine, foxmoth, tiger moth, and similar substances can cause severe reactions when introduced into the corneal or adnexal tissues. The caterpillar hair has spurs that are inclined toward the distal end, and because it is usually the thicker, basal end that penetrates, easy removal is almost impossible. The hair is brittle and the proximal end usually breaks, which helps it to penetrate by sharpening it. Toxins may also be released. The toxins may be produced by unicel-

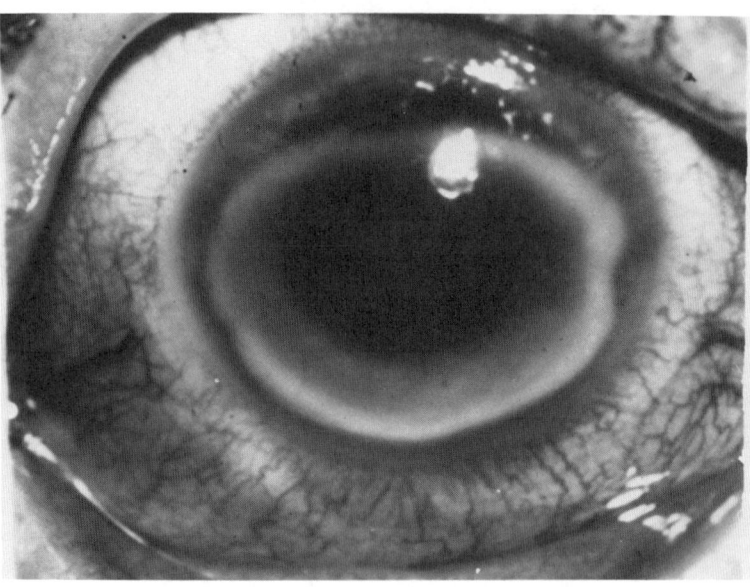

FIG. 4-25 Corneal immune ring after antigenic foreign body penetrated cornea.

lular glands attached to the walls of the hair cavity. The pathogenesis of the hypersensitivity reaction has not been explained.

A nummular keratitis develops around each hair, and conjunctival nodules form around the hairs. After several days the reaction quiets and remains quiescent for days or months. The foreign material may then migrate through the cornea into the inner eye, causing a severe inflammatory response. The best treatment is prevention (by avoiding contact with the hair and refraining from rubbing the eyes if a penetration has occurred). The only other effective treatment is removal of the hair with a curette after copious irrigation.

PERIPHERAL CORNEAL INFILTRATES. Peripheral infiltrates may occur in noninfectious states. Circulating immune complexes may alter vascular permeability, and this change may lead to the deposition of the immune complexes in the peripheral cornea [149, 150]. If the vascular permeability has already been altered by local disease, then immune complexes may be deposited at the alteration sites (the ocular Auer reaction).

Peripheral infiltrates may occur in such systemic diseases as temporal arteritis [151], inflammatory bowel disease [152], rheumatoid arthritis [153], psoriasis, Wegener's granulomatosis, lupus erythematosus, myasthenia gravis [17], periarteritis nodosa, and leukemia. The infiltrate appears first in the peripheral corneal stroma and is usually followed by ulceration of the epithelium. In several of the diseases, the limbal and scleral tissues become affected.

The rheumatoid marginal ulcer can be differentiated from the Mooren's ulcer. Women are more frequently involved; ocular pain is minimal or absent; a gray overhanging central edge to the ulcer is absent; a lucid interval is present; conjunctival, episcleral, and scleral hyperemia is minimal; and a history of rheumatoid arthritis is long standing.

Peripheral corneal infiltrates have also been noted after the intravenous introduction of chemicals [154].

Experimentally, immune complexes can produce recurrent interstitial keratitis in guinea pigs [155].

AMYLOIDOSIS. Amyloid, which is an amorphous, eosinophilic, glassy, hyaline deposit, ubiquitous in its distribution, does not provoke an inflammatory response. The functional impairment of the organ or tissue that it affects depends on the physical presence of amyloid in that area. In most organs, large amounts of amyloid appear to have little deleterious effect until the whole organ has been almost replaced.

Amyloid has a fibrillar structure when examined by electron microscopy; the fibrils are randomly oriented and consist of two or more aggregated filaments measuring 5.0 to 7.5 nm in diameter [156]. Amyloid also has a unique x-ray diffraction pattern indicative of a β-pleated molecular configuration [157]. Amyloid stains pink with hematoxylin and eosin, metachromatically with crystal violet or methyl violet, and positively with direct cotton dyes such as Sirius red. Congo red is one of the most widely used stains but is not specific as it also stains elastic tissue and dense bands of collagen. But when Congo-red–stained sections are viewed with a polarizing microscope, a unique red-green birefringence is seen. This characteristic is true of all amyloid regardless of its location, and staining with Congo red remains the single most useful histologic test of its presence.

A staining technique in which fluorochromes are used to produce secondary fluorescence has been described [158]. Thioflavin T reacts strongly with amyloid but lacks specificity; it also stains a number of other tissues [159] and reacts very strongly, in fact, with the juxtaglomerular apparatus [160].

The protein of amyloid may be an abnormal protein produced by genetically defective cells, by cells under stress, or by certain clones of plasma cells. The first amyloid protein to be characterized was associated with multiple myeloma and has been designated AL because of the light chain amino acid sequence. Most Bence Jones proteins can yield this type of immune amyloid after proteolytic digestion. AL is usually found in primary amyloidosis. A second group of amyloid fibril proteins share a common amino acid sequence distinct from the light chain. These proteins have been designated AA and are largely found in secondary amyloidosis and familial Mediterranean fever. In familial amyloid polyneuropathy another amyloid fibril protein (AF_p) and in medullary carcinoma of the thyroid yet another protein (APUD or AE_T) have been found. At least one amyloid protein associated with aging has been found (ASc_1).

The P component is a protein, distinct from the amyloid fibrillar proteins that have been found in association with a variety of amyloid subtypes [161].

These different types of amyloid should give us clues to the pathogenesis of amyloid deposition, but so far amyloidosis remains a disease of unknown cause. It was originally thought to be a degeneration but is now believed to be related to immune and nonimmune mechanisms.

Nomenclature has been a problem with amyloidosis. Presently, as previously noted, the nonimmune type is usually designated as AA or AP and the immune type as AL. If the amyloid is present in the serum, then the prefix *S* is employed (i.e., SAL).

Nonimmune amyloid may be derived from the reticuloendothelial cells [162]. It may be an abnormal accumulation of filaments normally present in the extracellular spaces in small amounts throughout the body. Under a wide variety of stimuli, such as infection, inflammation, neoplasia, enzymatic defects, or immunologic stimulation, the amyloid is either overproduced or undermetabolized. This process can be genetically determined. The amyloid fibril formation is the obvious, visible abnormality, the principal defect lying in the ground substance in which the amyloid is deposited [163].

It has been implied that complement, or some other product of inflammation, may participate in the origin of this nonimmune type of amyloid [164], which is distinguished by being devoid of threonine and cysteine, low in proline, and rich in arginine [165]. This amyloid protein is linked with the presence of antigenically related protein in the circulating plasma [166].

Amyloid may also be of Ig origin and derive from the polymerized fragments of Ig light chains [167]. Antisera to amyloid of this type cross-react with Bence Jones protein [168] and have an identical amino acid sequence [169]. The Bence Jones proteins [168] in the urine of multiple myeloma patients are intact light chains. Amyloid, on the other hand, is formed from incomplete light chains, largely from their terminal ends. Amyloid fibrils can be formed in vitro by the proteolytic digestion of homogeneous light chains, and it has been suggested that the formation of this immune type of amyloid in vivo depends on the local concentration and consequent polymerization of identical light-chain fragments.

In patients with amyloidosis, nonspecific Ig abnormalities (elevated serum levels of IgG, IgA, and IgM) often occur [170]. IgM has also been found in the skin lesions of patients with systemic amyloidosis [171].

An association between Crohn's disease and amyloidosis has been noted [172], and the two diseases may be immunologically related.

Although in this chapter local diseases affecting the external ocular tissues are discussed (systemic diseases are discussed in Chapter 5), for the sake of continuity all forms of amyloidosis are discussed here.

Primary systemic amyloidosis is diagnosed by excluding other possibilities, and it must then be proven that the condition is not secondary amyloidosis. Muscles, skin, nerves, and blood vessels are affected predominantly, and vascular deposits may be found in sites that are typically those of secondary systemic amyloidosis (e.g., the liver, spleen, kidneys, and adrenal glands) [173].

Primary systemic amyloidosis shows a wide variety of clinical lesions. Heart failure resulting from amyloidosis of heart muscle is a frequent cause of death. Macroglossia associated with amyloid infiltration of the muscles of the tongue is relatively common, and digestive disorders may be related to amyloidosis of intestinal muscle. Chronic sensomotor polyneuropathy is common, and among other manifestations are paresthesia, loss of the sensation of pain and temperature, and impairment of deep tendon reflexes. The peripheral nerves are sometimes palpable. If the sacral autonomic nerves and ganglia are affected, disturbances of bowel and bladder function may follow [174]. Amyloid has also been found in the cervical sympathetic ganglia, and amyloid neuropathy may explain some of the pupillary abnormalities that have been reported [175, 176]. Purpura is a common manifestation when there is amyloid in the walls of blood vessels [177], and in this form of amyloidosis there may also be occult plasma-cell dyscrasias. The amyloid in these conditions is the immune type and is deposited pericollagenously [178].

It has been estimated that 8 percent of patients with this form of amyloidosis have ocular lesions. The lids are affected more often than other ocular tissues and are sometimes the most affected site in the body [179–182]. There may be lid as well as conjunctival hemorrhages [183]. The lesions are papules or plaques and resemble those of xanthelasma. They are usually small, symmetric, smooth, waxy, yellow, and either discrete or confluent. There is no itching associated with them and the hemorrhages give the affected areas a purple color.

Amyloid lesions in the skin of the lids is virtually diagnostic of the primary systemic form of the disease. Local amyloid deposits have been found in the levator superioris muscle [184]; in the palpebral and bulbar conjunctiva; in the tarsus, cornea, sclera, iris, vitreous, retina, choroid [185], optic nerve, and peripheral ocular nerves; and in the orbital fat and ocular muscles [186]. Occlusion of the choriocapillaris [187] and external ophthalmoplegia [188] have both been reported.

Heredofamilial amyloidosis is of several types. The Portuguese type has a dominant inheritance pattern, and the patients have amyloid deposits in the nerves. The clinical course is surprisingly consistent. The disease begins in most patients in their 20s or 30s with an insidious onset of paresis of the lower extremities, absent deep tendon reflexes, and atrophy. They usually die 10 or 20 years later with cachexia, intercurrent infection, or cardiovascular collapse. Almost all organ systems are ultimately affected.

The ocular signs and symptoms are the result of (1) neuropathy secondary to amyloid deposits in the optic nerve, (2) vascular fragility and obstruction from amyloid deposition in the vessel walls, (3) impairment of function and structural distortion referable to the mass of amyloid that has been deposited, and (4) vitreous opacification.

The common eye signs are unequal pupils; poor light and convergence reactions; pupils with irregular outlines; proptosis; ptosis; thick-

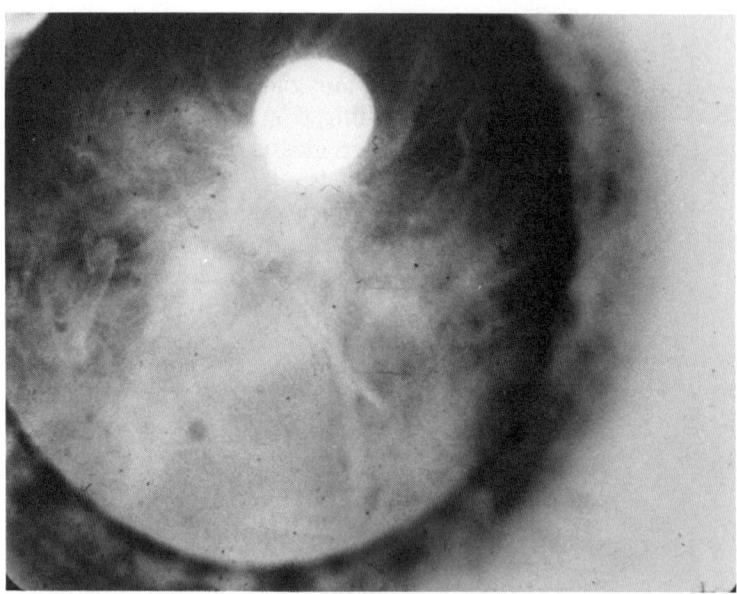

FIG. 4-26   Amyloid deposits in the vitreous.

ening of the lids; and hemorrhage into the lids, conjunctiva, sclera, and retina. Perhaps the most important ocular sign in this type of amyloidosis is the vitreous veil (Fig. 4-26). These veils, or opacities, range from small, localized, clinically unimportant deposits to lesions that affect the entire vitreous, severely impair vision, and preclude examination of the retina. Gray, beadlike or plaquelike infiltrates of amyloid may also be seen along the retinal arterioles. When viewed microscopically, the amyloid is seen to extend from the adventitia of the retinal vessels into the vitreous. Removal of most of the affected vitreous is the only treatment, and there may be recurrences [188, 189]. Common as the vitreous opacities are, they are apparently not pathognomonic of the familial types of amyloidosis because they have also been described in primary nonfamilial systemic amyloidosis [178].

One amyloid nephropathy is associated with Mediterranean fever. It has a recessive inheritance pattern and would more accurately be classified as a "familial secondary systemic amyloidosis." There is also a familial amyloid cardiopathy and a familial cutaneous amyloidosis. Familial amyloid nephropathy has a dominant inheritance pattern and causes nephropathy, deafness, and glaucoma.

Patients with familial medullary thyroid carcinoma have amyloid deposits in the thyroid gland, corneal vascularization, and associated pheochromocytomas.

Secondary systemic amyloidosis is the type most often encountered in general medicine. It has been found in more than 20 percent of postmortem studies of patients with chronic diseases. When viewed microscopically, the kidneys, spleen, liver, adrenal glands, and blood vessels are found to be the tissues most often affected. The clinical lesions are proteinemia, the nephrotic syndrome, uremia, and hepatosplenomegaly. Amyloid has been seen in the eye only rarely in this type of amyloidosis.

The systemic disorders complicated by amyloidosis are the following:

Chronic infectious diseases

Tuberculosis
Hansen's disease (leprosy)
Syphilis
Osteomyelitis
Pyelonephritis
Bronchiectasis
Trachoma

Chronic inflammatory diseases

Rheumatoid arthritis and related disorders
Reiter's syndrome [190]
Regional enteritis
Ulcerative colitis
Whipple's disease

Neoplasms

Hodgkin's disease
Multiple myeloma
Renal cell carcinoma
Medullary carcinoma of the thyroid gland

Metabolic disease: diabetes mellitus

Other diseases

Dysproteinemia
Chronically infected burns
Hypogammaglobulinemia
Multiple blood transfusions

The amyloid in secondary amyloidosis may be the nonimmunoglobulin type or the light-chain type, and according to the type, the deposits are in the perireticulin area or the pericollagenous area, respectively. A fine-needle biopsy of the subcutaneous fat is a simple and reliable diagnostic procedure [191].

Amyloidosis associated with aging may be classified as either primary or secondary. One study showed that almost 90 percent of patients more than 60 years of age who died from senile dementia had amyloid deposits in the brain, pancreas, and heart [192]. Animal experiments have also shown an association between amyloidosis and aging [193]. Cardiac amyloidosis, once thought to be an unimportant and incidental occurrence, is now known to cause serious symptoms in many patients [194]. The

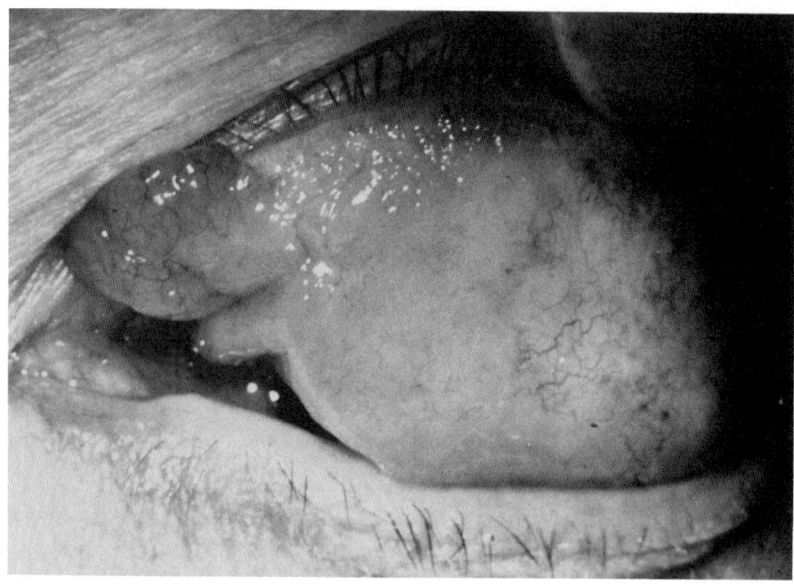

FIG. 4-27 Amyloid deposits in palpebral conjunctiva.

pathogenesis of amyloid deposition in old age is not understood, however.

As a local disease, amyloidosis may occur in either of two forms. It may be an incidental degenerative process associated with pathologic states (the secondary localized form), or a clinical entity *sui generis* (the primary localized form). Both κ and λ light chains were identified in abundance in resection of amyloid tissue in the conjunctiva [195]. This finding of AL protein suggests that some forms of localized nonfamilial ocular amyloidosis involves the accumulation of proteins similar to immunoglobulins. Schaldenbrand and Keren [196] found IgD amyloid in the conjunctiva.

Primary Localized Amyloidosis. Primary localized amyloidosis is usually bilateral. The lacrimal gland or orbit may be involved [197]. When the conjunctiva is affected, the victims are young adults between 20 and 30 years of age, and the deposits begin at the fornix and extend to the bulbar and palpebral conjunctiva. The lesions affect the epithelium, substantia propria, blood vessels, tarsal plate, levator muscle, and Tenon's capsule [198–201]. Conjunctival amyloidosis is often asymptomatic and may be present for years before the patient seeks medical attention. The first complaints are swelling of the eyelids and occasionally ptosis or epiphora.

Typically there is a discrete, nontender, nonulcerating, yellow, waxy, rubbery, firm, subconjunctival mass (Fig. 4-27). The conjunctival surface is usually smooth. Occasionally it is friable and from time to time may even bleed. If the tarsal plate and adjacent muscular and subcutaneous layers are infiltrated, the eyelid may be thickened and eversion difficult.

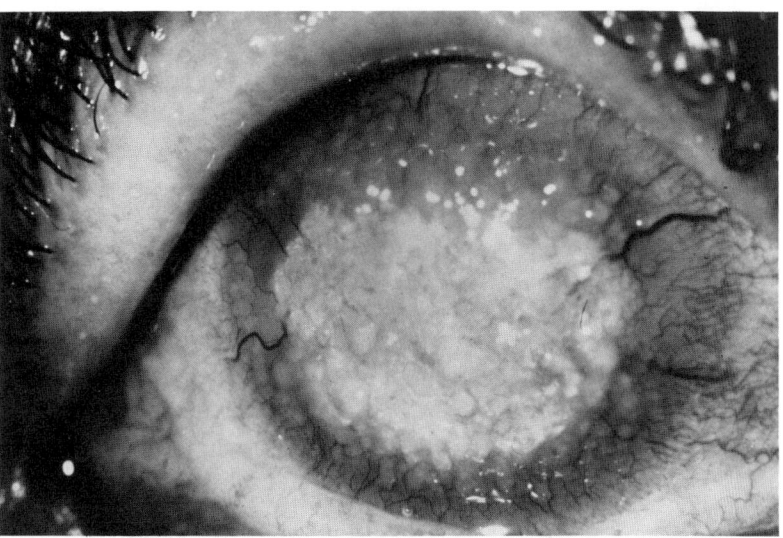

FIG. 4-28 Gelatinous droplike dystrophy.

The ptosis usually is due to the weight of the amyloid mass but can sometimes be due to amyloid deposits in the levator muscle. Conjunctival hemorrhagic lymphangiectasia and occlusion of the orbital veins were seen in one patient with conjunctival amyloidosis [202]. As a rule these patients are healthy and free from amyloidosis elsewhere. The localized ocular disease has its parallel in localized primary amyloidosis of other organs such as the larynx, lung, and heart.

Although corneal amyloidosis is usually the result of direct extension from the conjunctiva, recently primary corneal amyloid disease has been reported. For example, the Japanese have described a *gelatinous droplike dystrophy* characterized by bilateral, axially placed, multiple, subepithelial deposits of amyloid [203, 204]. Raised gelatinous masses give the lesion a mulberrylike surface. The peripheral corneas are usually clear and free of vascularization, and there may be an associated autosomal inheritance pattern. Similar lesions have been reported in the United States (Fig. 4-28). Some cases have been sporadic [205]; others have shown a recessive inheritance pattern [206, 207]. The amyloid may be derived from fibroblasts or the basal cells of the corneal epithelium [208, 209].

Lattice dystrophy of the cornea may be a localized form of familial amyloidosis. The amyloid is in the stromal lesions of the disease [210, 211], the deposits appearing in the first decade of life. The nonimmune type of amyloid (AA) has been seen in this disease process [212–214]. Both sexes are equally affected, and the disease has an autosomal dominant inheritance pattern. The initial deposits are axially placed and bilateral, and the peripheral corneas remain clear and avascular. These early deposits are in the anterior stroma, but all layers are ultimately affected. The branching, linear opacities widen and become more opaque as the patient ages (Fig. 4-29). Central opacities develop as time goes on, and

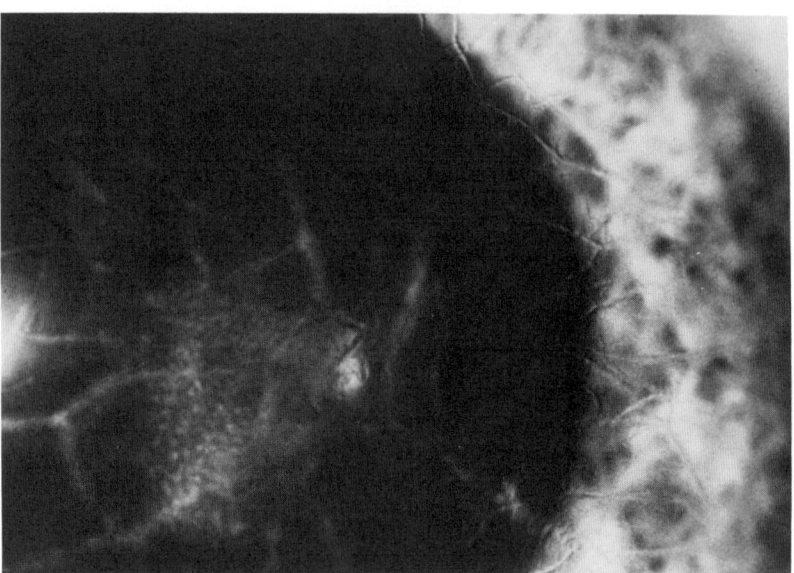

FIG. 4-29 Lattice dystrophy. Note branching linear opacities.

the visual acuity may be seriously compromised by the fourth decade of life. The anterior deposits may affect the basement membrane, and attacks of recurrent erosion occur. Keratoplasty is usually highly successful, and recurrences in the donor graft are rare and usually do not affect the integrity and clarity of the grafted tissue.

Reports indicate that there may be a variant of lattice dystrophy that develops in early adulthood and is associated with systemic amyloid deposition in the skin, central nervous system, and internal organs [215–217].

In polymorphic stromal dystrophy amyloid has been detected [218, 219], and the entity is now more properly designated polymorphic amyloid degeneration.

Secondary Localized Amyloidosis. Corneal amyloidosis is usually secondary to other ocular disease or to corneal trauma. Some of the conditions with which corneal amyloid deposits are associated are trachoma [220] (probably the most important of the associations), conjunctival sarcoidosis [221], neoplasms [222], lipoid proteinosis [174], leprosy [223], phlyctenulosis, lipoidal degeneration, and keratoconus [224]. According to one team of observers [224], the amyloid deposits in the cornea seem to occur in the following three forms according to their location: (1) as subepithelial masses resembling degenerated pannus (Fig. 4-30); (2) as lamellar deposits occurring only in the deep corneal stroma; and (3) as perivascular deposits associated with corneal vascularization. The authors concluded that secondary localized amyloidosis should be suspected in all patients with corneal scarring and opacification because it was present in 3.5 percent of all of the corneas submitted to their laboratory.

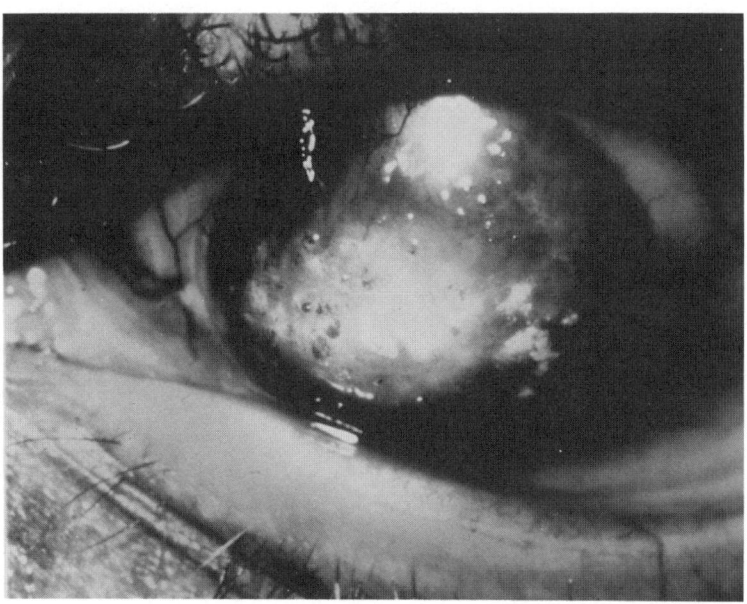

FIG. 4-30   Secondary localized amyloid deposits in the cornea.

The clinical appearance of the corneal lesion depends on the primary disease as well as on the subsequent amyloid deposition. Corneal opacification, vascularization, and a yellowish discoloration are common features of most of the primary entities.

The treatment of systemic amyloidosis is not discussed in this book. The treatment of localized amyloidosis is usually surgical, but the operation should be performed only when function is threatened. Owing to the infiltrating nature of amyloid, complete excision is usually not possible, and recurrence can be expected [225]. Radiation therapy may be employed in conjunction with operation [226].

The mass of amyloid can be removed to alleviate vision-impairing ptosis. Keratoplasty is successful when the amyloid deposits are in an avascular cornea, as is the case in localized primary amyloidosis (i.e., lattice dystrophy or gelatinous droplike dystrophy). In localized secondary amyloidosis, the highly vascularized corneas run an increased risk of graft rejection. If vision is seriously impaired by amyloid deposits in the vitreous, much of the vitreous can be removed and replaced. Unfortunately, the deposits may recur in the new material [227]. In localized secondary amyloidosis, treatment of the underlying disease may halt the deposition of new amyloid.

EPISCLERITIS AND SCLERITIS. The inflammatory response of the sclera and episclera tends to be granulomatous. The ground substance usually undergoes fibrinoid necrosis and an abnormal precipitation of mucopolysaccharides.

Episcleritis. Two types of episcleritis are nodular and diffuse. The cause

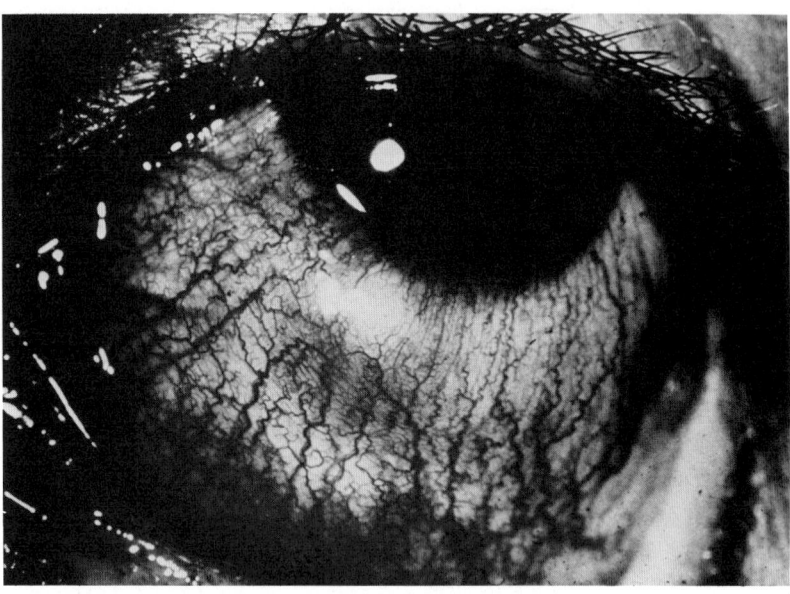

FIG. 4-31   Nodular episcleritis.

of the disease, whether nodular or diffuse, is unknown, but it may be an immune response to episcleral tissues. Episcleritis is on rare occasions associated with rheumatoid arthritis and even more rarely with other systemic diseases.

NODULAR EPISCLERITIS. Patients with nodular episcleritis tend to be older (in the 40s to 50s) than those with diffuse episcleritis [228]. The disease is chronic and recurrent and usually runs a benign course. The nodule is dark red or purple, sensitive to touch, and fixed to the sclera. It is a mass of large mononuclear cells, giant cells, lymphocytes, and plasma cells, sometimes with central necrosis. The conjunctiva can be moved over the lesion, which rarely ulcerates. The lesion lasts 4 to 6 weeks, and then pales, flattens, and absorbs, sometimes leaving an atrophic scar (Fig. 4-31).

Nodular episcleritis must be differentiated from phlyctenulosis. Compared with nodular episcleritis the phlyctenule runs a more acute course (10–14 days), causes more symptoms, and the conjunctiva cannot be moved over it. Unlike the episcleritic nodule, at an early stage the phlyctenule contains predominantly lymphocytes and macrophages, and once necrosis starts, polymorphonuclear leukocytes increase in number and become the predominant cell.

DIFFUSE EPISCLERITIS. In this form of the disease, there is diffuse congestion and edema of an area of episcleral tissue and of the conjunctiva over the area. The disease is usually localized to one quadrant, is evanescent in nature, and tends to recur at regular intervals bilaterally. Attacks usually last from hours to days, and the symptoms may be minimal (Fig. 4-32). The same inflammatory cells seen in nodular episcleritis (large

4. REACTIONS LIMITED TO THE EXTERNAL EYE

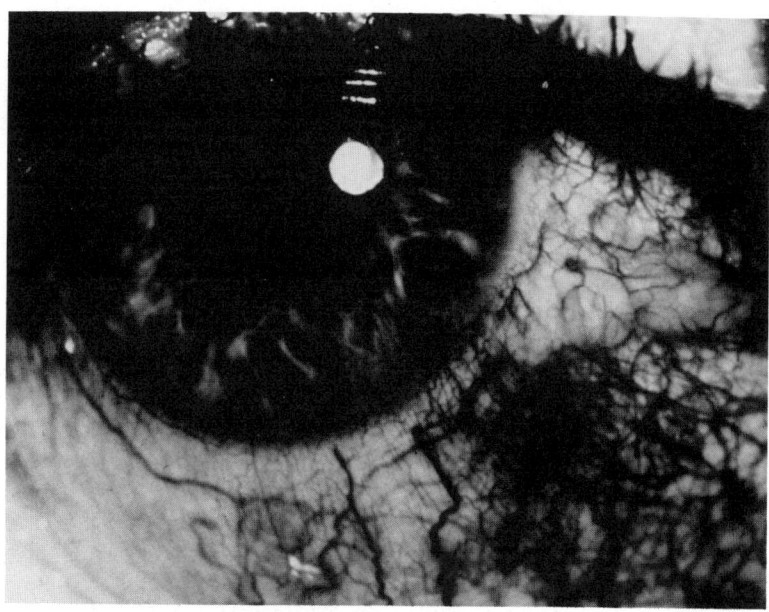

FIG. 4-32   Diffuse episcleritis limited to one quadrant.

mononuclear cells, giant cells, lymphocytes, and plasma cells) are scattered throughout the affected tissue.

The treatment of both forms of episcleritis is the local application of potent corticosteroid preparations. Regrettably, both forms of the disease are all too often unresponsive. (The use of systemic corticosteroids is not warranted.)

Scleritis. There are five types of scleritis: anterior scleritis, brawny scleritis, sclerokeratitis, and the two necrotizing types (i.e., necrotizing nodular scleritis and scleromalacia perforans). Whatever their type, most cases of scleritis are associated with systemic disease (predominantly rheumatoid arthritis).

Anterior scleritis occurs principally in young women aged 30 and older and is usually bilateral. There is a diffuse anterior dark reddish or purple swelling. Pinhead-sized, yellowish white nodules appear periodically. The lesion is very tender, severely painful, and cannot be moved by lid pressure. There is concurrent uveitis. The disease may last for weeks or months, and staphylomas and sclerokeratitis sometimes develop late in its course. The sequelae of this troublesome disease are scleral thinning, punched-out scleral areas, peripheral corneal opacification, and vascularization.

Anterior scleritis can be distinguished from episcleritis by the following differences: the lesion of episcleritis is usually unilateral and localized, reddish, only slightly tender, mildly or moderately painful, and can be moved by lid pressure. It may blanch when in contact with 1 : 1,000 epinephrine (which the scleral lesion never does), and there is usually no

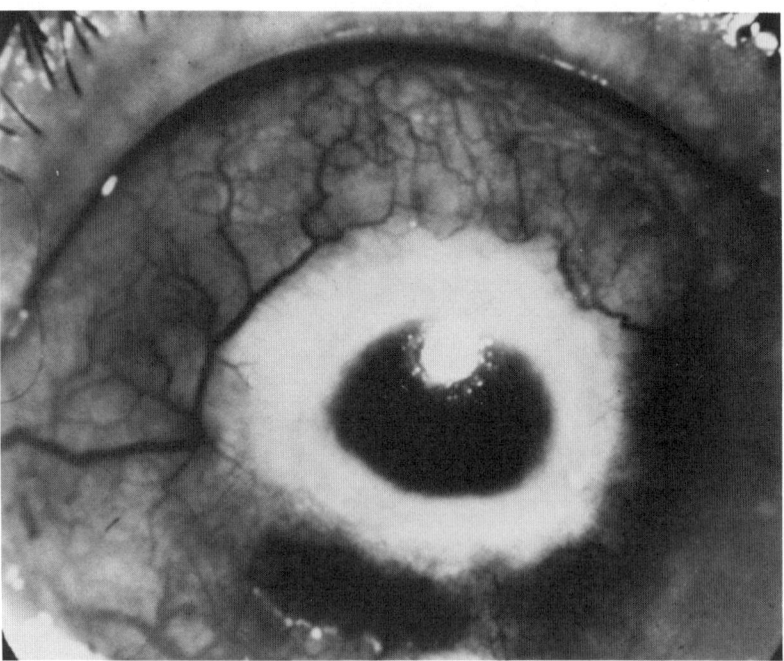

FIG. 4-33 Active extensive sclerokeratitis.

associated uveitis. The sequelae, if any, are minimal. In contrast the lesions of scleritis are usually bilateral and diffuse, reddish purple, very tender and painful; they cannot be moved by lid pressure and sequelae occur [228].

Brawny scleritis is a severe form of anterior scleritis. It occurs in elderly women (usually with rheumatoid arthritis) and may lead to loss of vision. The histologic changes are the changes seen in rheumatoid nodules.

Sclerokeratitis may accompany anterior or brawny scleritis or may occur by itself. It is often treated with local or systemic corticosteroids and occasionally with other immunosuppressive agents [229] (Figs. 4-33, 4-34).

Necrotizing nodular scleritis and *scleromalacia perforans,* both of which are bilateral, occur principally in women in their 50s or older. Both conditions may be due to ischemia or to an immune response to scleral mesenchyme, and trauma may initiate them, perhaps by altering the scleral antigen.

In necrotizing nodular scleritis there are repeated attacks of disease in which several raised nodules with yellow centers may appear and may ulcerate (Fig. 4-35). Uveitis complicates the picture, and there is severe pain. In scleromalacia perforans the yellow necrotic nodules (located usually between the limbus and the equator; Fig. 4-36) often slough over a period of several months, leaving scleral defects (Fig. 4-37). The globe may perforate. Altogether the prognosis of both entities is poor.

In episcleritis of all forms, as well as the benign forms of scleritis, the

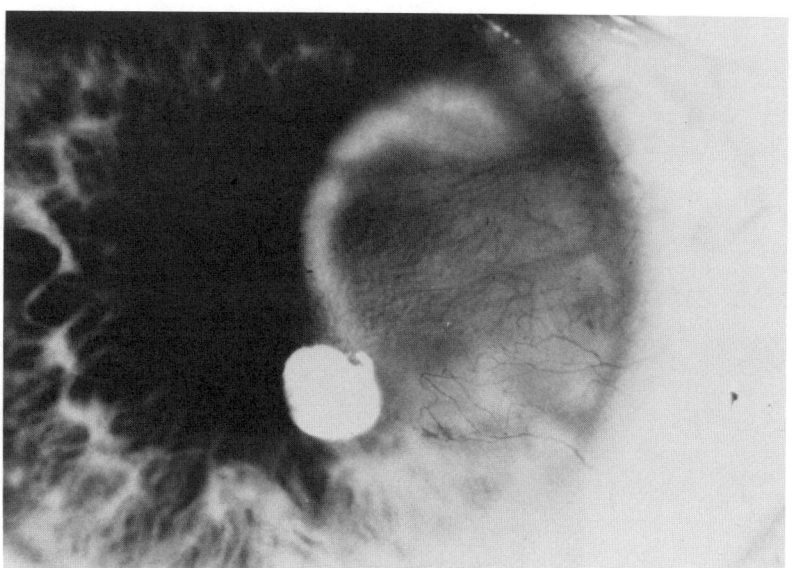

FIG. 4-34   Corneal sequelae after attack of sclerokeratitis.

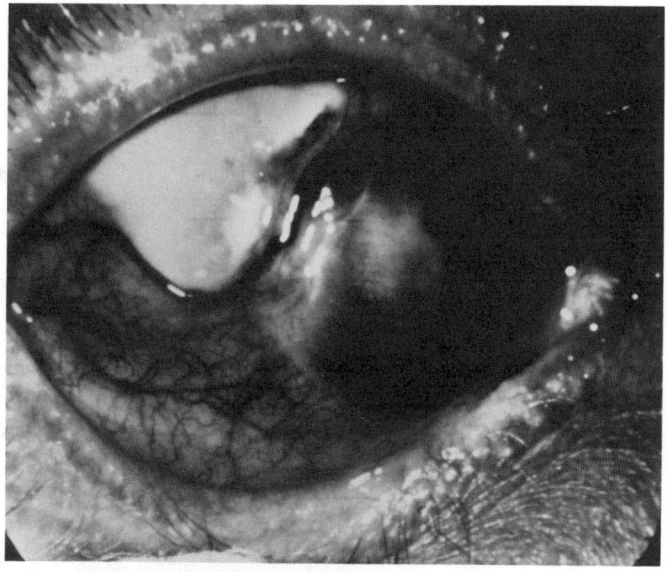

FIG. 4-35   Necrotizing nodular scleritis. Area of sclera ready to slough.

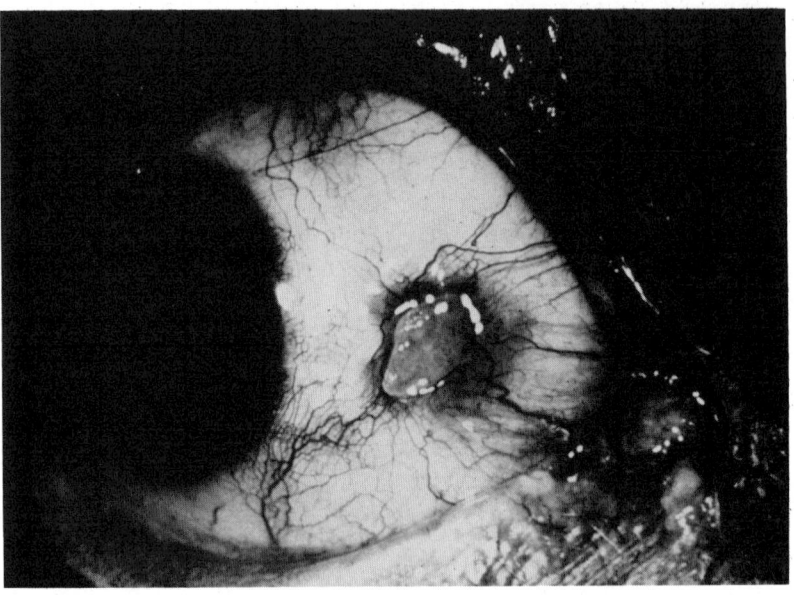

FIG. 4-36   Scleromalacia perforans.

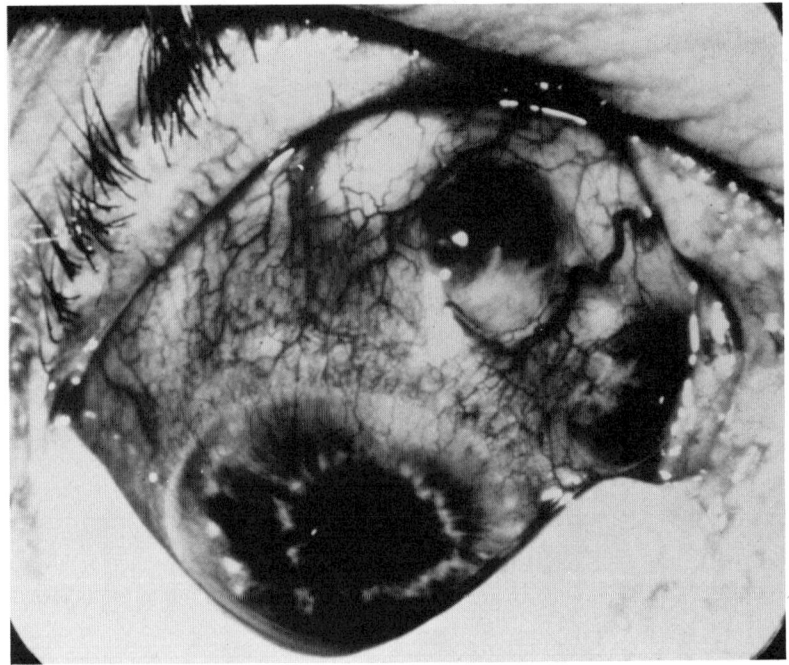

FIG. 4-37   Scleral thinning as sequelae of scleromalacia perforans.

vasculature overlying the sclera is dilated and the blood flow extremely rapid. In necrotizing scleritis there are gross vascular abnormalities involving the venules of the episclera, and the flow of blood in the small venules become slowed. In patients in whom the blood flow is rapid, nonsteroidal anti-inflammatory agents (i.e., oxyphenbutazone, indomethacin, ibuprofen) are effective. Local therapy is ineffective. When the blood flow is decreased systemic corticosteroid therapy is indicated [230].

Systemic corticosteroids seem at first to be effective but later may lose their efficacy [231]. Scleral and fascia lata grafts have been performed in attempts to give the internal ocular tissue a new protective covering. They have had only limited success, however [232, 233]. Unfortunately, the disease process can recur in the newly grafted tissue.

CELL-MEDIATED IMMUNE REACTIONS

Phlyctenulosis

Phlyctenae (blisters) used to be associated almost entirely with hypersensitivity to tuberculoprotein, and there was a higher prevalence in poor families living in unhygienic, crowded conditions than in more affluent segments of the population. But in the United States more phlyctenulosis seems to be associated with hypersensitivity to staphylococcal antigens than with hypersensitivity to tuberculoprotein.

CAUSE. Phlyctenulosis is the result of hypersensitivity to a previous infection with an agent to which the host can produce a delayed-hypersensitivity type of skin reaction [234]. The eye lesion is a CMI response to the foreign protein that has been presented to the conjunctival sac either endogenously or exogenously.

Experimental phlyctenulosis can be produced by instilling tuberculoprotein into the conjunctival sacs of sensitized animals or human volunteers [235]. In human beings it can be produced also by injecting tuberculin subcutaneously [236]. (The lesions produced by sensitizing rabbits with bovine serum albumin, crushing the conjunctiva with large-toothed forceps, and then instilling bovine serum albumin topically onto the cornea, are probably immune-complex–mediated lesions [237] even though they resemble phlyctenules.)

Phlyctenulosis often occurs in the first two decades of life, and only rarely later in life, and this may be explained by the high degree of CMI responsiveness present early in life and the relatively low degree present late in life. This factor could also account for the frequency of phlyctenulosis in patients with clinically inactive tuberculosis (whose cellular immunity may be normal) and its infrequency in patients with clinically active tuberculosis (whose cellular immunity may be depressed).

Hypersensitivity to tuberculoprotein and staphylococcal antigen has been widely recognized as causing phlyctenulosis, but there are also less frequent causes, such as *Candida albicans*, *Coccidioides immitis*, the agent of lymphogranuloma venereum [238], and *Leishmania* sp. [239]. Although tuberculosis is now an infrequent cause of the eye disease in the United States, it is still important to rule it out in any patient with phlyctenulosis. Hypoparathyroidism alone or with Addison's disease is often associated with phlyctenulosis, and local inflammatory conditions (increased vascular permeability brings more effector [T-lymphocytes] cells to the external ocular tissue) may trigger phlyctenule formation, but how they do so is not yet understood.

CLINICAL FEATURES. In the initial attack of phlyctenulosis, from whatever cause, the lesion appears at the limbus and only in later attacks does it occur on the conjunctiva and cornea. The phlyctenule begins as a small, round, or oval lesion 1 to 3 mm in diameter. It is hard, red, elevated, and surrounded by a zone of hyperemia. Within 2 or 3 days a grayish white center develops and then ulcerates; within 10 to 12 days the lesion disappears. Scarring is limited to the cornea and leaves a pathognomonic scar, limbus-based and triangular. The staphylococcal type of phlyctenule usually runs a slightly longer course than a phlyctenule owing to tuberculoprotein.

The limbus is usually also the site of recurrent lesions, but the cornea, the bulbar conjunctiva, and very rarely the tarsal conjunctiva may also have phlyctenules. The rare tarsal phlyctenules are firmer than the bulbar phlyctenules [240] and are most likely to occur near the lid border [241]. Several phlyctenules may develop during a single attack, and as many as 15 have been seen on the cornea all at the same time. The corneal phlyctenule is an amorphous infiltrate, usually gray at first but yellowish later when necrosis occurs.

In corneal phlyctenulosis, pannus usually develops. Recurrent lesions appear close to the limbal blood vessels or to the older pannus left by previous corneal phlyctenules. In this way the pannus progresses centrally with each recurrence. It is usually irregular and often located inferiorly. In rare instances, a central phlyctenule may not vascularize, perhaps because of the distance of the necrotic process from the limbal blood vessels. If it is the necrotic cells that "signal" for polymorphonuclear leukocyte invasion, then the amount of necrosis and its distance from the limbus become crucial determinants of the leukocytic response. The same necrotic stimulus will in fact cause less neovascularization as the stimulus moves centrally.

The scarring associated with corneal phlyctenules is usually superficial but sometimes reaches the deep stroma. The scar is typically triangular with its apex toward the cornea. Rarely, in recurrences, Salzmann's nodular corneal degeneration may arise. Corneal perforations owing to tuberculous phlyctenules are more common in blacks and Eskimos than in Caucasians, possibly because the blacks and Eskimos, many of whom suffer from malnutrition, mildly active tuberculosis, and other wasting diseases [242], are more likely to be immunosuppressed. (Corneal perforation in staphylococcal phlyctenulosis has been reported but is extremely rare [242].) A single phlyctenule at the corneal margin usually ulcerates quickly. The tissue surrounding the ulceration is necrotic and loaded with polymorphonuclear leukocytes, appearing as a yellow area of infiltration [243].

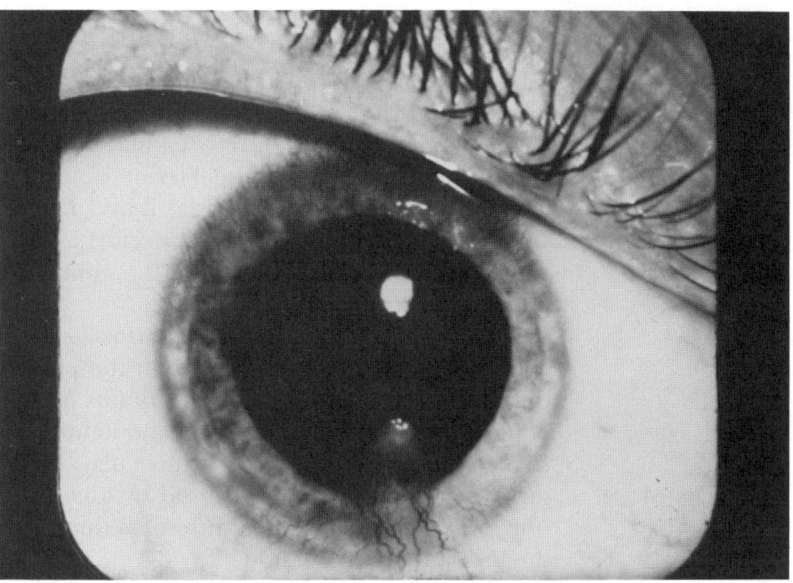

FIG. 4-38   Fascicular keratitis associated with corneal phlyctenule.

Although the most common cause of fascicular keratitis in the United States today is herpes simplex virus, a corneal phlyctenule may also lead to a somewhat elevated, fascicular keratitis that flattens after the acute process subsides (Fig. 4-38).

HISTOPATHOLOGIC FEATURES. The cellular reaction of the phlyctenule is a typical delayed-hypersensitivity reaction, that is, a focal subepithelial infiltration of small round cells and a few macrophages. When the central epithelium of the phlyctenule undergoes necrosis, large numbers of polymorphonuclear leukocytes come to the area, the cells infiltrating between the epithelium and Bowman's layer and overflowing beneath Bowman's layer. The epithelium, basement membrane, and Bowman's layer all undergo necrosis, and the subsequent vascularization is thus beneath the corneal epithelium.

The symptoms associated with conjunctival phlyctenules are usually minimal, for example, tearing and mild irritation. Corneal phlyctenules, on the other hand, cause severe symptoms that include tearing, photophobia, and pain. The photophobia and pain are severe in the tuberculoprotein-induced disease, much milder in the staphylococcal disease.

The other ocular diseases with which phlyctenulosis can be confused are nodular episcleritis, pingueculitis, rosacea keratoconjunctivitis, limbal vernal keratoconjunctivitis, herpetic keratoconjunctivitis, and trachoma.

1. *Nodular episcleritis* lasts for 2 to 3 weeks, does not ulcerate, does not leave a scar, and is often associated with rheumatoid disease.

2. *Pingueculitis* does not ulcerate and lasts a variable length of time (approximately 3 weeks).
3. *Rosacea keratoconjunctivitis* is usually associated with facial rosacea and dilatation of the conjunctival and lid margin vessels. The limbal excrescences and pannus of rosacea may resemble phlyctenular corneal lesions, but the rosacea corneal lesion is never fascicular, has a narrow base at the limbus, and widens as it invades the cornea proper (spade shaped). The pannus is located inferiorly. There may be an associated staphylococcal infection of the lids, conjunctiva, or cornea. The tear pH may be alkaline.
4. *Limbal vernal keratoconjunctivitis* is associated with the following differentiating features: giant papillae in the palpebral and conjunctiva; a thick, sticky, white exudate; a gelatinous mass at the limbus; Horner's points; eosinophils in scrapings; and itching.
5. In *herpetic keratoconjunctivitis,* fascicular keratitis is associated with fewer symptoms than are caused by a comparable process owing to phlyctenulosis, perhaps because of reduced or absent sensation over the herpetic corneal lesion.
6. *Pannus trachomatosus* is usually located superiorly and is more regular than the pannus of phlyctenulosis. The superior palpebral conjunctiva usually shows other distinctive signs of trachoma, for example, follicular hypertrophy, papillary hypertrophy, stellate scars, and Arlt's line.

TREATMENT. Phlyctenulosis owing to tuberculoprotein is extremely responsive to topical corticosteroids. The symptoms are relieved dramatically within 24 hours, and the lesions disappear within 48 hours [244, 245]. The phlyctenulosis caused by staphylococcal disease is much less responsive to corticosteroids, which are perhaps not even indicated; the milder symptoms, the limited course of the untreated disease, its unresponsiveness to steroids, and the side effects of topical administration of steroids would seem to militate against their use.

The concomitant bacterial (staphylococcal) blepharoconjunctivitis should be treated as well. Conjunctival and lid margin material should be subjected to culture and antibiotic sensitivity tests, and an appropriate antibiotic ointment should then be applied.

Whenever feasible, the hygiene and dietary health of the affected patients should be improved, and if there is underlying systemic disease, it too should be treated.

Graft Rejection

The corneal graft reaction is the subject of Chapter 6.

Contact Dermatitis

Contact dermatitis is the commonest of all skin diseases and is especially important in industry. Everyone is susceptible to it whether he or she has a history of allergies, but it occurs more commonly in allergic persons. It more often affects women than men [246] and occurs in persons of all ages (it has been seen in a 4-week-old infant). Statistically significant associations between some agents that cause contact dermatitis and HLA antigens (B7, A3) have been reported [246a].

The molecular structures with an amine or choline group at the para *(P)* position of a benzene ring (e.g., cosmetics, dyes, anesthetics, sulfonamides) and the structures with pyrimidine nuclei (idoxuridine or IDU) seem to be effective sensitizers. Other excitants are photodevelopers, soaps, rubber compounds, insecticides and fungicides, explosives, oils, resins and waxes, weeds, flowers, and certain foods [247, 248]. It is not always the major pharmacologically active component of a preparation that is the sensitizer; preservatives and vehicles may also be at fault. Parabens [249], thimerosal, and even such seemingly innocuous vehicles as lanolin and petrolatum can act as sensitizers.

Numerous topically applied ophthalmic drugs can sensitize. Neomycin, atropine, IDU, gentamicin, and thimerosal are most likely to do so. Less frequent sensitizers are sulfonamides, chloramphenicol, homatropine, scopolamine, silver, zinc, and benzalkonium [250]. Nonpharmacologic substances that can sensitize are soap, hair dye, nail polish, scented cosmetics, perfumes, powders, shampoos, hair sprays, all types of eye makeup, and cleaning fluid for spectacles [251].

The major barriers to the percutaneous penetration of drugs are the lipids of the keratin layer [252], which explains the clinical observation that ointments and other lipid-soluble preparations are more apt to cause sensitization than are water-soluble preparations. The lipids of the stratum corneum, and possibly of the granular layer, exist as complex hydrophilic mixtures [253]. Ointments may act to defat the skin and to deprive it of its ability to retain water. The result of this is increased drug penetration because of dryness, flaking, and scaling.

In search for the cause of a contact dermatitis, a careful history must be taken. Consideration of the patient's occupation and hobbies may be helpful, and the patient may be asked to keep a diary. A record of seasonal variations in the dermatitis and of any differences in symptoms referable to the days of the week can provide clues to the identity of the sensitizer.

The standard confirmatory test is the *patch test*. This procedure is usually performed on the volar aspect of the forearm or on the back. The material to be tested is applied to the skin and covered by a small piece of impermeable material (e.g., Saran wrap), which is held in place with nonallergenic tape. Readings are taken at 24 and 48 hours, preferably approximately 30 minutes after removing the dressing to allow time for pressure-induced effects to subside. The skin changes indicating a positive reaction mimic the skin changes induced by the contact dermatitis. False-negatives and false-positives can occur [254], and the patch test sometimes causes a flare-up of a quiescent lesion.

A study of this reaction by Flax and Caulfield [255] showed that after an initial vasodilation, the skin was infiltrated with lymphocytes, and that this reaction was followed in 2 to 10 hours by vacuolar degeneration of the overlying epithelium.

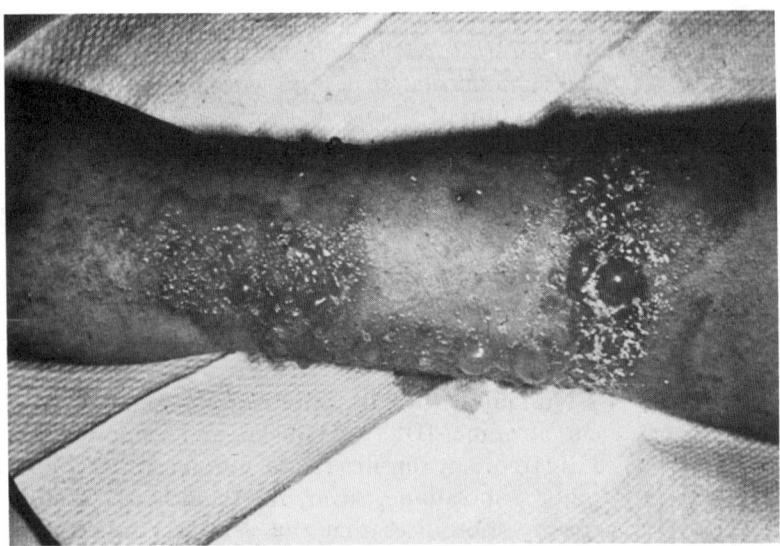

FIG. 4-39 Contact dermatitis on forearm.

The pattern of contact dermatitis may help determine the sensitizer. Sharply demarcated lesions are caused by adhesive tape (Fig. 4-39), and nickel, linear streaks are often caused by plants. Spreading lesions may be caused by cosmetics, poison oak, or poison ivy, and unilateral ocular lesions may be caused by eye drops.

PATHOGENESIS. There are two types of contact dermatitis, irritant (the more common) and allergic. Irritant contact dermatitis is caused by damage to the skin from excessive moisture or from acids, alkalis, resins, or chemicals that can injure the skin if they are in contact with it long enough. Allergy plays no role. In contrast, allergic contact dermatitis occurs in sensitized persons. Before the chemical agent can initiate an allergic response, it has to combine with a protein (behaving as a hapten), which may be either a soluble epithelial component [256] or a serum protein [257]. Because conjugation of the hapten with tissue protein appears to take place in the subepidermal dermis, and possibly in the superficial stroma of the conjunctiva, it is crucial that the inciting substance be able to penetrate the epidermis or conjunctival epithelium.

The thinness of the conjunctiva and of the skin of the eyelids makes these tissues more susceptible than others to the development of contact allergy. That the response is primarily cell-mediated can be deduced from the following: (1) The reaction takes approximately 24 hours to reach maximum severity; (2) passive transfer of a given hypersensitivity can be accomplished by lymphocytes and not by serum; and (3) patients with congenital B-cell deficiency can develop contact dermatitis.

Sensitization requires at least 5 to 10 days for potent sensitizers but may require months for weak sensitizers. After the initial sensitization, the interval between a second exposure to the allergen and the appearance of disease is 24 to 48 hours. Once established, sensitization tends to persist for life, with the possible exception of sensitivity to poison oak and poison ivy.

Reexposure to the allergen at a new site can sometimes produce a flare-up of the dermatitis at the original site several days later. It is not understood why it is that the original site is predisposed to such a recurrence without direct contact with the hapten. Systemic reexposure can also elicit a flare-up of the disease at its original site, and on rare occasions can cause diffuse contact dermatitis.

In studies of the role of the prostaglandins in allergic contact dermatitis, it has been learned that PGE can induce delayed-onset inflammation and a dusky erythema of the skin that persists for up to 10 hours.

The role of eosinophils and basophils in contact dermatitis has not been clearly defined. Some authors have stated that eosinophils are not found in the condition [258], but the authors and others have shown the eosinophils and basophil situation to be both complex and variable. For example, Dvorak and associates [259, 260] found recently that contact dermatitis lesions in both guinea pigs and human beings contained large infiltrations of basophils.

CLINICAL FEATURES. Topical ophthalmic drops that cause dermatitis of the lids always cause allergic conjunctivitis first. Contact dermatitis of the lids without conjunctivitis is nearly always caused by a substance that has reached the lids without having been instilled into the conjunctival sac. In both circumstances, the earliest signs usually appear along the course of the natural flow of the tears and drugs, that is, the inferior or inferonasal areas of the conjunctiva and the nasal aspect of the lower eyelid. The cardinal symptom is itching. Biomicroscopic examination shows small flakes of fibrin and scales of epidermis on the periocular tissue. The conjunctivitis tends to be diffuse and papillary, and there may be a mucoid or lightly mucopurulent exudate. Punctal edema, stenosis, and occlusion may occur. In severe cases there may be some mild keratinization of the conjunctival tissue.

Both punctate and coarse epithelial keratopathy develops. Much of the epithelium is degenerated, and heaps and swirls of opaque epithelium can lead to large erosions. Pseudodendrites, which are in fact opaque, degenerated epithelium that has assumed a linear or somewhat dendritiform configuration [261], may appear. Rarely, marginal corneal ulcerations occur [262], and there may be superficial pannus. Thimerosal in contact lens solutions can frequently cause such severe changes.

HISTOPATHOLOGIC FEATURES. The histopathologic features of contact dermatitis are intraepidermal vesicles and bullae, intercellular and intracellular edema, lymphocytes, plasma cells, neutrophils in the epidermis, and hyperemia and edema of the upper part of the dermis [263, 264]. Perivascular infiltrates, composed largely of lymphocytes but with some neutrophils and plasma cells, are also seen in the dermis. Acanthosis, parakeratosis, and hyperkeratosis appear late.

Cytologic study of the conjunctiva shows lymphocytes, plasma cells, a few neutrophils, and various abnormalities (including degenerative changes) of the epithelial cells. Several or all of the following degenerative changes may occur: cellular enlargement, prominent and multiple nucleoli, clumping of chromatin, multinucleation, and toxic granules. The toxic granules are large, basophilic granules.

TREATMENT. Elimination or avoidance of the offending substance is the best treatment for contact dermatitis. Mechanical irritation, soaps, and cleansers are to be avoided as well. Creams or ointments containing corticosteroids are useful in the dry, subacute, and chronic stages, but probably should be avoided in the early phase. Systemic corticosteroids are not necessary.

The condition may worsen even during corticosteroid therapy if contact with the offending agent is not eliminated. Rarely, in fact, the corticosteroids may even cause a contact dermatitis [250]. Because secondary infection is a common complication, the use of corticosteroids must in any event be instituted with caution. It may be necessary to prepare the therapeutic agent (i.e., the corticosteroid) in a fresh solution without a preservative. Antihistamines have no effect on contact dermatitis, which is expected in a disease the pathogenesis of which depends largely on the CMI response.

REFERENCES

1. Thygeson, P., and Dawson, C. R. Pseudotrachoma caused by molluscum contagiosum virus and various chemical irritants. *Excerpta Medica, International Congress Series* 222:1894, 1970.
2. Patten, J. T., Cavanaugh, H. D., and Allansmith, M. R. Induced ocular pseudopemphigoid. *Am. J. Ophthalmol.* 82:272, 1976.
3. Nettleship, E. Chronic serpiginous ulcer of the cornea. *Trans. Ophthalmol. Soc. U.K.* 22:103, 1902.
4. Linn, J. G. Chronic serpiginous ulcer of the cornea. *Am. J. Ophthalmol.* 32:691, 1949.
5. Duke-Elder, S. *System of Ophthalmology, Vol. 7.* St. Louis: Mosby, 1965, p. 916.
6. Wood, T. O., and Kaufman, H. E. Mooren's ulcer. *Am. J. Ophthalmol.* 71:417, 1971.
7. Salamon, S. M., Mondino, B. J., and Zaidman, G. W. Peripheral corneal ulcers, conjunctival ulcers and scleritis after cataract surgery. *Am. J. Ophthalmol.* 93:334, 1982.
8. Hall, J., Smolin, G., and Wilson, F. M., II. Soluble antigens of the bovine cornea. *Invest. Ophthalmol.* 13:304, 1974.
9. Holt, W. S., and Kinoshita, J. H. The soluble proteins of the bovine cornea. *Invest. Ophthalmol.* 12:114, 1973.
10. Berger, B. Demonstration of a tissue-specific antigen in bovine corneal epithelium by immunodiffusion. *Acta Ophthalmol.* 49:790, 1971.
11. Murray, P. L., and Rahi, A. H. S. Pathogenesis of Mooren's ulcer. *Br. J. Ophthalmol.* 68:182, 1984.
12. Brown, S. I., Mondino, B. J., and Rabin, B. S. Autoimmune phenomenon in Mooren's ulcer. *Am. J. Ophthalmol.* 82:835, 1976.
13. Shaap, O. L., Feltkamp, T. E. W., and Breebaart, A. C. Circulating antibod-

ies to corneal tissue in a patient suffering from Mooren's ulcer. *Clin. Exp. Immunol.* 5:365, 1969.
14. Mondino, B. J., Brown, S. I., and Rabin, B. S. Cellular immunity in Mooren's ulcer. *Am. J. Ophthalmol.* 85:788, 1978.
15. Kietzman, B. Mooren's ulcer in Nigeria. *Am. J. Ophthalmol.* 71:417, 1968.
16. Foster, C. S., Kenyon, K. R., Greiner, J., and Greineder, D. K. The immunopathology of Mooren's ulcer. *Am. J. Ophthalmol.* 88:149, 1979.
17. Tabbara, K. F. The Role of the Conjunctiva in Peripheral Corneal Disease. In G. R. O. O'Connor (Ed.), *Immunologic Diseases of the Mucous Membranes.* New York: Masson, 1980.
18. Frayer, W. C. The histopathology of perilimbal ulceration in Wegener's granulomatosis. *Arch. Ophthalmol.* 64:58, 1960.
19. Kawaguchi, F. J. Histologic findings in rodent ulcer. *J. Clin. Ophthalmol.* 14:103, 1960.
20. Brown, S. I. Mooren's ulcer. *Br. J. Ophthalmol.* 59:670, 1975.
21. Brown, S. I., and Mondino, B. J. Therapy of Mooren's ulcer. *Am. J. Ophthalmol.* 98:1, 1984.
22. Friede, R. Medicamental and operative treatment of serpiginous corneal ulcer. *Acta Ophthalmol.* 26:509, 1948.
23. Aronson, S. B., et al. Pathogenetic approach to therapy of peripheral corneal inflammatory disease. *Am. J. Ophthalmol.* 70:65, 1970.
24. Joondeph, H. C., et al. Mooren's ulcer. *Ann. Ophthalmol.* 8:187, 1976.
25. Gifford, S. R. Rodent or Mooren's ulcer of the cornea. *Arch. Ophthalmol.* 10:800, 1933.
26. Kline, B. C. Pili, plasmids, and microbial virulence. *Mayo Clin. Proc.* 51:3, 1976.
27. Chattopadhyay, B. Gentamicin-resistant *Pseudomonas aeruginosa. Lancet* 1:1054, 1975.
28. Baughn, R. E., and Bonventre, P. F. Cell-mediated immune phenomena induced by lymphokines from splenic lymphocytes of mice with chronic staphylococcal infection. *Infect. Immun.* 11:313, 1975.
29. Smith, B. G., and Johnson, H. M. The effect of staphylococcal enterotoxins on the primary in vitro immune response. *J. Immunol.* 15:575, 1975.
30. Mudd, S., and Shayegani, M. Delayed-type hypersensitivity to *S. aureus* and its uses. *Ann. N.Y. Acad. Sci.* 236:244, 1974.
31. Palestine, A. G., Meyers, S. M., Fauci, A. S., and Gallin, J. I. Ocular findings in patients with neutrophil dysfunction. *Am. J. Ophthalmol.* 95:598, 1983.
32. Kim, H. B., and Ostler, H. B. Marginal corneal ulcer due to β streptococcus. *Arch. Ophthalmol.* 95:454, 1977.
33. Leibold, A. M., and Suie, T. In vitro effects of sulfacetamide. *Am. J. Ophthalmol.* 45:383, 1958.
34. Gordon, D. M. Gentamicin sulfate in external eye infections. *Am. J. Ophthalmol.* 69:300, 1970.
35. Smolin, G., et al. Effect of systemic corticosteroids on antibody-forming cells in the eye and draining lymph nodes. *Ann. Ophthalmol.* 9:1417, 1977.
36. Smolin, G., and Okumoto, M. Staphylococcal blepharitis. *Arch. Ophthalmol.* 95:812, 1977.
37. Gifford, S. R., and Hund, C. F. Ring abscess. *Arch. Ophthalmol.* 1:494, 1929.
38. Mondino, B. J., et al. Corneal rings with gram-negative bacteria. *Arch. Ophthalmol.* 95:2222, 1977.
39. Standish, M. Diphtheric conjunctivitis. *Trans. Am. Ophthalmol. Soc.* 7:694, 1896.

40. Howard, H., and James, W. Membranous conjunctivitis with loss of eyeballs. *J.A.M.A.* 93:1783, 1929.
41. Gifford, H. The pneumococcus as a frequent cause of acute catarrhal conjunctivitis. *Arch. Ophthalmol.* 25:314, 1896.
42. Francois, J., and Victoria-Troncoso, V. Ligneous conjunctivitis. *Am. J. Ophthalmol.* 65:673, 1968.
43. Spaeth, G. L. Chronic membranous conjunctivitis. *Am. J. Ophthalmol.* 64:300, 1967.
44. Hogan, M. J. Conjunctivitis with membrane formation. *Am. J. Ophthalmol.* 30:1495, 1947.
45. Firat, T. Ligneous conjunctivitis. *Am. J. Ophthalmol.* 78:679, 1974.
46. Parinaud, H. Infective conjunctivitis of animal origin. *Ann. Oculistique* 10:252, 1889.
47. Margileth, A. M., et al. Cat-scratch disease. *J.A.M.A.* 252:928, 1984.
48. Hadfield, T. L., et al. Electron microscopy of the cat-scratch disease bacillus. *J. Infect. Dis.* 152:643, 1985.
49. Wear, D. J., et al. Cat-scratch disease bacilli in the conjunctiva of patients with Parinaud's oculoglandular syndrome. *Ophthalmology* 92:1282, 1985.
50. Anderson, R. A. Oculoglandular tularemia. *J. Iowa Med. Soc.* 21:24, 1970.
51. Francis, E. Oculoglandular tularemia. *Arch. Ophthalmol.* 28:711, 1942.
52. Archer, D., and Bird, A. Primary tuberculosis of the conjunctiva. *Br. J. Ophthalmol.* 51:679, 1967.
53. McGrath, H., and Singer, J. Ocular sporotrichosis. *Am. J. Ophthalmol.* 35:102, 1952.
54. Wood, T. R. Ocular coccidioidomycosis. *Am. J. Ophthalmol.* 64:69, 1967.
55. Wong, S. P., and Grayson, J. T. Local and Systemic Antibody Response to Trachoma Eye Infection in Monkeys. In R. L. Nichols (Ed.), *Trachoma and Related Disorders Caused by Chlamydial Agents.* London: Excerpta Medica, 1971, p. 217.
56. Isa, A. H. The Antibody Response to Chlamydial Agents. In R. L. Nichols (Ed.), *Trachoma and Related Disorders Caused by Chlamydial Agents.* London: Excerpta Medica, 1971, p. 196.
57. Murray, E. S., Charbonnet, L. T., and MacDonald, A. B. Immunity to chlamydial infections of the eye. *J. Immunol.* 110:1518, 1973.
58. Isa, A. H., et al. Experimental inclusion conjunctivitis in man. *J. Immunol.* 101:1154, 1968.
59. Collier, L. H., and Blyth, W. A. Immunogenicity of experimental trachoma vaccine in baboons. *J. Hyg. (Lond.)* 64:513, 1966.
60. Dawson, C. R., and Schachter, J. Trachoma—Antibiotic or vaccine. *Invest. Ophthalmol.* 13:85, 1974.
61. Cho-Chou, K., and Grayston, T. J. Studies on delayed hypersensitivity with trachoma organisms. *J. Immunol.* 112:540, 1974.
62. Jawetz, E., et al. Immunoglobulin Nature of Antibodies in Chlamydial Infections. In R. L. Nichols (Ed.), *Trachoma and Related Disorders Caused by Chlamydial Agents.* London: Excerpta Medica, 1971.
63. Silverstein, A. M., and Prendergast, R. A. Lymphofollicular Hyperplastic Responses in Ectopic Locations. In K. Lindahl-Kiessling, G. Alm, and M. Hanna (Eds.), *Morphological and Functional Aspects of Immunity.* New York: Plenum Press, 1971.
64. Silverstein, A. M. Immunologic modulation of infectious disease pathogenesis. *Invest. Ophthalmol.* 13:560, 1974.

65. Kaufman, H. E., Kanai, A., and Ellison, E. D. Herpetic iritis. *Am. J. Ophthalmol.* 71:465, 1970.
66. Witmer, R., and Iwamoto, T. Electron microscope observation of herpeslike particles in the iris. *Arch. Ophthalmol.* 79:331, 1968.
67. Shimomura, Y., et al. HSV-1 quantitation from rabbit neural tissues after epinephrine-induced reactivation. *Invest. Ophthalmol. Vis. Sci.* 1:121, 1985.
68. Openshaw, H. Latency of herpes simplex virus in ocular tissue in mice. *Infect. Immun.* 39:960, 1983.
69. Pollack, F., et al. Immune host response to corneal grafts sensitive to herpes simplex virus. *Invest. Ophthalmol.* 15:188, 1976.
70. McCulley, J. P., et al. Collagenolytic activity in experimental herpes simplex keratitis. *Arch. Ophthalmol.* 84:516, 1970.
71. Laibson, P. R., and Kibrick, S. Reactivation of herpetic keratitis in rabbits. *Arch. Ophthalmol.* 77:244, 1967.
72. Walton, J. M. A., Ivayi, L., and Lehner, T. Cell-mediated immunity in *Herpesvirus hominis* infections. *Br. Med. J.* 1:723, 1972.
73. Bloomfield, S. E., and Lopez, C. Herpes infections in the immunosuppressed host. *Ophthalmology* 87:1226, 1980.
74. Easty, D. L., Maine, R. N., and Jones, B. R. Cellular immunity in herpes simplex keratitis. *Trans. Ophthalmol. Soc. U.K.* 93:171, 1973.
75. Glasgow, L. A. Interrelationship of interferon and immunity during viral infections. *J. Gen. Physiol.* 56:212, 1970.
76. Mackenzie, A. M. R. Variations in interferon production by lymphocytes from patients with chronic lymphatic leukemia. *J. Clin. Pathol.* 25:768, 1972.
77. Pollifoff, R., Cannavale, P., and Dixon, P. Herpes simplex virus infections in rabbit eyes. *Arch. Ophthalmol.* 88:52, 1972.
78. Galin, M. A., Chowchuveck, E., and Kronenberg, B. Therapeutic use of inducers of interferon on herpes simplex keratitis in humans. *Ann. Ophthalmol.* 8:72, 1976.
79. Jones, B. R., et al. Topical therapy of ulcerative herpetic keratitis with human interferon. *Lancet* 2:128, 1976.
80. Pollikoff, R., Dipuppo, A., and Cannavale, P. Vesicular stomatitis virus infection in rabbit eyes. *Invest. Ophthalmol.* 8:488, 1969.
81. Smolin, G., et al. Use of recombinant interferon to prevent recurrent herpesvirus shedding. *Curr. Eye Res.* 31:1069, 1984.
82. Mayer, M., et al. Recombinant human interferon alpha D in HSV-1 recurrences in the rabbit. *Invest. Ophthalmol. Vis. Sci.* 26:237, 1985.
83. Zimmerman, T. J., et al. HLA types and recurrent corneal herpes simplex infection. *Invest. Ophthalmol.* 16:756, 1977.
84. Meyers, R. L. Immunology of herpes simplex virus infection. *Int. Ophthalmol. Clin.* 15:37, 1975.
85. Easty, D. L., Maine, R. N., and Jones, B. R. Cellular immunity in herpes simplex keratitis. *Trans. Ophthalmol. Soc. U.K.* 93:171, 1973.
86. Wilton, J. M. A., Ivanyi, L., and Lehner, T. Cell-mediated immunity in herpesvirus hominis infections. *Br. Med. J.* 1:723, 1972.
87. Gange, R. W., et al. Cellular immunity and circulating antibody to herpes simplex virus in subjects with recurrent herpes simplex lesions and controls as measured by the mixed leukocytes migration inhibition test and complement fixation. *Br. J. Dermatol.* 97:539, 1975.
88. Meyers, R. L., and Pettit, T. H. The pathogenesis of corneal inflammation due to herpes simplex virus. *J. Immunol.* 111:1031, 1973.

89. Russell, R. G., et al. Role of T-lymphocytes in the pathogenesis of herpetic stromal disease. *Invest. Ophthalmol.* 25:938, 1984.
90. Kaufman, H. E. Treatment of viral diseases. *Int. Ophthalmol. Clin.* 4:334, 1964.
91. Metcalf, J. F., and Kaufman, H. E. Herpetic stromal keratitis—Evidence for cell-mediated immunopathogenesis. *Am. J. Ophthalmol.* 82:827, 1976.
92. Sery, T. W., Richman, M. W., and Nagy, R. M. Experimental disciform keratitis. *J. Allergy* 38:338, 1966.
93. Henson, D., et al. Ultrastructural localization of herpes simplex virus antigens on rabbit corneal cells using sheep antihuman IgG antihorse ferritin hybrid antibodies. *Invest. Ophthalmol.* 13:819, 1974.
94. Laibson, P. R., et al. Corneal infiltrates in epidemic keratoconjunctivitis. *Arch. Ophthalmol.* 84:36, 1970.
95. Kiernan, J. P., Schanzlin, D. J., and Leveille, A. S. Stevens-Johnson syndrome associated with adenovirus conjunctivitis. *Am. J. Ophthalmol.* 92:543, 1981.
96. Boisjoly, H. M., Woog, J. J., and Pavan-Langston, D. Prophylactic topical cyclosporine in experimental herpetic stromal keratitis. *Arch. Ophthalmol.* 102:1804, 1984.
97. Balfour, Jr., H. H., et al. Acyclovir halts progression of herpes zoster in immunocompromised patients. *N. Engl. J. Med.* 308:1448, 1983.
98. McGill, J., Chapman, C., Copplestone, A., and Maharasingam, M. A review of acyclovir treatment of ocular herpes zoster and skin infections. *J. Antimicrob. Chemother.* 12:45, 1983.
99. Felber, T. D., Smith, E. B., and Knox, J. Photodynamic inactivation of herpes simplex. *J.A.M.A.* 223:289, 1973.
100. Rapp, F., and Duff, R. *In vitro* cell transformation by herpes viruses. *Fed. Proc.* 31:1660, 1972.
101. Kern, A. B., and Schiff, B. L. Smallpox vaccinations in the management of recurrent herpes simplex. *J. Invest. Dermatol.* 33:99, 1959.
102. Goldman, L. Reactions of autoinoculation for recurrent herpes simplex. *Arch. Dermatol.* 84:1025, 1961.
103. Scriba, M. Animal studies on the efficacy of vaccination against recurrent herpes. *Med. Microbiol. Immunol.* 171:33, 1982.
104. Fulginiti, V. A., et al. Therapy of experimental vaccinial keratitis. *Arch. Ophthalmol.* 74:539, 1965.
105. Smolin, G., and Okumoto, M. Human transfer factor in the treatment of guinea pig herpetic keratitis. *Ann. Ophthalmol.* 8:427, 1976.
106. Renoux, G., and Renoux, M. Action immunostimulante de dérivé du phenylimidothiazole sur les cellules spleniques. *Acad. Sci.* 274:756, 1972.
107. Symoens, J., and Brugman, J. Treatment of recurrent aphthous stomatitis and herpes with levamisole. *Br. J. Med.* 4:592, 1974.
108. Kint, A., and Verlinden, L. Levamisole for recurrent herpes labialis. *N. Engl. J. Med.* 291:308, 1974.
109. David, J. R. The elusive humors of the lymphocyte mediators of delayed hypersensitivity. *J. Allergy* 47:237, 1971.
110. Baram, P., and Cardoulis, W. Studies on rhesus-monkey nondialyzable and dialyzable transfer factor. *Transplant. Proc.* 6:209, 1974.
111. Smolin, G., Tabbara, K., and Okumoto, M. Guinea pig herpes simplex keratitis treated with lymphocyte extract. *Am. J. Ophthalmol.* 78:921, 1974.
112. Pallin, O., Lundmark, K. M., and Brege, K. G. Interferon in severe herpes

simplex of the cornea. *Lancet* 1:1187, 1976.
113. Paque, R. E., and Dray, S. Transfer of delayed hypersensitivity to nonsensitive human leukocytes with rhesus monkey lymphoid RNA extracts. *Transplant. Proc.* 6:203, 1974.
114. Rosenthal, S. R. BCG and the lympho-reticulo-endothelial system. *Recent Results Cancer Res.* 47:2228, 1974.
115. Hotterman, O. A., Casale, G. P., and Klein, E. Tumor cell destruction by macrophages. *J. Med.* 3:305, 1972.
116. Larson, C. L., et al. *Herpesvirus hominis* type 2 infections in rabbits. *Infect. Immun.* 6:465, 1972.
117. Scott, M. T. *Corynebacterium parvum* as an immunotherapeutic anticancer agent. *Semin. Oncol.* 1:367, 1974.
118. Pinckard, R. N., Weir, D. M., and McBride, W. H. Effects of *C. Parvum* in immunologic unresponsiveness to bovine serum albumin in the rabbit. *Nature* 215:870, 1967.
119. Sher, N. A., Chaparos, S. D., and Greenberg, L. E. The effect of BCG and *C. parvum* on the mortality from *S. aureus* septicemia in mice. *Proc. Am. Assoc. Cancer Res.* 16:71, 1975.
120. Cohen, B. E., and Cohen, I. K. Vitamin A: Adjuvant and steroid antagonist in the immune response. *J. Immunol.* 111:1376, 1973.
121. Cohen, B. E., and Elin, R. J. Vitamin A–induced nonspecific resistance to infection. *J. Infect. Dis.* 129:597, 1974.
122. Goldstein, A. L., et al. Hormonal influence on the reticuloendothelial system. *J. Reticuloendothel. Soc.* 23:253, 1978.
123. Pivetti-Pezzi, P., et al. Thymic factor therapy for herpetic keratitis. *Ann. Ophthalmol.* 17:327, 1985.
124. Schmidt, K. L., and Mueller-Eckhardt, C. Agranulocytosis, levamisole, and HLA-B27. *Lancet* 2:85, 1977.
125. Graber, H., Takacs, L., and Vedrody, K. Agranulocytosis due to levamisole. *Lancet* 2:1248, 1976.
126. Smolin, G., Okumoto, M., and Friedlaender, M. Treatment of herpetic keratitis with levamisole. *Arch. Ophthalmol.* 96:1078, 1978.
127. Friedlaender, M., Okumoto, M., and Smolin, G. Levamisole treatment of herpetic reinfection. *Am. J. Ophthalmol.* 86:245, 1978.
128. Rytel, M. W., et al. Therapy of cytomegalovirus retinitis with transfer factor. *Cell. Immunol.* 19:821, 1975.
129. Stevens, D. A., et al. Immunotherapy in recurrent coccidioidomycosis. *Cell. Immunol.* 12:37, 1974.
130. Schulkind, M. L., et al. Transfer factor in the treatment of a case of chronic mucocutaneous candidiasis. *Cell. Immunol.* 3:606, 1972.
131. Pearsall, N. N., Sundsmo, J. S., and Weiser, R. S. Lymphokine toxicity for yeast cells. *J. Immunol.* 110:1444, 1973.
132. Krahenbuhl, J. L., Rosenberg, L. T., and Remington, J. S. The role of thymus-derived lymphocytes in the *in vitro* activation of macrophages to kill *Listeria Monocytogenes*. *J. Immunol.* 111:992, 1973.
133. Klesius, P. H., Kelley, L. N., and Trujillo, P. R. Leukocyte stimulation, enhanced phagocytosis of staphylococcus. *Proc. Soc. Exp. Biol. Med.* 140:397, 1972.
134. Smolin, G., Okumoto, M., and Belfort, R., Jr. The treatment of experimental herpetic keratitis with BCG. *Can. J. Ophthalmol.* 10:385, 1975.
135. Smolin, G., et al. Effect of immunization with attenuated *Mycobacterium bovis* on experimental herpetic keratitis. *Immunol. Abstr.* 1:98, 1976.

136. Jawetz, E., Melnick, J. L., and Adelberg, E. A. (Eds.). *Medical Microbiology.* Los Altos, Calif.: Lange, 1966, p. 135.
137. Bigley, N. J. (Ed.). *Immunologic Fundamentals.* Chicago: Year Book, 1975, pp. 1, 140.
138. Howard, D. H., Otto, V., and Gupta, R. K. Lymphocyte-mediated cellular immunity in histoplasmosis. *Infect. Immun.* 4:605, 1971.
139. Canales, L., et al. Immunological observations in chronic mucocutaneous candidiasis. *Lancet* 2:567, 1969.
140. Chilgren, R. A., et al. Chronic mucocutaneous candidiasis, deficiency of delayed hypersensitivity and selective antibody defect. *Lancet* 2:688, 1967.
141. Wong, V. G., and Kirkpatrick, C. H. Immune reconstitution in keratoconjunctivitis and superficial candidiasis. *Arch. Ophthalmol.* 92:335, 1974.
142. La Force, F. M., et al. Inhibition of leukocyte candidiacidal activity by serum from patients with disseminated candidiasis. *J. Lab. Clin. Med.* 86:657, 1975.
143. Thygeson, P., and Okumoto, M. Keratomycoses: A preventable disease. *Trans. Am. Acad. Ophthalmol. Otolaryngol.* 78:433, 1974.
144. Kaufman, H. E., and Wood, R. M. Mycotic keratitis. *Am. J. Ophthalmol.* 59:993, 1965.
145. Getnick, R. A., and Rodrigues, M. M. Endogenous fungal endophthalmitis in a drug addict. *Am. J. Ophthalmol.* 77:680, 1974.
146. Greene, W. H., and Wiernik, P. H. Candida endophthalmitis. *Am. J. Ophthalmol.* 74:1100, 1972.
147. Chandler, J. W., Kalina, R. E., and Milan, D. G. Coccidioidal choroiditis following renal transplantation. *Am. J. Ophthalmol.* 74:1080, 1972.
148. Berson, E. L., et al. Topical corticosteroids and fungal keratitis. *Invest. Ophthalmol.* 6:512, 1967.
149. Howes, E. L., Jr., and McKay, D. G. Comparison of the ocular effects of circulating endotoxin and immune complexes. *J. Immunol.* 114:734, 1975.
150. Howes, E. L., Jr., and McKay, D. G. Circulating immune complexes. *Arch. Ophthalmol.* 93:365, 1975.
151. Gerstle, C. C., and Friedman, A. H. Marginal corneal ulceration as a presenting sign of temporal arteritis. *Ophthalmology* 87:1173, 1980.
152. Schulman, M. F., and Sugar, A. Peripheral corneal infiltrates in inflammatory bowel disease. *Ann. Ophthalmol.* 12:190, 1980.
153. Michels, M. L., et al. Rheumatoid arthritis and sterile corneal ulceration. *Arthritis Rheum.* 27:606, 1984.
154. Baum, J. L., and Bierstock, S. R. Peripheral corneal infiltrates following intravenous injection of diatrizoate meglumine. *Am. J. Ophthalmol.* 85:613, 1978.
155. Kopeloff, L. M. Recurrent immunologic interstitial keratitis. *Arch. Pathol. Lab. Med.* 100:74, 1976.
156. Shirahama, T., and Cohen, A. S. High resolution electron microscopic analysis of the amyloid fibril. *J. Cell. Biol.* 33:679, 1967.
157. Eanes, E. D., and Genner, G. G. X-ray diffraction studies on amyloid filaments. *J. Histochem. Cytochem.* 16:673, 1968.
158. Vassar, P. S., and Culling, C. F. A. Fluorescent stains with special reference to amyloid and connective tissues. *Arch. Pathol.* 68:487, 1959.
159. Rogers, P. R. Screening for amyloid with thioflavin T fluorescent material. *Am. J. Clin. Pathol.* 44:59, 1965.
160. Lehner, T. Juxtaglomerular apparatus staining with thioflavin T fluorochrome and its confusion with amyloid. *Nature* 206:738, 1965.
161. Cohen, H. J., and Crawford, J. Disorders of Amyloid Deposition. In A. S.

Cohen (Ed.), *Pathology of Immunoglobulins: Diagnostic and Clinical Aspects.* New York: Liss, 1982, p. 293.
162. Telium, G. Origin of Amyloidosis from PAS-positive Reticuloendothelial Cells *In Situ* and Basic Factors in Pathogenesis. In E. Mandema, et al. (Ed.), *Amyloidosis.* Amsterdam: Excerpta Medica, 1968, p. 37.
163. Cohen, A. S. Amyloidosis. *N. Engl. J. Med.* 277:522, 1967.
164. McAdam, K. P. W. J., et al. Association of amyloidosis with erythema nodosum leprosum reactions and recurrent neutrophil leucocytosis in leprosy. *Lancet* 2:572, 1975.
165. Benditt, E. P., and Ericksen, N. Chemical classes of amyloid substances. *Am. J. Pathol.* 65:231, 1971.
166. Levin, M., Pras, M., and Franklin, E. C. Immunologic studies of the major nonimmunoglobulinprotein of amyloid. *J. Exp. Med.* 138:373, 1973.
167. Glenner, G. G., et al. Amyloid fibril proteins. *Science* 171:1150, 1971.
168. Glenner, G. G., et al. The creation of amyloid fibers from Bence Jones protein *in vitro. Science* 1974:712, 1971.
169. Glenner, G. G. The pathogenetic and therapeutic implications of the discovery of the immunoglobulin origin of amyloid fibers. *Hum. Pathol.* 3:157, 1972.
170. Cathcart, E. S., et al. Immunoglobulins and amyloidosis. *Am. J. Med.* 52:93, 1972.
171. Garcia, R. L., and Backe, J. T. IgM in skin lesions of systemic amyloidosis. *J.A.M.A.* 237:1598, 1977.
172. Galmiche, J. P., et al. L'Association maladie de Crohn-amylose. *Nouv. Presse Med.* 6:105, 1977.
173. Brownstein, M. H. The clinical spectrum of amyloidosis. *Med. Times.* 96:232, 1968.
174. Brownstein, M. H., Elliott, R., and Helwig, E. B. Ophthalmologic aspects of amyloidosis. *Am. J. Ophthalmol.* 69:423, 1970.
175. Fisher, H., and Preuss, F. S. Primary systemic amyloidosis with involvement of the nervous system. *Am. J. Clin. Pathol.* 21:758, 1951.
176. Goldman, M. J., and Gerstl, B. Primary systemic amyloidosis. *Calif. Med.* 61:36, 1949.
177. Brownstein, M. H., and Hashimoto, K. Macula amyloidosis. *Arch. Dermatol.* 106:50, 1972.
178. Ferry, A. P., and Lieberman, T. W. Bilateral amyloidosis of the vitreous body. *Arch. Ophthalmol.* 94:982, 1976.
179. Beebe, R. T., Propp, S., and Scharfman, W. B. Chronic purpura due to amyloidosis. *Trans. Am. Clin. Climatol.* 64:18, 1953.
180. Propp, S., et al. Atypical amyloidosis associated with nonthrombocytopenic purpura and plasmocyte hyperplasia of the bone marrow. *Blood* 9:397, 1954.
181. Hallen, J., and Rudin, R. Pericollagenous amyloidosis. *Acta Med. Scand.* 179:483, 1966.
182. Goltz, R. W. Systematized amyloidosis. *Medicine* 31:381, 1952.
183. Purcell, J. J., Birkenkamp, R., Tsai, C. C., and Riner, R. N. Conjunctival involvement in primary systemic nonfamilial amyloidosis. *Am. J. Ophthalmol.* 95:845, 1983.
184. Liesegang, T. J. Amyloid infiltration of the levator palpebrae superioris muscle. *Ann. Ophthalmol.* 15:610, 1983.
185. Schwartz, M. F., et al. An unusual case of ocular involvement in primary systemic nonfamilial amyloidosis. *Ophthalmology* 89:394, 1982.

186. Macoul, K. L., and Winter, F. C. External ophthalmoplegia. *Arch. Ophthalmol.* 79:182, 1968.
187. Ts'o, M. O., and Bettman, J. W., Jr. Occlusion of choriocapillaris in primary nonfamilial amyloidosis. *Arch. Ophthalmol.* 86:281, 1971.
188. Chambers, R. A., Medd, W. E., and Spencer, H. Primary amyloidosis. *Q. J. Med.* 27:207, 1958.
189. Kasner, D., et al. Surgical treatment of amyloidosis of the vitreous. *Trans. Am. Acad. Ophthalmol. Otolaryngol.* 72:410, 1968.
190. Bleehen, S. S., Everall, J. D., and Tighe, J. R. Amyloidosis complicating Reiter's syndrome. *Br. J. Vener. Dis.* 42:88, 1966.
191. Westermark, P., and Stenkvist, B. A new method for the diagnosis of systemic amyloidosis. *Arch. Intern. Med.* 132:522, 1973.
192. Schwartz, P. Senile cerebral, pancreatic, insular and cardiac amyloidosis. *Trans. N.Y. Acad. Sci.* 27:393, 1965.
193. Cohen, A. S. Constitution and Genesis of Amyloid. In G. W. Richter and M. A. Epstein (Eds.), *International Review of Experimental Pathology*, Vol. IV. New York: Academic, 1965, p. 159.
194. Buerger, L., and Braunstein, H. Senile cardiac amyloidosis. *Am. J. Med.* 28:357, 1960.
195. Borodic, G. E., et al. Immunoglobulin deposition in localized conjunctival amyloidosis. *Am. J. Ophthalmol.* 98:617, 1984.
196. Schaldenbrand, J. D., and Keren, D. F. IgD amyloid in IgD-A monoclonal conjunctival amyloidosis. *Arch. Pathol. Lab. Med.* 107:626, 1983.
197. Lucas, D. R., Knowx, F., and Davies, S. Apparent monoclonal origin of lymphocytes and plasma cells infiltrating ocular adnexal amyloid deposits. *Br. J. Ophthalmol.* 66:606, 1982.
198. Elles, N. B. Amyloid disease of the conjunctiva. *Trans. Am. Ophthalmol. Soc.* 42:262, 1944.
199. Halasa, A. H. Amyloid disease of the eyelid and conjunctiva. *Arch. Ophthalmol.* 74:298, 1965.
200. Mathur, S. P., and Mathur, B. P. Conjunctival amyloidosis. *Br. J. Ophthalmol.* 43:765, 1959.
201. Smith, M. E., and Zimmerman, L. E. Amyloidosis of the eyelid and conjunctiva. *Arch. Ophthalmol.* 75:42, 1966.
202. Jensen, J. E. Localized amyloidosis in relation to conjunctival hemorrhagic lymphangiecstasia and occlusion of the orbital veins. *Acta Ophthalmol.* 61:254, 1983.
203. Matsui, M., Ito, K., and Akiya, S. Histochemical and electron microscopic examinations on so-called gelatinous drop-like dystrophy of the cornea. *Folia Ophthalmol. Jpn.* 23:466, 1972.
204. Nagati, S., Tanishima, T., and Sakomoto, T. A case of primary gelatinous drop-like corneal dystrophy. *Jpn. J. Ophthalmol.* 16:107, 1972.
205. Ramsey, M. S., and Fine, B. S. Localized corneal amyloidosis. *Am. J. Ophthalmol.* 73:560, 1972.
206. Stock, E. L., and Kielar, R. A. Primary familial amyloidosis of the cornea. *Am. J. Ophthalmol.* 82:266, 1976.
207. Kirk, H. Q., et al. Primary familial amyloidosis of the cornea. *Trans. Am. Acad. Ophthalmol. Otolaryngol.* 77:411, 1973.
208. Takahashi, T., Kondo, T., Isobe, T., and Okada, S. A case of corneal amyloidosis. *Acta Ophthalmol.* 61:150, 1983.
209. Ohnishi, Y., Shinoda, Y., Ishibashi, T., and Taniguchi, Y. The origin of amyloid in gelatinous drop-like corneal dystrophy. *Curr. Eye Res.* 2:225, 1983.

210. Smith, M. E., and Zimmerman, L. E. Amyloid in corneal dystrophies. *Arch. Ophthalmol.* 79:407, 1968.
211. Bowen, R. A., et al. Lattice dystrophy of the cornea as a variety of amyloidosis. *Am. J. Ophthalmol.* 70:822, 1970.
212. Mondino, B. J., et al. Protein AA and lattice corneal dystrophy. *Am. J. Ophthalmol.* 89:377, 1980.
213. Wheeler, G. E., and Eiferman, R. A. Immunohistochemical identification of the AA protein in lattice dystrophy. *Exp. Eye Res.* 36:181, 1983.
214. Mondino, B. J., et al. Primary familial amyloidosis of the cornea. *Am. J. Ophthalmol.* 92:732, 1981.
215. Meretoja, J. Familial systemic paramyloidosis with lattice dystrophy of the cornea, progressive cranial neuropathy, skin changes and various internal symptoms. *Ann. Clin. Res.* 1:314, 1969.
216. Meretoja, J. Comparative histopathology and clinical findings in eyes with lattice corneal dystrophy of 2 different types. *Ophthalmologica* 165:15, 1972.
217. Meretoja, J., and Teppo, L. Histopathologic findings of familial amyloidosis with cranial neuropathy as the principal manifestation. *Acta Pathol. Microbiol. Scand. Sec. A*79:432, 1971.
218. Mannis, M. J., et al. Polymorphic amyloid degeneration of the cornea. *Arch. Ophthalmol.* 99:1217, 1981.
219. Krachmer, J. H., Dubord, P. J., Rodrigues, M. M., and Mannis, M. J. Corneal posterior crocodile shagreen and polymorphic amyloid degeneration. *Arch. Ophthalmol.* 101:54, 1983.
220. Smaltino, M. Contributo all conoscenza delle degenerazioni corneali nel trachoma. *Boll. Ocul.* 16:126, 1937.
221. Bernath, G. Amyloidosis in malignant tumors. *Acta Morphol.* 2:137, 1956.
222. Duke-Elder, W. S. *Textbook of Ophthalmology.* St. Louis: Mosby, 1965.
223. Rodrigues, M., and Zimmerman, L. L. Secondary amyloidosis in ocular leprosy. *Arch. Ophthalmol.* 85:277, 1971.
224. McPherson, S. D., Jr., Kiffney, G. T., Jr., and Freed, C. C. Corneal amyloidosis. *Trans. Am. Ophthalmol. Soc.* 64:148, 1966.
225. Groniowski, J. Orbital amyloidosis. *Acta Ophthalmol.* 43:725, 1965.
226. Pecora, J. L., Sambursky, J. S., and Vargha, Z. Radiation therapy in amyloidosis of the eyelid and conjunctiva. *Ann. Ophthalmol.* 14:194, 1982.
227. Irvine, A. R., and Char, D. H. Recurrent amyloid involvement in the vitreous body after vitrectomy. *Am. J. Ophthalmol.* 82:705, 1976.
228. Watson, P. G. Diseases of the Sclera and Episclera. In D. Duane (Ed.), *Clinical Ophthalmology.* Hagertown, Md.: Harper and Row, 1980. Vol. 4 Chapter 23, pp. 1–39.
229. Brubaker, R., Font, R. L., and Shepherd, E. M. Granulomatosis sclerouveitis. *Arch. Ophthalmol.* 86:517, 1971.
230. Watson, P. G., and Bovey, E. Anterior segment fluorescein angiography in the diagnosis of scleral inflammation. *Ophthalmology* 92:1, 1985.
231. Sevel, D. Necrogranulomatous scleritis. *Am. J. Ophthalmol.* 64:1125, 1967.
232. Merz, E. H. Scleral reinforcement with aortic tissue. *Am. J. Ophthalmol.* 62:763, 1964.
233. Torchia, R. H., Dunn, R. E., and Pease, P. J. Fascia lata grafting in scleromalacia perforans. *Am. J. Ophthalmol.* 66:705, 1968.
234. Fransden, E. Eye disease following BCG vaccination. *Acta Ophthalmol.* 57:13, 1959.
235. Kuniya, Y. Über die frage nach der Kenntnis der experimentellen phlyktane. *Acta Soc. Ophthalmol. Jpn.* 39:32, 1935.

236. Igersheimer, J., and Prinz, W. Gedanken und untersuchungen zur pathogenese der phlyctänlaren augenentzundungen und zum schicksal skrofuloser augen patienten. *Arch. Ophthalmol.* 105:640, 1921.
237. Davis, P. L., and Watson, J. I. Experimental conjunctival phlyctenulosis. *Can. J. Ophthalmol.* 4:183, 1969.
238. Thygeson, P. Observations on nontuberculosis phlyctenular keratoconjunctivitis. *Trans. Am. Acad. Ophthalmol. Otolaryngol.* 58:128, 1954.
239. Jeffrey, M. P. Ocular diseases caused by nematodes. *Am. J. Ophthalmol.* 40:41, 1953.
240. De Schweinitz, C. E. *Diseases of the Eye.* Philadelphia: Saunders, 1917, p. 211.
241. Thygeson, P. Etiology and treatment of phlyctenular keratoconjunctivitis. *Am. J. Ophthalmol.* 34: 1217, 1951.
242. Ostler, H. B. Corneal perforation in nontuberculous phlyctenular keratoconjunctivitis. *Am. J. Ophthalmol.* 79:445, 1975.
243. Ostler, Y. B., and Lanier, J. D. Phlyctenular keratoconjunctivitis with special reference to the staphylococcus type. *Trans. Pac. Coast Otoophthalmol. Soc.* 55:237, 1974.
244. Thygeson, P., and Fritz, M. H. Cortisone in phlyctenular keratoconjunctivitis. *Am. J. Ophthalmol.* 34:357, 1951.
245. Stefferson, E. H., et al. Topical cortisone in the treatment of anterior segment eye disease. *Am. J. Ophthalmol.* 34:345, 1957.
246. Waldbott, G. *Contact Dermatitis.* (American Lecture Series.) Springfield, Ill.: Thomas, 1953.
246a. Wilson, F. M. II. Adverse external ocular effects of topical ophthalmic therapy. *Trans. Am. Ophthalmol. Soc.* 81:854, 1983.
247. Sulzberger, M. B. *Dermatologic Allergy.* Springfield, Ill.: Thomas, 1940.
248. Baer, R. L., and Witten, V. H. Allergic Eczematous Contact Dermatitis: A Review of Selected Aspects for the Practitioner. In *Year Book of Dermatology.* Chicago: Year Book, 1956, 1957, pp. 7–38 (Part I) and 7–46 (Part II).
249. Aeling, J. L., and Nuss, D. D. Systemic eczematous contact-type dermatitis medicamentosa caused by parabens. *Arch. Dermatol.* 110:640, 1974.
250. Theodore, F. H., and Schlossman, A. *Ocular Allergy.* Baltimore: Williams & Wilkins, 1958.
251. Taub, S. J. Cosmetic allergies. *Eye Ear Nose Throat Mon.* 55:33, 1976.
252. Malkinson, F. D. Permeability of the stratum corneum. In W. Montagna and W. C. Lobitz, Jr. (Eds.), *The Epidermis.* New York: Academic, 1961.
253. Bluefarb, S. M. *Scope Monograph on Dermatology.* Kalamazoo, Mich.: Upjohn, 1972.
254. Gellin, G. A. *Occupational Dermatosis.* Chicago: American Medical Association, 1972.
255. Flax, M. H., and Caulfield, J. B. Cellular and vascular components of allergic contact dermatitis. *Am. J. Pathol.* 43:1031, 1963.
256. Salvin, S., and Smith, R. F. The specificity of allergic reactions. *J. Exp. Med.* 114:185, 1961.
257. Gell, P. G. H., and Benacerraf, B. Studies on hypersensitivity. *J. Exp. Med.* 113:571, 1961.
258. Allansmith, M. R. Ocular Allergy. In B. Golden (Ed.), *Ocular Inflammatory Disease.* Springfield, Ill.: Thomas, 1974.
259. Dvorak, H. F., and Dvorak, A. M. Basophilic leukocytes. *Clin. Hematol.* 4:651, 1975.
260. Dvorak, H. F., et al. Cutaneous basophil hypersensitivity. *J. Exp. Med.* 132:558, 1970.

261. Wilson, F. M., II. Personal communication, 1985.
262. Thygeson, P. Marginal corneal infiltrates and ulcers. *Trans. Am. Acad. Ophthalmol. Otolaryngol.* 51:198, 1947.
263. Fitzpatrick, T. B., et al. *Dermatology in General Medicine.* New York: McGraw-Hill, 1971.
264. Yanoff, M., and Fine, B. S. *Ocular Pathology: A Text and Atlas.* Hagerstown, Md.: Harper & Row, 1975.
265. Fedukowicz, H., Wise, G. N., and Zaret, M. M. Toxic conjunctivitis due to antibiotics. *Am. J. Ophthalmol.* 40:849, 1955.

5 SYSTEMIC IMMUNOLOGIC DISEASES AFFECTING THE EXTERNAL EYE

PEMPHIGUS AND PEMPHIGOID

Pemphigus Vulgaris

Ocular pemphigus and pemphigoid have erroneously been considered to be the same entity by certain authors in the past.

Pemphigus vulgaris is characterized by the occurrence of intraepithelial bullae over all the body surfaces. The areas affected most severely are the skin, mouth, and eyes. With rupture of the bullae, which is always quite painful, there is a discharge of serous fluid. The resulting ulcerated areas are susceptible to secondary infection, and if these infections are not adequately treated, death may occur from septicemia.

The disease primarily affects individuals in the middle-age group, and of all the ethnic groups plagued by this malady, Jews seem to have been the hardest hit. This group's susceptibility may be related to the possession of common HLA antigens among certain groups of European Jews who have tended to marry within the confines of a few families. Indeed, Park and Terasaki [1] have shown that over 90 percent of Jewish patients suffering from pemphigus vulgaris possess the HLA DRW4 gene. One can only speculate that in this group, at least, a common immunogenetic factor predisposes these patients to develop this particular problem. Perhaps, the possession of a particular HLA gene, coupled with exposure to a particular environmental stimulus, brings about the onset of the disease. Many patients affected by the disease have been exposed to domestic animals or their by-products. Thus pemphigus seems to have affected more than its share of butchers, tanners, sausage makers, and the like. This characteristic has led to the speculation that the disease may be caused by an epizootic virus, but as yet, none has been isolated.

Pemphigus is associated with the presence of circulating IgG antibodies directed against an intercellular antigen. Such antibodies can often be demonstrated in high titer at the time of onset of an attack. They appear to have a destructive effect on the cement substance that binds cells together in the prickle cell layer. Hashimoto et al [2] have shown that plasminogen activators, which are serine proteinases that catalyze the conversion of plasminogen to plasmin, are liberated by epithelial cells following the attachment of pemphigus autoantibodies to the surfaces of the cell membranes. These proteinases break down the intercellular cement substances that ordinarily keep epithelial cells in contact. This destruction results in acantholysis (a separation and contraction of these cells), ultimately leading to an intraepithelial bulla. The basement membrane remains covered by at least a thin layer of epithelium, and this layer may prevent fibrous tissue elements from entering the lesion and causing scars. Scarring therefore usually does not occur.

Lesions on the eye most often affect the skin of the lid, but may also affect the conjunctiva, particularly on the nasal side of the bulbar conjunctiva. The bursting of these bullae is painful, but the lesion generally heals without serious visual sequelae, provided that secondary infection is suppressed with local or systemic antimicrobials. *Staphylococcus* is the most common bacterial invader in these situations.

Antibodies to the intercellular antigen in the prickle cell layer can be demonstrated by fluorescent antibody techniques. For this purpose, either normal or abnormal epithelium can be used. For example, serum from the affected patient can be placed on frozen sections of rat esophagus and allowed to react with the tissue. After washing off all unbound protein, the location of the antibodies can be demonstrated by adding fluorescein-tagged duck antihuman IgG to the preparation and by viewing it under an ultraviolet microscope. The intercellular fluorescence in the prickle cell layer is characteristic and diagnostic (Fig. 5-1). The circulating antibodies characteristic of pemphigus vulgaris do not fix complement.

TREATMENT. Prior to the advent of corticosteroid therapy, pemphigus vulgaris was almost universally fatal. With the use of systemic corticosteroids the course of the lesions is significantly modified, and this benefit has led to the widespread use of oral prednisone in the therapy of the disease. Many patients become relatively resistant to corticosteroid therapy after prolonged use, and, when higher doses are required, the secondary effects of steroids become more troublesome. Demineralization of bone, hypertension, and secondary diabetes are commonly encountered complications. For this reason, immunosuppressive therapy has been attempted in some cases [3] with promising results. In cases where immunosuppressive therapy must be interrupted because of unacceptable side effects [3a], plasmapheresis has proved valuable as a supplementary therapy. In such cases, the removal of antibodies that are directly causative of the disease makes sense. However, plasmapheresis is not only expensive, it is also frought with multiple complications of its own: the induction of thromboses, tetany, hepatitis, and other problems.

5. DISEASES AFFECTING THE EXTERNAL EYE

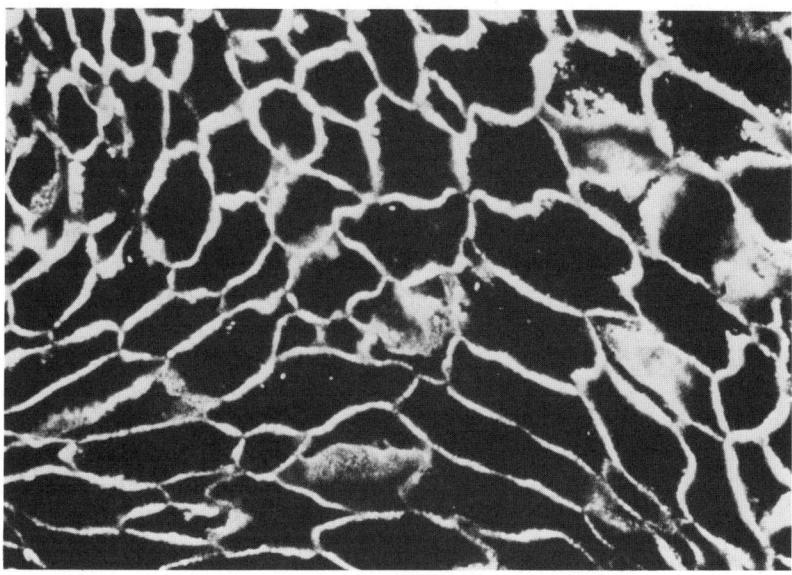

FIG. 5-1 Intercellular fluorescence in pemphigus vulgaris. Ultraviolet light. (× 312 before reduction). (Courtesy of Dr. Troy E. Daniels, University of California, San Francisco.)

Cicatricial Pemphigoid

Cicatricial pemphigoid, variously referred to as benign mucous membrane pemphigoid, ocular pemphigoid, essential shrinkage of the conjunctiva, or cicatricial pemphigoid, may have disastrous effects on the eye. It is a "benign" disease only in the sense that it usually does not cause death. In addition to the conjunctiva, the mucous membranes of the mouth, rectum, vagina, pharynx, and esophagus are often involved. Strictures of the esophagus have resulted in the death of several patients; thus the sequelae of the disease are not altogether benign.

Cicatricial pemphigoid is probably the best name for this disease. The relationship of cicatricial lesions of the mucous membranes to cicatricial bullae of the skin ("bullous pemphigoid") remains unknown, although both seem to exhibit a similar immunohistopathologic picture. A bulla is produced under the epithelium of the mucous membrane or skin. When the bulla ruptures, fibrous tissue from the underlying corium may invade the lesion, and scarring is virtually inevitable. In the case of the conjunctiva, the touching of two surfaces that have been denuded of their epithelium may result in symblepharon formation and ultimate obliteration of the conjunctival fornices. As the formation of fibrous tissue progresses, symblepharon formation becomes more extensive, passing from the palpebral to the bulbar conjunctiva. The inferior fornix is always involved more profoundly than the superior fornix. The desmosomal attachments of the basal layers of the epithelium to the basement membrane appear to be lysed by an immunologic process that results in cellular destruction. Autoantibodies of both the IgG and IgA type have been described in pemphigoid [4], and in the case of the former, fixation of IgG to the basement membrane may be followed by the binding of complement to that site. This action sets the stage for the attraction of polymorphonuclear leukocytes and monocytes to the area. When the former release their lytic enzymes in the affected tissue, additional necrosis occurs.

A number of variants of bullous pemphigoid have been described, some of which may be confused with dermatitis herpetiformis. One of these, designated IgA bullous pemphigoid [5], is characterized by linear deposits of IgA in the lamina lucida of the basement membrane. Dermatitis herpetiformis is a pruritic bullous disease in which the deposits of IgA are usually *granular* in distribution, and the deposits are found beneath the basement membrane. Both conditions may be responsive to dapsone therapy.

Although antibody can be shown to be bound to the affected basement membrane, the detectability of circulating autoantibody is highly variable, ranging from 2 percent to 80 percent in various reports [5, 6]. Furthermore, the disease cannot be transmitted by passive transfer of serum from affected individuals. This finding has led Griffith et al. [7] to assume that pemphigoid is attributable to an insoluble antigen attached to the basement membrane of the epithelium and that a subsequent antibody-mediated complement-dependent reaction produces cytotoxic (type II) reactions at the tissue site (Fig. 5-2).

Ahmed et al. [8] found elevated levels of immune complexes in 31 percent of the blister fluids that they examined among patients with bullous pemphigoid, whereas only 17 percent of the sera from these same patients showed such complexes. Anti-basement membrane zone antibody was found in 57 percent of the precipitated complexes from the blister fluids. The authors suggested that the majority of the immune complexes are formed in situ.

Many questions remain unanswered concerning the etiology of cicatricial pemphigoid. Mondino et al. [9] found an association between HLA-B12 and the disease, but only in 44 percent of the patients. A decrease in the number of circulating T-cells has been reported among pemphigoid patients [10], but the nonspecific suppressor functions of the patients' suppressor T-cells appear to be intact [11]. Perhaps there is an antigen-specific defect in suppressor function.

The late sequelae of cicatricial pemphigoid include not only the obliteration of the fornices but the destruction of mucus-producing elements in the conjunctiva (goblet cells) [12]. This lack of mucus results in an unstable tear film and a rapid breakup of any films that are established. Ultimately the orifices of the ductules leading from the lacrimal glands to the superior fornix are obliterated and severe dryness of the eyes results. This condition, coupled with damage to the cornea from inturned lashes (trichiasis and entropion), ultimately leads to severe corneal damage with a dry, irregular surface and vascularization.

5. DISEASES AFFECTING THE EXTERNAL EYE

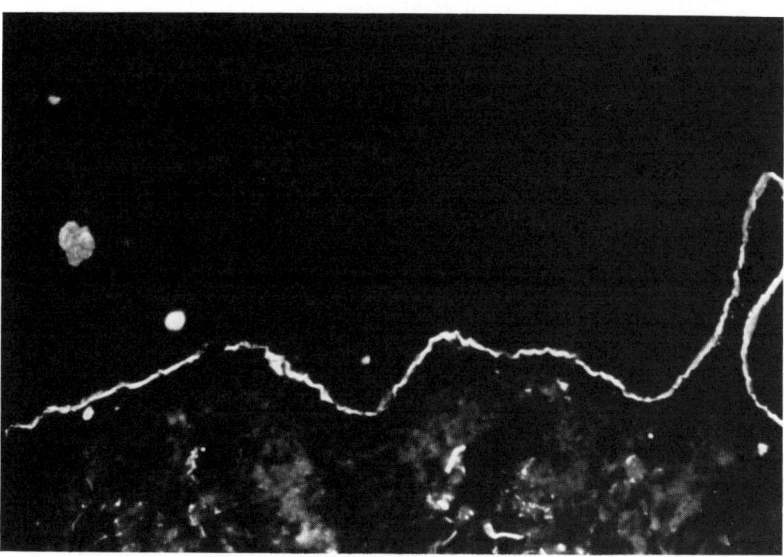

FIG. 5-2 Fluorescence of the basement membrane of the epithelium in cicatricial pemphigoid. Ultraviolet light. × 156. (From T. E. Daniels, Immunopathology of Recurrent Aphthous Ulcers and Bullous Diseases of the Mouth—A Review. In G. R. O'Connor (Ed.), *Immunologic Diseases of the Mucous Membranes.* New York, Masson, 1980. p. 104. © 1980 Masson Publishing USA, Inc. NY. Reproduced with permission.)

TREATMENT. Treatment of cicatricial pemphigoid has been manifestly unsuccessful in the hands of most practitioners. The disease seems to take its own inexorable course, whatever the treatment applied. One study from the Mayo Clinic [13] suggested that the use of subconjunctivally administered depot-steroids might halt the course of the disease. This use of steroids has not been universally successful by any means. Corticosteroid drops may decrease the papillary inflammation that accompanies the early stages of the disease, but they are of little avail in the later stages. The use of immunosuppressive agents, such as cyclophosphamide, offers some hope for the treatment of this otherwise disastrous autoimmune disease, and Foster, et al. [14] have had considerable success with the combined use of cyclophosphamide and systemically administered corticosteroids. A certain segment of the cicatricial pemphigoid population also appears to respond well to dapsone at initial dosages of 100 to 150 mg per day. Rogers et al. [15] found that this segment could be easily identified after an initial therapeutic trial of 12 weeks.

SARCOIDOSIS

Sarcoidosis is an enigmatic systemic disease that often attacks the external eye as well as many other tissues of the body. The characteristic lesion is a noncaseating granuloma composed of epithelioid cells, giant cells,

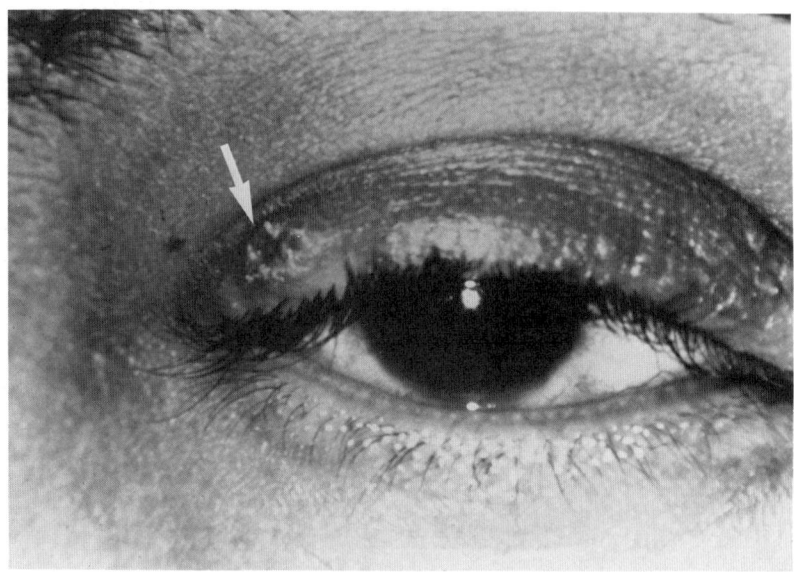

FIG. 5-3 Dermal lesions of sarcoidosis (*arrow*) on the upper lid of a patient suffering from sarcoid uveitis. (From G. R. O'Connor: Ocular Sarcoidosis. In E. A. Klein (Ed.), *Symposium on Medical and Surgical Diseases of the Retina and Vitreous.* St. Louis: Mosby, 1982. Reproduced with permission.)

and lymphocytes. The cause of sarcoidosis is unknown, but it behaves very much like an infection, closely resembling tuberculosis in many ways. It would appear that the macrophagic components of the sarcoid lesion have been directed to the tissue site to eliminate some particulate matter, be it infectious or otherwise. Viruses [16], atypical mycobacteria [17], mycoplasma [18], and other infectious agents have all been suspected, but there is no conclusive evidence that any of these agents is causative of the disease. Certain ethnic groups appear to have a predilection for the disease. In the United States, blacks are affected more commonly than other racial or ethnic groups, while in Europe, Scandinavians appear to be more prone to the disease. Here again, common genetic factors may influence the prevalence of the disease in certain groups, but Merritt et al [19] have been unable to find an HLA association with sarcoid.

The principal manifestations of sarcoidosis in the external eye consist of nodular lesions of the skin of the eyelids (Fig. 5-3), conjunctival nodules (Fig. 5-4), calcific band keratopathy, and infiltration of the lacrimal glands leading to keratoconjunctivitis sicca. The presentation of a nodule in the conjunctiva may provide material for a positive biopsy, sparing the patient some of the more invasive procedures that are commonly used by chest surgeons (endotracheal biopsy, bronchial lavage, or scalene node biopsy). Such nodules are generally a little larger than a conjunctival follicle and instead of being transparent, they usually appear slightly opaque and whitish-yellow (Fig. 5-4). Histologic sectioning of such nod-

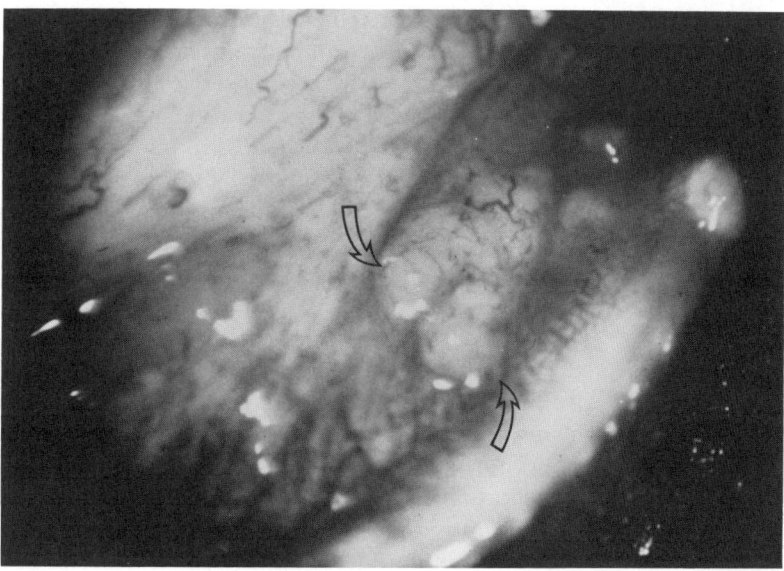

FIG. 5-4 Cluster of sarcoid nodules (*arrows*) on the inferior palpebral conjunctiva of a patient suffering from sarcoid uveitis. (From G. R. O'Connor: Ocular sarcoidosis. In E. A. Klein (Ed.), *Symposium on Medical and Surgical Diseases of the Retina and Vitreous*. St. Louis: Mosby, 1982. Reproduced with permission.)

ules generally reveals noncaseating granulomata so characteristic of the disease. Giant cells are usually present along with epithelioid cells and lymphocytes. Biopsy of nodules of the skin shows essentially the same findings except that the epidermal surface is keratinized.

Calcific band keratopathy in sarcoidosis may appear as a result of two processes.

1. It may be related to the hypercalcemia that often accompanies the disease, and in this case the calcific deposits are usually intracellular.
2. It may follow the development of a chronic iridocyclitis, and in this case the deposits are usually extracellular.

Extracellular deposits have been seen repeatedly in the infantile variety of ocular sarcoidosis, which has sometimes been confused with the iridocyclitis of juvenile rheumatoid arthritis. Both may be characterized by pauci-articular arthritis and chronic iridocyclitis with calcific band keratopathy. In the case of sarcoidosis, a positive chest roentgenogram, a positive gallium scan, or elevated levels of serum angiotensin converting enzyme and serum lysozyme may make the diagnosis (see Chapter 2).

Infiltration of the lacrimal glands in sarcoidosis may result in tear deficiency, and this problem may make itself manifest in either the acute febrile form of the disease known as uveoparotid fever (Heerfordt's syndrome) or in the chronic form of the disease. Crick et al. [20] found that almost half of their patients with sarcoidosis revealed evidence of tear deficiency, as detected by the Schirmer strip or by rose bengal staining of the cornea and conjunctiva. The infiltrative process that causes the dry eye syndrome in sarcoidosis is, in effect, so similar to that which causes keratoconjunctivitis sicca in the rheumatoid diseases that biopsy may occasionally be indicated. Lip biopsy may eventually replace lacrimal gland biopsy, as it has in Sjögren's syndrome, provided that a uniform pattern of cellular infiltration can be demonstrated in the labial glands, as suggested by Penneau et al [21].

The origin of sarcoidosis remains obscure, and its manifestations are highly variable. Many patients suffering from the disease manifest cutaneous anergy; i.e., a battery of commonly applied skin-test antigens, such as mumps, *Trichophyton, Candida,* and streptokinase-streptodornase, produces negative reactions at the end of 48 hours. Anergy is by no means universal, however, since 10 to 15 percent of sarcoid patients respond normally to skin-test antigens. The anergy of sarcoid is taken as an indication of defective T-cell activity, but this defect is not complete. The lymphocytes of patients with sarcoidosis "liberate macrophage migration inhibition factor" (MIF) when exposed to extracts of sarcoid tissue [22], and as Rahi and Garner [23] state, this reaction may be the basis of the positive Kveim test in sarcoidosis. Obtunded T-cell responses may ultimately account for the fact that these patients are prone to develop chronic infections such as tuberculosis. Their B-cell responses, on the other hand, are said to be normal. Such patients often exhibit an exaggerated IgG peak on immunoelectrophoresis [24, 25] but the cause of this remains unexplained. Faure et al [26] have suggested that the excessively high levels of immunoglobulins observed in the sera of certain patients suffering from sarcoidosis may be related to a decrease in the number of circulating suppressor T cells.

TREATMENT. Ocular sarcoidosis affecting the anterior segment of the eye alone is best treated by the local application of corticosteroid drops and cycloplegics. If the iritis is acute and severe, long-acting cycloplegics such as atropine 1% or scopolamine 0.25% should be used twice a day. After the pain and photophobia have subsided, long-acting cycloplegics should be stopped, and short-acting dilators such as tropicamide 1% should be applied instead, two or three times a day. This latter form of therapy prevents synechia formation by keeping the pupil moving.

The posterior lesions of ocular sarcoidosis must be treated by systemic corticosteroids or by the judicious use of periocular injections of depot corticosteroids. The chorioretinal infiltrates and vasculitic lesions appear to respond well to orally administered corticosteroids at levels of 60 to 100 mg per day. Optic nerve lesions also appear to improve under this form of therapy, although irreversible damage to the nerve fibers often occurs before therapy can be instituted. Since sarcoidosis is a chronic disease that cannot be permanently arrested by corticosteroid therapy, it is best to give systemic corticosteroids in short courses lasting only a few weeks or months. Long-term therapy at maintenance levels of 30 to 40 mg per day may cause serious side effects that might otherwise be

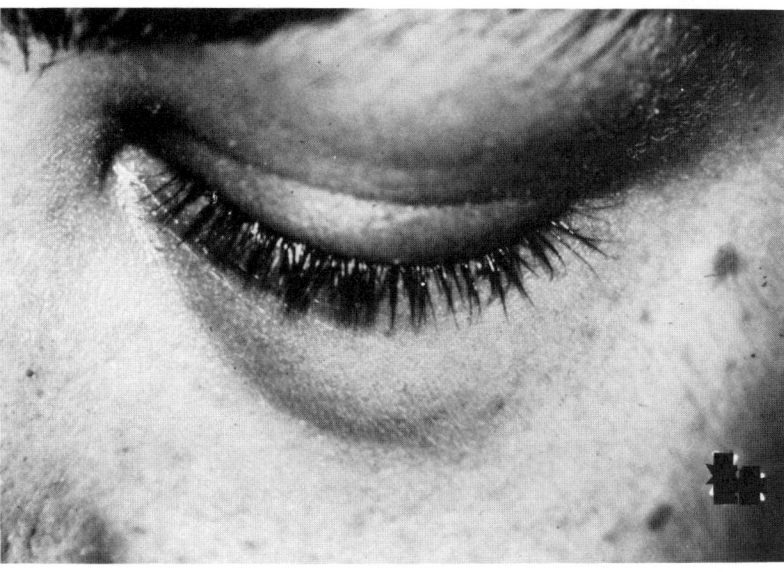

FIG. 5-5   Acute swelling of the upper and lower lids in a patient suffering from anaphylactoid reaction to shellfish protein.

avoided. This precaution is particularly applicable to children whose growth and development may be retarded considerably by long-term steroid administration.

GENERALIZED ANAPHYLACTOID RESPONSES

Urticarial reactions to various allergens often express themselves most dramatically in the periorbital tissues, particularly in the skin of the lids. This characteristic may be due, in part, to the high concentrations of mast cells in this area. It may also be related to the looseness with which the skin of the lids is attached to the underlying structures. When urticaria affects the periorbital skin, the lower lid is generally more prominently affected than the upper (Fig. 5-5) and this difference may reflect the effect of gravity on the extravasated fluid.

Anaphylactoid reactions in the external ocular structures are characteristic of type I hypersensitivity reactions. They sometimes occur with frightening rapidity, but are always self-limited and retreat without leaving any signs of scarring. The usual route of entrance of the allergen is the respiratory tract or the gastrointestinal tract. Animal danders are among the most common offenders, but foodstuffs such as citrus fruits and shellfish may produce the same kind of reaction. With regard to food allergies, the simultaneous ingestion of alcoholic beverages and the food to which the patient is allergic may increase the absorption of allergen and trigger the reaction.

Patients afflicted by these peculiar forms of allergy come to recognize the signs and symptoms early in the course of the disease. The same target organ may be attacked again and again, e.g., the periorbita of the left eye. A patient who is allergic to oysters may be able to ingest one or two without developing symptoms, but if this act is accompanied by the ingestion of alcohol, puffiness of the lids develops within a few minutes.

The state of denaturation of the allergen may be important. Individuals allergic to eggs may be able to eat them in baked form (as in pastries) but are unable to ingest them as fried eggs or scrambled eggs. In other individuals, even heat denaturation fails to inactivate the antigen, and these individuals are generally sensitive to extremely small amounts of antigens. Certain nut oils concealed in candy or baked goods may act as highly offensive antigens in this sense, and the patient must learn by trial and error the things that he can or cannot eat.

Periorbital edema may sometimes be related to hereditary angioneurotic edema, a disease due to a deficiency of a serum factor that ordinarily inhibits C_1 esterase [27]. Hereditary angioneurotic edema is usually associated with marked dermatographia as well.

TREATMENT. The symptoms of anaphylactoid reactions consist primarily of swelling and itching of the lids. They may be relieved by the injection of epinephrine (0.5 ml of 1 : 10,000 adrenalin) or by the ingestion of antihistaminics such as Periactin (4 mg). Relief provided by antihistaminics, however, may be some time in coming because the receptors occupied by histamine cannot be taken over immediately by the histamine-blocking agents. Cold compresses applied to the affected area will generally help to reduce the swelling.

STEVENS-JOHNSON SYNDROME

The Stevens-Johnson syndrome, thought of as a severe form of erythema multiforme that affects the mucosae as well as the skin, is believed to represent an immune complex (type III) disease. It is characterized by fever and malaise, by the development of papular skin rash and bullae affecting the limbs and face, and by ulcerative lesions of the mucosae, particularly those of the mouth, genitalia, and conjunctivae. The skin lesions may have the appearance of an "iris" or "bull's eye" with a deeply colored center surrounded by a zone of lighter pigmentation.

The symptoms may begin several days or weeks after the ingestion of a particular drug. Sulfonamides and barbiturates have been incriminated most often, but various other medications have also been implicated in the pathogenesis of the disease. It is assumed that the offending medication acts as a hapten, combining with autologous tissue protein in such a way as to form an autoantigen. This autoantigen stimulates antibody formation, which in turn accounts for the deposition of immune complexes in the microvasculature of the skin and mucous membranes. Kazmierowski and Wuepper [28] have demonstrated these complexes in the superficial blood vessels of the skin. Microthrombi form there, and necrosis of both the vessel wall and the surrounding tissue may occur. Mononuclear cells, rather than polymorphonuclear leukocytes, characteristically accumulate in the dermis and in the conjunctival stroma.

Wuepper et al [29] believe that the physicochemical nature of the accumulated immune complexes determines the type of cell that migrates into the lesion. Whereas neutrophilic granulocytes attracted by C3b accumulate in lesions known as "leukocytoclastic vasculitis," erythema multiforme (and its mucosal counterpart, Stevens-Johnson syndrome) appear to be different. It is suggested that the immune complexes in the latter case bear C3d, as modified by C3b inactivator and B1H globulin. This substance is attractive to mononuclear cells rather than neutrophilic granulocytes.

While drugs have generally been blamed for the development of the disease, it is known to occur in the absence of drug therapy. It has developed in the wake of herpes simplex infection [30], and has been observed in association with measles infection, smallpox vaccination, and malignancy [31]. Thus, the tissue damage that ultimately contributes to autoantigen formation may be of multiple origins.

Recurrent cycles of lesions characterize the disease. These occur at intervals of about 2 weeks, but most of the lesions will generally have appeared by the end of 6 weeks [31]. Recurrences after this time are rare, although the late sequelae of the disease (e.g., loss of fingernails or progressive cicatricial changes in the conjunctiva) may continue to plague the patient for years. The recurrent cycles of lesions in the early period are of particular interest in view of the postulated immune complex origin of the disease. Recurrence of symptoms would seem, indeed, to be rather characteristic of a number of immune complex diseases, including lupus erythematosus, rheumatoid arthritis, and the iritis caused by serum sickness [32]. Maximum antibody formation generally takes place at about 10 to 14 days after injection of an antigen. It may be that the cyclic recurrences of erythema multiforme correspond to waves of antibody formation in individuals harboring significant amounts of sequestered autoantigen.

The conjunctiva is one of the principal targets of the disease. Bullous lesions occur principally on the palpebral conjunctivae and these lesions may rupture, leaving ulcerated surfaces that are prone to secondary infection. The scarring that almost always takes place may produce symblepharon and obliteration of the fornices, as in cicatricial pemphigoid. Depending on the extent of the scarring, dryness of the eye may become a problem. Cicatrization of the ductules leading into the upper fornix from the lacrimal gland may cause a loss of the aqueous component of tears, but more commonly the mucous content of the tears decreases owing to destruction of the goblet cells. In severe cases of scarring, trichiasis and entropion may supervene, giving rise to corneal opacity.

TREATMENT. Corticosteroids used both locally and systemically may modify the course of the disease in its early stages, whereas they are of no avail after symblepharon formation has occurred. Irrigation of the conjunctival fornices with balanced salt solutions and lysis of any symblephara that have formed (with a sterile glass rod) are generally recommended, but these procedures are often very painful and impracticable. Use of local antibiotics to prevent secondary infection is also indicated, provided that the patient has no history of hypersensitivity to the antibiotic. In the late stages of the disease, when shrinkage of the fornices and further damage to the cornea are feared, limited help may be provided by the wearing of a scleral contact lens.

MULTIPLE MYELOMA

Multiple myeloma is a malignant neoplasm that stems from the uncontrolled proliferation of a specific clone of B lymphocytes. Both mature and immature plasma cells may be produced in great numbers. Those that reach maturity secrete immunoglobulins of only one class; i.e., a given multiple myeloma may produce IgG, IgA or IgE, but it will not produce mixtures of these immunoglobulins. This fact is the basis for the name *monoclonal gammopathy* that is often applied to multiple myeloma. Studies on patients with multiple myeloma have provided the only means of investigating certain immunoglobulins that are normally present in small quantities in the serum, as is certainly the case with IgE (whose normal serum level is listed at 0.003 mg/dl) [33].

The disease may produce widespread infiltrations in many parts of the body, including the conjunctiva and cornea. In addition, lytic lesions may erode the bone of the orbit, while tumefactions in the posterior orbit may cause papilledema and cranial nerve palsies.

The principal changes in the anterior segment of the eye consist of protein-filled cysts of the nonpigmented epithelium of the ciliary body, crystalline deposits in the cornea and conjunctiva, and tortuosity of the conjunctival vessels [34]. The latter is a nonspecific change that tends to make itself evident in any of the syndromes associated with hyperviscosity of the serum. Thus, Waldenström's macroglobulinemia may be accompanied by similar changes in both the conjunctival and retinal vessels.

The crystalline deposits that occur in the cornea and conjunctiva are, however, highly characteristic. They are generally needlelike and polychromatic and are localized in the anterior half of the cornea. While Grayson [35] notes that the crystals are present in the corneal epithelium, Aronson and Shaw [36] stated that the epithelium was spared, and Pinkerton and Robertson [37] indicated that the anterior stroma of the cornea was involved rather than the epithelium. The paraprotein of multiple myeloma appears to bind copper [38], and this quality may account for the dustlike deposits of copper that are seen in Descemet's membrane centrally and on the anterior lens capsule. Other abnormalities include hypercalcemia, and this condition may produce calcific band keratopathy in some individuals [39].

TREATMENT. The treatment of multiple myeloma is essentially the treatment of the systemic disease. Various forms of cytotoxic chemotherapy have been attempted [40], but the disease is invariably fatal. Calcific band keratopathy, when it occurs in conjunction with multiple myeloma, can be treated by removal of the corneal epithelium and exposure of the deposits of calcium salts to 0.37 M disodium edetate.

SJÖGREN'S SYNDROME

In 1933, the Swedish ophthalmologist, Henrik Sjögren [41], described a syndrome consisting of (1) keratoconjunctivitis sicca, (2) xerostomia, and (3) a connective tissue disease. Rheumatoid arthritis was the connective tissue disorder most often observed by Sjögren, but the syndrome was made to include such entities as lupus erythematosus, scleroderma, and dermatomyositis. Clearly, the syndrome represents only one segment of a broad category of autoimmune diseases that may include Hashimoto's thyroiditis, psoriatic arthritis, polyarteritis nodosa, progressive systemic sclerosis, and even lymphoreticular neoplasms. It is useful at the outset, however, to differentiate primary Sjögren's syndrome from secondary Sjögren's syndrome. The former is seen by itself (i.e., xerostomia and keratoconjunctivitis sicca alone); the latter occurs in association with some other autoimmune disease such as rheumatoid arthritis or lupus erythematosus. Primary Sjögren's syndrome occurs almost exclusively in females, whereas the male/female ratio is almost 1.0 in secondary Sjögren's syndrome. Primary Sjögren's syndrome has a definite association with HLA B8 and DW3; secondary Sjögren's syndrome has not. Both forms, however are associated with B-cell antigens Ia-172 and Ia-350 [42], and both forms show identical histopathologic changes in the lacrimal and salivary glands.

In parallel with infiltrative lesions of the salivary glands, the lacrimal glands show destructive changes resulting in focal degeneration of the acini, destruction of the ductular epithelium, and eventual replacement of these structures by fibrous connective tissue. The infiltrates are composed of lymphocytes and histiocytes, and the severity of infiltration in any given biopsy specimen may be graded according to the criteria of Tabbara et al [43]. With progression of the disease, there is marked atrophy of the lacrimal (and salivary) glands, leaving only small islands of epimyoepithelial cells in the midst of a mass of fibrous connective tissue.

Antibodies to salivary duct antigens can be found in the serum of the majority of patients [44], but the significance of these antibodies is not clear since some normal individuals also have these antibodies [45]. Furthermore, Anderson et al. [46] found that patients with high levels of these antibodies actually showed less destructive changes in their salivary glands and lacrimal glands than patients who exhibited no antibodies. They questioned whether these antibodies might play a protective role by blocking certain receptor sites on the target tissue. There is evidence that T lymphocytes may also participate in the destructive changes that occur in Sjögren's syndrome, for Berry et al. [47] found leukocyte migration inhibition test positive in two-thirds of their patients when extracts of parotid gland were used as the challenge antigen. Furthermore, Adamson et al. [48] in their analysis of the lymphocyte subsets in inflammatory infiltrates of the salivary glands in primary Sjögren's syndrome found that 75 percent of the lymphocytes were T cells, the majority being OKT4 positive. More than 50 percent of the T cells were also Ia positive, i.e., positive for activation antigens. Significant differences were found between the characteristics of the circulating blood lymphocytes of these patients and the characteristics of the lymphocytes in their inflammatory lesions.

As in most inflammatory autoimmune diseases it seems likely that multiple immunologic mechanisms are at play. Many patients with Sjögren's disease are positive for rheumatoid factor, a macroglobulin antibody directed against their own IgG. Yoshinoya et al [49] showed that elevated levels of immune complexes could be demonstrated in patients with Sjögren's syndrome and that both IgM and IgG rheumatoid factor made substantial contributions to these complexes in both primary and secondary Sjögren's syndrome. Many show the presence of antinuclear antibodies in their serum, although those who do are mainly in the lupus group [50]. Moutsopoulos et al. [42] found that 88 percent of patients with primary Sjögren's syndrome had antibodies to the extractable nuclear antigen SS-A, while 58 percent of patients with lupus erythematosus and 0 percent of patients with rheumatoid arthritis showed antibodies to the same antigen. Manthorpe et al. [51] showed that 45 percent of patients with the primary syndrome had antibodies to the nuclear antigen SS-B (Ha) while only 14 percent of patients with the secondary syndrome had these antibodies. Thus, there are clear differences between the different varieties of the syndrome, based, perhaps, on the possession of HLA-DW2 or HLA-DW3.

It seems clear that patients with Sjögren's syndrome produce multiple autoantibodies, indicating hyperreactivity of their B-cell system at a polyclonal level. The cause of this immunoregulatory failure is unknown in humans, but mouse models of Sjögren's syndrome seem to show that multiple autoantibodies are present even at birth in animals with a genetic predisposition to the disease. Among these antibodies are antibodies that are specifically cytotoxic to T-suppressor cells [52]. Thus, the loss of suppressor T cells may be fundamental, at least in the primary form of Sjögren's syndrome and in the form associated with lupus.

Sjögren's syndrome strikes a predominantly female, middle-aged group of patients. The ocular symptoms range from mild dryness of the eyes with minor burning and itching to incapacitating inflammation and severe foreign body sensation. Severe keratoconjunctivitis sicca is characterized by a filamentary keratitis with scrolls of desquamated epithelium adhering to the cornea. Because of the decreased aqueous component, the tear volume is reduced. Such patients will show only minimal wetting of a Schirmer strip placed in the inferior conjunctival cul-de-sac. As if in compensation for decreased aqueous component, mucus is secreted abundantly, tending to become inspissated with continued evaporation. These fragments of dried mucus also contribute to the foreign body sensation of which most patients complain. Occasionally, bacterial ulceration of the cornea occurs because of the compromised vitality of the corneal epithelium. When the ocular picture is full blown, there is little difficulty in making a diagnosis. The cornea loses its natural luster; filaments and dried mucus are present on the cornea; and the eyes may be grossly hyperemic from an associated papillary conjunctivitis. Under these circumstances the Schirmer test may show only a millimeter or two of wetting in 5 minutes' time.

With incipient disease, the signs may be much more subtle. A normal or nearly normal tear film may be present, but it will be laden with debris. The tear meniscus observed between the mucocutaneous border of the lower lid and the surface of the bulbar conjunctiva may be interrupted in only one or two places. Under such circumstances, the testing of the tears for their lysozyme content may be helpful in making the diagnosis. The lysozyme content of the tears is contributed almost exclusively by the lacrimal gland. Furthermore, lysozyme levels tend to decrease before there is a marked deficit in tear volume. Thus, a decrease in tear lysozyme, as measured by the method of de Luise, et al. [53] is a good indication of early sicca syndrome.

Biopsy of the lacrimal gland is sometimes difficult to perform and may occasionally give rise to draining fistulas, particularly when performed through the skin of the upper lid. Since the pathologic events that occur in the lacrimal gland are generally mirrored by events occurring simultaneously in the salivary glands, biopsy of the labial salivary glands has provided a convenient substitute for lacrimal gland biopsy. As Tabbara et al. [43] have demonstrated, their technique for assaying the submucosal salivary glands of the lower lip provides good evidence of simultaneous lacrimal gland dysfunction. The correlation between the depression of tear lysozyme content and the severity of histopathologic findings in the salivary glands is particularly impressive.

TREATMENT. The initial loss of tear volume noted by patients with keratoconjunctivitis sicca can be compensated for by the use of tear substitutes. A large number of commercial preparations are now available, most of them utilizing methyl cellulose or polyvinyl alcohol as a base. It is sometimes difficult to tell in advance which ones will afford the greatest relief. One finds the most efficacious ones by trial and error.

The wearing of moisture-chamber spectacles helps to prevent evaporation, but may reduce vision owing to a film of condensed water vapor on the inside of the lens. Considerable adjustment is sometimes necessary with these devices.

Punctal occlusion may sometimes be helpful as a means of preserving whatever natural moisture the patient has. It must be remembered, however, that Sjögren's syndrome is a potentially reversible disease. More than one patient who has undergone permanent occlusion of the lacrimal puncta has developed epiphora when the disease has gone into remission. This sequela has been particularly troublesome among males treated by punctal occlusion. Temporary occlusion with silicone plugs has given some idea of what can be expected from this form of treatment.

There are some indications that alternate-day systemic steroid therapy can reverse the destructive process that is going on in the lacrimal gland when such therapy is given early [54]. Clearly nothing can be gained by use of these agents in the later cicatricial stages of the disease. Steroid therapy is still being evaluated for its efficacy and safety.

REFERENCES

1. Park, M. S., and Terasaki, P. I. HLA DRW4 in 91% of Jewish pemphigus vulgaris patients. *Lancet* 2:441, 1979.
2. Hashimoto, K., et al. Anti-cell surface pemphigus autoantibody stimulates plasminogen activator activity of human epidermal cells: A mechanism for the loss of epidermal cohesion and blister formation. *J. Exp. Med.* 157:259, 1983.
3. Roenigk, H. R., and Deodhar, S. Pemphigus treatment with azathioprine. *Arch. Dermatol.* 107:353, 1973.
3a. Blaszczyk, M., et al. Plasmapheresis as a supplementary treatment in pemphigus. *Arch. Immunol. Ther. Exper.* 29:763, 1981.
4. Sams, W. M., and Logan, W. S. The skin as reflector of immunologic diseases. In G. E. Ehrlich, (Ed.), *Oculocutaneous Manifestations of Rheumatic Diseases*. Basel: Karger, 1973. P. 98.
5. Jones, R. R., and Goolamali, S. K. IgA bullous pemphigoid, a distinct blistering disorder. *Br. J. Dermatol.* 102:719, 1980.
6. Bean, S. F. Cicatricial pemphigoid: immunofluorescent studies. *Arch. Dermatol.* 110:552, 1974.
7. Griffith, M. R., et al. Immunofluorescent studies in mucous membrane pemphigoid. *Arch. Dermatol.* 109:195, 1976.
8. Ahmed, A. R., et al. Immune complexes in pemphigus and bullous pemphigoid. *Dermatologica* 166:175, 1983.
9. Mondino, B. J., et al. HLA antigens in ocular cicatricial pemphigoid. *Arch. Ophthalmol.* 97:479, 1979.
10. Mondino, B. J., et al. T and B lymphocytes in ocular cicatricial pemphigoid. *Am. J. Ophthalmol.* 92:536, 1981.
11. King, A. J., et al. Suppressor cell function is preserved in pemphigus and pemphigoid. *J. Invest. Dermatol.* 79:183, 1982.
12. Mondino, B. J., and Brown, S. I. Ocular cicatricial pemphigoid. *Ophthalmology* 88:95, 1981.
13. Hardy, K., et al. Benign mucous membrane pemphigoid. *Arch. Dermatol.* 104:467, 1971.
14. Foster, C. S., et al. Immunosuppressive therapy for progressive ocular cicatricial pemphigoid. *Ophthalmology* 89:340, 1982.
15. Rogers, R. S., et al. Treatment of cicatricial (benign mucous membrane) pemphigoid with dapsone. *J. Am. Acad. Dermatol.* 6:215, 1982.
16. Byrne, E. B., et al. Serological hyperreactivity to Epstein-Barr virus and other viral antigens in sarcoidosis. In K. Iwai and Y. Hosada (Eds.), *Proceedings of the Sixth International Conference on Sarcoidosis*. Baltimore: University Park, 1974. P. 218.
17. Barth, C. L., et al. Isolation of an acid-fast organism from the aqueous humor in a case of sarcoidosis. *Henry Ford Hosp. Med. J.* 27:127, 1979.
18. Jansson, E. Isolation of *Mycoplasma* from sarcoid tissue. *J. Clin. Pathol.* 25:837, 1972.
19. Merritt, J. C. HLA-A, -B, and -DR antigenic factors in ocular sarcoidosis. *Am. J. Ophthalmol.* 96:396, 1983.

20. Crick, R., Hoyle, C., and Smellie, H. The eyes in sarcoidosis. *Br. J. Ophthalmol.* 45:461, 1961.
21. Penneau, M., et al. Diagnostic histologique de la sarcoidose par biopsie des glandes salivaires accessoires labiales. *Nouv. Presse. Med.* 7:4239, 1978.
22. Jones-Williams, W., et al. The Kmif (Kveim-induced macrophage migration inhibition factor) test in sarcoidosis. *J. Clin. Pathol.* 25:951, 1972.
23. Rahi, A. H. S., and Garner, A. *Immunopathology of the Eye.* Oxford, England: Blackwell, 1976. P. 305.
24. Patnode, R. A., Allin, R. C., and Carpenter, R. L. Serum immunoglobulin levels in sarcoidosis. *Am. J. Clin. Pathol.* 45:398, 1966.
25. Saint-Remy, J. R., et al. Variations in immunoglobulin levels and circulating immune complexes in sarcoidosis. Correlation with extent of disease and duration of symptoms. *Am. Rev. Resp. Dis.* 127:23, 1983.
26. Faure, M., et al. Numeration of T cell subsets in sarcoidosis using monoclonal antibodies: decreased levels of peripheral blood T cells with suppressor T cell phenotype. *Dermatologica* 165:88, 1982.
27. Donaldson, V. H., and Evans, R. R. A biochemical abnormality in hereditary angioneurotic edema: absence of serum inhibitor of C_1-esterase. *Am. J. Med.* 25:37, 1963.
28. Kazmierowski, J. A., and Wuepper, K. D. Erythema multiforme: immune complex vasculitis of the superficial cutaneous microvasculature. *J. Invest. Dermatol.* 71:366, 1978.
29. Wuepper, K. D., et al. Immune complexes in erythema multiforme and the Stevens-Johnson syndrome. *J. Invest. Dermatol.* 74:368, 1980.
30. Britz, M., and Sibulkin, D. Recurrent erythema multiforme and herpes genitalis (type 2). *J.A.M.A.* 233:812, 1975.
31. Ostler, H. B., Conant, M. A., and Groundwater, J. Lyell's disease the Stevens-Johnson syndrome, and exfoliative dermatitis. *Trans. Am. Acad. Ophthalmol. Otolaryngol.* 74:1254, 1970.
32. Theodore, F. H., and Lewson, A. C. Bilateral iritis complicating serum sickness. *Arch. Ophthalmol.* 21:828, 1939.
33. Allansmith, M. R., and O'Connor, G. R. Immunoglobulins: structure, function, and relation to the eye. *Surv. Ophthalmol.* 14:367, 1970.
34. Orellana, J., et al. Ocular manifestations of multiple myeloma, Waldenström's macroglobulinemia, and benign monoclonal gammopathy. *Surv. Ophthalmol.* 26:157, 1981.
35. Grayson, M. *Diseases of the Cornea.* St. Louis: Mosby, 1979. P. 367.
36. Aronson, S. B., and Shaw, R. Corneal crystals in multiple myeloma. *Arch. Ophthalmol.* 61:541, 1959.
37. Pinkerton, R. M. H., and Robertson, D. M. Corneal and conjunctival changes in dysproteinemia. *Invest. Ophthalmol.* 8:357, 1969.
38. Lewis, R. A., Falls, H. F., and Troyer, D. O. Ocular manifestations of hypercupremia associated with multiple myeloma. *Arch. Ophthalmol.* 93:1050, 1975.
39. Wilson, K. S. Band keratopathy in hypercalcemia of myeloma. *J. Can. Med. Assoc.* 126:1314, 1982.
40. Tirelli, U., et al. Combination chemotherapy for multiple myeloma with melphalan, prednisone, cyclophosphamide, vincristine, and carmustine (BCNU) (M-2 Protocol). *Cancer Treat. Rep.* 66:1971, 1982.
41. Sjögren, H. Zur Kenntnis der Keratoconjunctivitis sicca (keratitis filiformis) bei Hypofunction der Tränendrüsen. *Acta Ophthalmol.* (Suppl.) 2:1, 1933.
42. Moutsopoulos, H. M., et al. Sjögren's syndrome (Sicca syndrome): Current issues. *Ann. Int. Med.* 92:212, 1980.

43. Tabbara, K. F., Ostler, H. B., and Daniels, T. E. Sjögren's syndrome a correlation between ocular findings and labial salivary gland histology. *Trans. Am. Acad. Ophthalmol. Otolaryngol.* 78:467, 1974.
44. Feltkamp, T. E. W., and van Rossu, A. L. Antibodies to salivary duct cells, and other autoantibodies, in patients with Sjögren's syndrome and other idiopathic autoimmune diseases. *Clin. Exp. Immunol.* 3:1, 1968.
45. Bertram, V., and Halberg, P. Organ antibodies in Sjögren's syndrome. *Acta Allergol. (Kbh.)* 20:462, 1965.
46. Anderson, L. G., Tarpley, T. M., and Talal, N. Cellular-versus-humoral responses to salivary gland in Sjögren's syndrome. *Clin. Exp. Immunol.* 13:335, 1973.
47. Berry, H., Bacon, P. A., and Davis, J. D. Cell-mediated immunity in Sjögren's syndrome. *Ann. Rheum. Dis.* 31:298, 1972.
48. Adamson, T. C., et al. Immunohistologic analysis of lymphoid infiltrates in primary Sjögren's syndrome using monoclonal antibodies. *J. Immunol.* 130:203, 1983.
49. Yoshinoya, S., et al. Detection and partial characterization of immune complexes in patients with rheumatoid arthritis plus Sjögren's syndrome and with Sjögren's syndrome alone. *Clin. Exp. Immunol.* 48:339, 1982.
50. Heaton, J. M. Sjögren's syndrome and systemic lupus erythematosus. *Br. Med. J.* 1:466, 1959.
51. Manthorpe, R., et al. Antibodies to SS-B in chronic inflammatory connective tissue diseases. Relationship with HLA-DW2 and HLA-DW3 antigen in primary Sjögren's syndrome. *Arthritis Rheum.* 25:662, 1982.
52. Theofilopoulos, A. N., et al. Distribution of lymphocytes identified by surface markers in murine strains with lupus erythematosuslike syndromes. *J. Exp. Med.* 149:516, 1979.
53. De Luise, W. P., et al. Quantitation of tear lysozyme levels in dry-eye disorders. *Arch. Ophthalmol.* 101:634, 1983.
54. Tabbara, K. F., and Frayha, R. A. Alternate-day steroid therapy for patients with primary Sjögren's syndrome. *Ann. Ophthalmol.* 15:358, 1983.

6 CORNEAL GRAFT REACTION

The attempt to replace a diseased cornea by a graft of healthy tissue from a donor has often been frustrated by the tendency of the recipient to reject the graft. It is the purpose of this chapter to discuss (1) the basic immunologic mechanisms that participate in this rejection, (2) the clinical course and histologic features of the rejection, and (3) the treatment of the rejection.

The transplantation of living tissue creates two distinct kinds of problems. The first are problems concerned directly with the act of transplantation; these problems are largely technical and are not discussed in this text. The second kind of problems are related to the graft's incompatibility with its new host.

That the destruction of allografts is clearly an immunologic phenomenon is indicated by the following observations:

1. If the basis of rejection were immunologic, a second contact with the same corneal antigen would be expected to induce a more violent reaction than the first; and indeed, the rejection of a second graft from the same donor begins after a much shorter interval and progresses more rapidly than the first rejection.
2. A second rejection does not occur with all subsequent allografts but only with those from the original donor or an immunologically similar animal.
3. Corneal allografts enjoy a brief period of latency—approximately 2 weeks after a first graft—before rejection begins.
4. Rejection correlates with the amount of antigen introduced with the graft.
5. Neonatally thymectomized animals reject grafts with difficulty, but their capacity to do so is restored when they are injected with lympho-

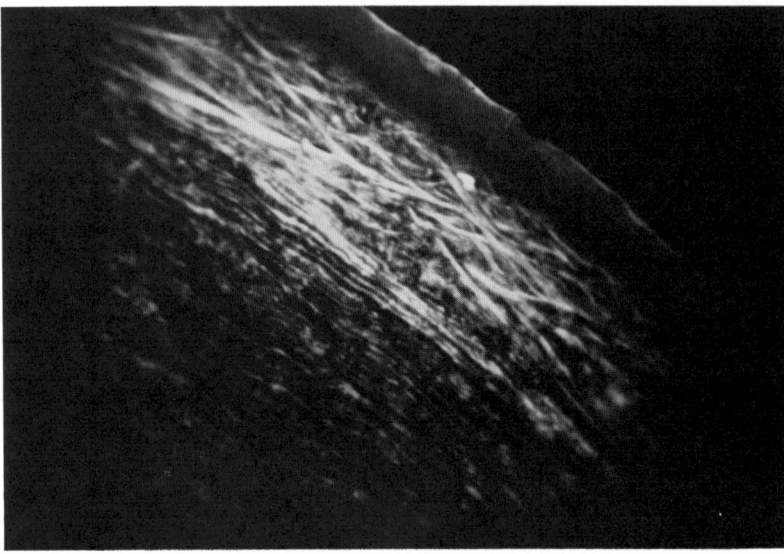

FIG. 6-1 Fluorescent antibody studies show serum proteins in corneal stroma but not in corneal epithelium.

cytes from a syngenesious normal donor, and this finding suggests that T cells play a role in rejection.
6. After rejection, many species—human beings, mice, rats, rabbits, chickens, and fish, for example—possess humoral antibodies specific for the donor of the graft [1].

BASIC IMMUNOLOGIC MECHANISMS OF REJECTION

Antigens

Tissue proteins are usually extracted experimentally by some form of mechanical disruption of the tissue in water, followed by centrifugation to separate the soluble proteins from the insoluble cellular elements. In attempts to define immunologically the soluble corneal antigens [2–6], corneal proteins have been extracted in this way and have then been tested by such techniques as paper electrophoresis, immunoelectrophoresis on agar, immunodiffusion, immunofluorescence, tannic-acid hemagglutination, and complement fixation.

In the bovine cornea, investigators have found from 6 to 15 antigens [7, 8]. Some of these were no doubt serum proteins, for although there are almost no serum proteins in the bovine corneal epithelium, the stroma contains bovine α globulin, β globulin, γ globulin, and albumin [9], with the albumin in smaller amounts centrally than peripherally [10] (Fig. 6-1). In one study of human corneas, immunoglobulins G and A were found at one-half and one-fifth their serum levels, respectively. In other studies the level of corneal IgG has been consistently in direct proportion to the level of serum IgG, but comparable studies of IgA levels have not been made. IgM is present less often than IgG and IgA and almost never in detectable amounts in the central cornea [11].

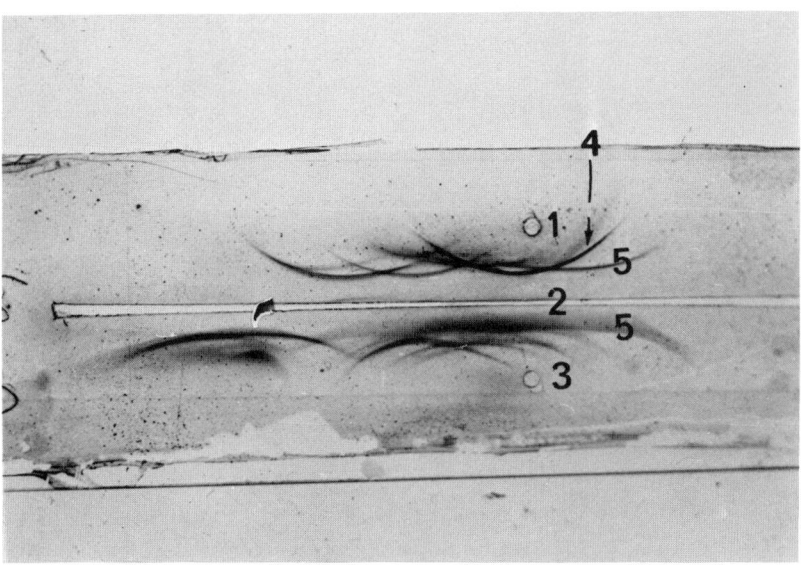

FIG. 6-2 Agar immunoelectrophoresis study with soluble bovine corneal antigen in top button (*1*), soluble bovine serum protein in bottom button (*3*), and antiserum to bovine serum protein in center well (*2*). Note protein line in cornea but not in serum (*4*), and several protein lines common to both cornea and serum (*5*). (Courtesy of Dr. Joan Hall.)

The tear film, which continuously bathes the cornea, contains prealbumin, ceruloplasmin, lactoferrin, secretory IgA, and lysozyme [12]. Holt and Kinoshita [13] described a protein that comprised approximately 40 percent of the soluble proteins in the bovine epithelium. It was also one of the two antigenic nonserum proteins in their unfractionated corneal extract. We too have noted this nonserum protein and have found it to be a strong antigen and present in moderately high concentrations (Figs. 6-2, 6-3). Remky [8] found the epithelium much more antigenic than the stroma. In his opinion a donor's stroma had almost no influence on the initiation of a graft rejection.

Some investigators [14] have shown serologically the organ specificity of the corneal antigens; others [15] their species specificity.

In addition to these soluble corneal antigens, some of which play a role in corneal graft rejection, we must consider other heterologous antigens, ABH (formerly ABO) blood-group antigens, and histocompatibility antigens.

The evidence suggests that bacterial cells, and group A streptococci in particular, may be a source of virtually unlimited quantities of antigen capable of modifying host reactions to allografts [16]. At least one staphylococcal antigen is known to have this effect.

By adsorption and elution experiments, investigators [17, 18] have found A and B blood-group antigens in the human cornea that correspond to the A and B antigens in red blood cells.

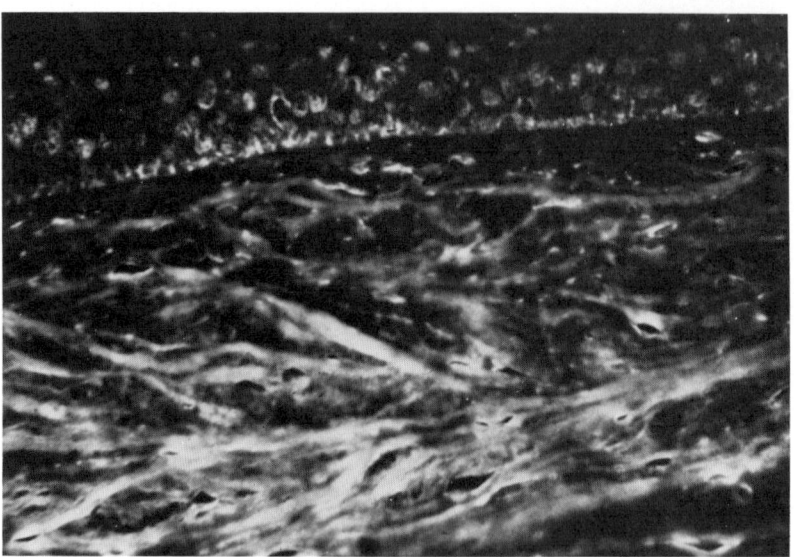

FIG. 6-3 Fluorescent-antibody studies performed with fluorescein-congugated antibovine epithelium antisera in normal rabbit cornea, showing organ-specific epithelial antigen in epithelium and in anterior stroma.

Initial studies reported on the absence of blood group antigens on human corneal endothelium [19], but more recent studies employing the ultrasensitive immunoperoxidase staining technique demonstrated the presence of blood groups A, B, and D (Rh) antigens on human corneal endothelial and epithelial cells [20]. Little antigen was present in the stroma.

There is no evidence that the ABH incompatibility is definitely correlated with graft rejection [21, 22].

The most exciting recent studies of the causes of corneal graft rejection deal with the histocompatibility antigens. These antigens are present on the surface of most body cells other than red blood cells, and their differences from person to person constitute the major reason that donor tissues cannot be freely transplanted to unrelated recipients without subsequent graft rejection. It was found that the sera from patients who had been given multiple transfusions often contained leukocyte-agglutinating antibodies that reacted with antigens present on the surfaces of human leukocytes [23, 24]. This finding led to the term *human leukocyte antigen* (HLA). The HLA can be typed by using sera with known human leukocyte antibody specificities.

Each chromosome carries genes in the form of DNA, and each gene determines the structure of specific protein polypeptide chains. The position of a gene along a chromosome is called the gene locus. Several genes may have the same locus and are then called alleles. The histocompatibility antigens are determined by four genes: One gene allele at each of two gene loci on each of the number 6 chromosomes (see Chap. 1).

More than 100 different antigens may be associated with these loci. Those whose separate identity is still debatable are called workshop (W) antigens.

The first histocompatibility locus is called HLA-A, the second HLA-C, and subsequent ones HLA-B and HLA-D. Most people have two alleles at each locus (i.e., they are heterozygous) [25, 26].

The HLA antigens located at locus A, B, or C are class I antigens and can be detected by serologic laboratory methods and are therefore also called serologically determined (SD) antigens. The HLA antigens located at the D locus are class II antigens and are determined by mixed lymphocyte cultures (MLC) and therefore are also called lymphocyte-defined (LD) antigens.

Recently serologically detected antigens associated with the D locus (DR) have been found in some tissues, and cellularly defined antigens have been identified at the HLA-A, B, and C loci (CD).

Genes located close to the HLA system control the immune responses, MLC reactions, and some aspects of the complement system [27, 28]. Immune response genes (Ir genes) determine how much antibody an individual will produce in response to a particular immunizing antigen [29]. The Ir genes influence T-cell function and may produce a protein called the *immune-associated antigen* (Ia or HLA-DR), which is detectable on the surface of B-lymphocytes, macrophages, dendritic cells, some T-lymphocyte subsets (i.e., suppressor cells), and in epidermal Langerhans' cells.

MLC reactions are immune cytotoxic reactions. They occur when non-compatible lymphocytes are mixed, and they differ from reactions owing to histocompatibility antigens. The lymphocyte activation observed in the MLC is believed to be the recognition phase of the graft reaction. The MLC locus is identified with the HLA-D locus [30]. MLC typing requires a set of lymphocytes of known MLC specificity and is therefore more difficult than HLA typing. Seven different MLC types have thus far been recognized. The MLC reactions are complex, and it is likely that MLC loci other than HLA-D also exist.

Class I antigens can be found regularly in cell culture derived from human corneal epithelium, stroma, or endothelium by the cytotoxic plating inhibition test [31, 32] or by using monoclonal antibodies in an indirect immunofluorescence assay. Class II antigens are not expressed [33]. Using sensitive immunoperoxidase techniques class I antigens have also been noted in human corneal epithelium, stroma, and endothelium of fresh donor buttons [34]. The corneal epithelium has the most antigen with the periphery having more than the center.

Class II antigens were found on cells scattered throughout both central and peripheral epithelium as well as the stroma [34]. The cells in the stroma with class II antigens (HLA-DR positive) appeared dendritic. The region of HLA-DR positivity in the stroma begins at a distance of 3.5 to 4.0 mm from the center [35]. HLA-DR positive cells (with Ia antigens) are present in the corneal epithelium. These Langerhans' cells are primarily present in the corneal periphery (Figs. 6-4, 6-5). Ia-positive cells

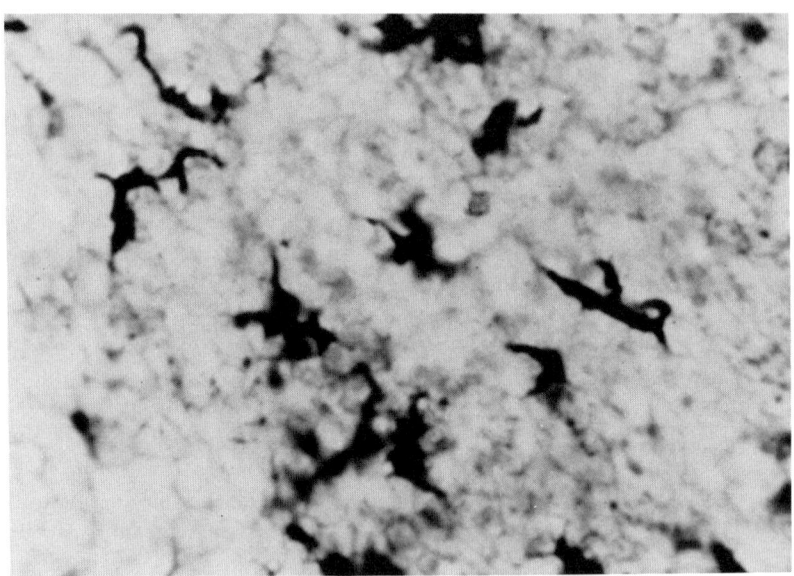

FIG. 6-4   Unstimulated Langerhans' cells at corneal limbus.

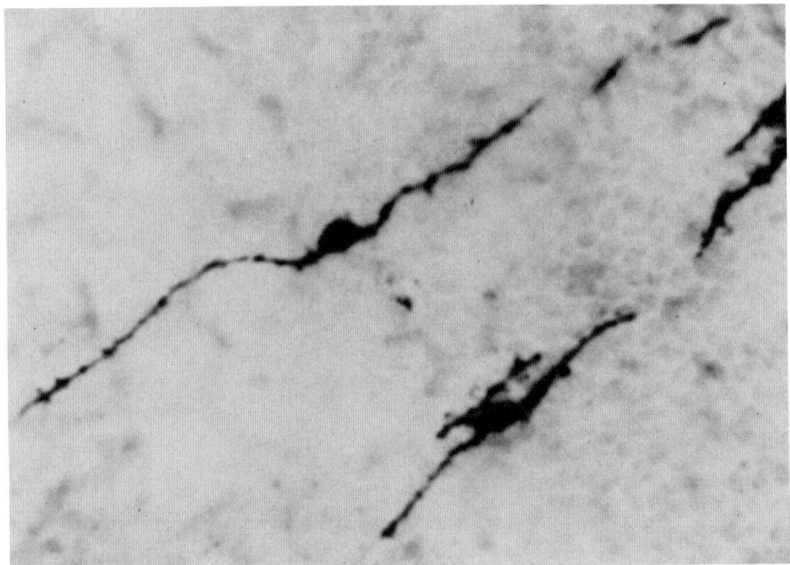

FIG. 6-5   Stimulated Langerhans' cells in streaming forms.

appear in the corneal endothelium during primary immunogenic uveitis, and class II antigens have been reported in the lower corneal endothelium after incubation with gamma interferon [36].

The specific antigenic stimuli that account for the corneal graft rejection must be better understood and are an exciting subject for future research.

Hypersensitivity Responses

An important unanswered question concerns the site where interaction between the graft antigen and the antigen-sensitive cells takes place. The conventional view is that sensitization begins when antigenic material from the graft percolates through peripheral lymphatics to the regional lymph nodes. Although no lymphatic vessels exist in avascular corneas, vascularized corneas apparently possess them [37, 38]. Because we know that intracorneally placed material can leave the cornea by way of these lymphatics and enter the regional lymph nodes, the assumption is that antigenic material can either diffuse from the cornea or exit through the lymphatic channels, enter the conjunctival lymphatics, and proceed to the lymph nodes (Fig. 6-6).

An alternative possibility, suggested by Medawar [39] is that sensitization may take place peripherally, possibly at the level of the graft's vascular endothelium. Activated lymphocytes may then traverse the graft parenchyma and travel by the lymphatic channels to the nodes where they generate the immunologic effector-cell population. Evidence of peripheral sensitization has been adduced from experiments with rat kidneys [40], and it is suggested that such sensitization may take place in all organ allografts whose blood supply has to be reestablished by surgical anastomosis. Evidence has been presented that passenger cells (i.e., leukocytes carried over in the vessels of skin and renal allografts) may play a major role in host sensitization [41, 42]. These cells contain leukocyte-defined antigens (HLA-D and DR in human beings; Ia in mice). It seems unlikely, however, that this type of sensitization plays a role in corneal graft rejection.

Two signals are required for T-cell activation. The source for signal 1 is the antigen on the surface of corneal tissue parenchyma—class I HLA antigens. The source for the second signal is cells that carry class II HLA antigens. These cells act as stimulators or antigen presenters or processors. These cells within the graft may constitute a major source of the tissue immunogenicity [43]. The passenger leukocytes just described may be a source of the second signal in most situations but in the cornea Langerhans' cells probably provide the source [44, 45]. Macrophages may also play some role in the initiation of the second signal.

Once sensitized, the host mounts an immunologic response that can manifest itself in several ways. In much of the work done on allograft rejection, transplants of skin or of solid tumors have been used because their fate is relatively easy to follow [46]. In these and the majority of corneal graft reactions, the cell-mediated immune (CMI) response plays the major role [47–49].

Corneal tissue from guinea pigs can induce cellular immunity in allo-

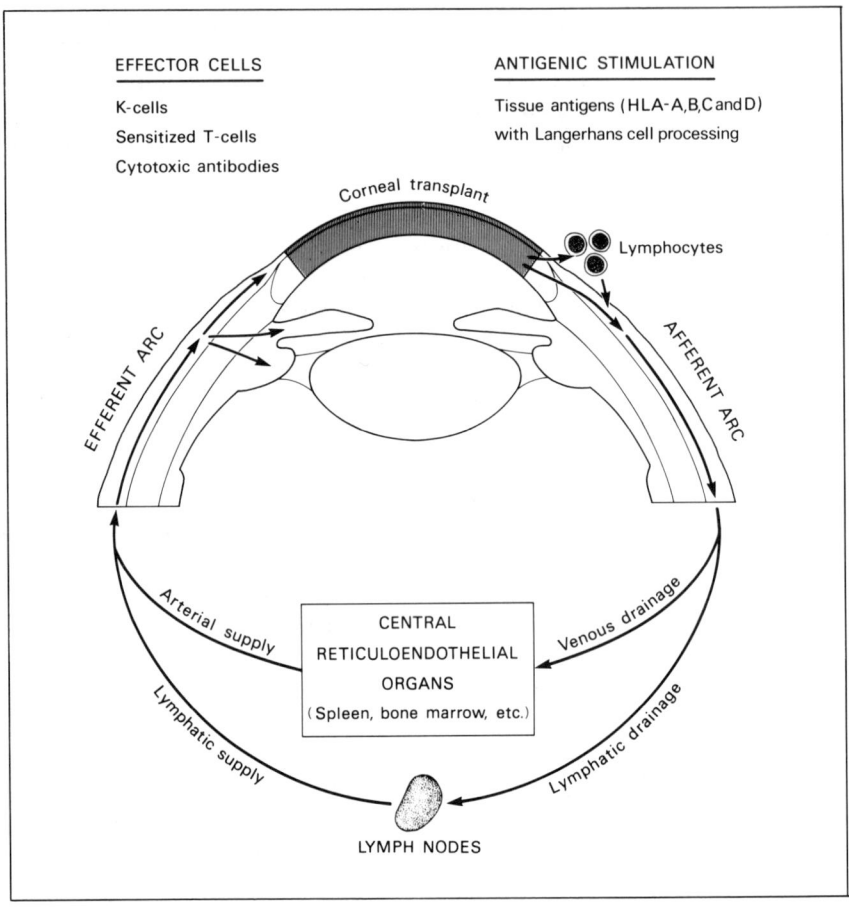

FIG. 6-6 Diagrammatic representation of afferent, central, and efferent arcs of corneal immune response.

geneic recipients, as shown by the production of migration inhibition factor (MIF), thymidine incorporation, skin testing, and passive transfer [48]. The MIF response reaches a peak 30 days after grafting and diminishes by 40 days. MIF activity, which is demonstrable in the aqueous humor of rabbits undergoing corneal xenograft or allograft rejection [50], is measurable when the earliest visible signs of clinical rejection appear, and it sometimes correlates with the severity of the rejection. When direct leukocyte migration inhibition (LMI) tests were performed with homologous corneal antigen in corneal transplant patients, persistent, increasing, or recurringly significant LMI always indicated eventual graft failure [51]. LMI factor can be produced by both T- and B-lymphocytes. The primary role of lymphoid cells in first rejections is consistent with the histologic features of early rejection, which show infiltration by a preponderance of mononuclear cells with only a few polymorphonuclear or plasma cells.

Cell transfer studies indicate that the activated lymphoid cells, identified as small lymphocytes, enter the circulation rapidly after their formation in the regional lymph nodes, and that they persist in the blood stream for hundreds of days [52, 53]. These small lymphocytes have a long life span and constantly recirculate from blood to lymph through the nodes. This finding of a long life span provides an explanation of the persistence of allograft sensitivity evoked by skin allografts. It also strengthens the view that the "second-set reaction" is an expression of a preexisting state of sensitivity rather than a reawakened one.

Critical experiments have shown that the vast majority of newly formed sensitized lymphocytes have no immunologic specificity. Thus the hitherto held and by no means unattractive view that the effector cells "home" specifically to the grafts responsible for their production may no longer be tenable [54]. Conflicting results have appeared in the literature, however.

Humoral antibodies have also played a role in certain organ transplant rejections [1]. In kidney grafting, a hyperacute rejection, characterized by the sludging of red cells and microthrombi in the glomeruli, can occur within minutes of transplantation. This reaction happens in patients with preexisting humoral antibodies owing to either blood-group incompatibility or presensitization by blood transfusions. An important component of the destructive process is a coagulopathy that always occurs within the graft and sometimes leads to systemic alterations resembling a disseminated intravascular coagulation. The acute early rejection is probably due to cell-mediated hypersensitivity, and the acute late rejection in immunosuppressed recipients is probably due to the binding of immunoglobulin and complement to the arterioles and glomerular capillaries [1]. This binding of immunoglobulin and complement has also followed heart transplants [55].

Humoral antibodies may also coat the grafted cells, making them susceptible to cytotoxic attack by normal unsensitized killer (K) cells [56, 57].

In corneal grafting, presensitization to HLA (indicated by elevation of the lymphocytotoxin level) has the same effect that it has in kidney grafting of sensitized recipients; for example, it increases the rejection rate [58]. The presence of lymphocytotoxic antibodies to corneal tissue in the peripheral blood can be detected in patients showing graft rejection [58–60]. Anticorneal antibodies are frequently formed after allografts in rabbits [61, 62] and the corneal endothelium of rabbits exposed to cytotoxic antibodies in the presence of complement shows cytotoxic damage [63]. In xenografts, soluble protein in the cornea sensitizes the host, and the graft reaction can be inhibited by lowering the systemic complement levels (with cobra venom and other substances). Ehlers and associates [64] reported a case in which rejection was probably only mediated by antibodies. In first allograft rejections, however, altering the systemic complement level does not affect the rejection [65]. In certain allograft and most xenograft reactions, polymorphonuclear leukocytes and plasma cells can be seen at the rejection site, suggesting the role of antibody and complement. The host leukocytes may contribute nonspecifically to enhance the destructive process.

In summary, the concept that HLA elicits a CMI response in the first corneal graft reaction is accurate. The roles of the other antigens in the cornea and the types of hypersensitivity elicited need to be more clearly defined, however. Clarification is needed not only in first rejections but also in the more complicated situations in which regrafting is done, the recipient beds are vascularized, or the corneas show preexistent antibodies.

Factors Affecting Rejection

As noted, lymphatics and regional lymph nodes play an important role in graft reactions [66]. Certain tissues, such as testes, brain, anterior chamber, lens, cornea, and hamster cheek pouch, are devoid of conventional lymphatic drainage; and they therefore support the growth of grafted tissues [67, 68]. Temporary interruption of lymphatic continuity in rabbits [69], or its permanent interruption in isolated guinea pig or rat-skin flaps [70], can delay or prevent host sensitization to skin allografts. When the chemical composition of the lymph draining an allograft site is altered by an increase in lysosomal enzymes, the draining lymph nodes are probably participating in some way in the survival of the allograft [71]. Adoptive transfer experiments suggest that skin allograft immunity is first demonstrable in the regional lymph nodes [72].

In comparable work on the participation of the lymphatic drainage and the regional lymph nodes in corneal immunologic reactions, lymphatics in both the conjunctiva and the vascularized cornea have been demonstrated [37, 73, 74]. The degree of corneal lymphatization influences the host's ability to recognize nonself corneal antigen, and the degree of corneal vascularization influences the host's ability (1) to recognize the antigen and (2) to bring effector lymphoid cells to the site of rejection.

It is estimated that the incidence of graft rejection in vascular corneal beds is 10 to 12 percent. This incidence increases as vascularization of the bed increases. In one study [65], hosts with avascular corneal beds rejected 3.5 percent of their grafts in an average of 10 months; hosts with mildly vascularized corneal beds rejected 13.3 percent of their grafts in 4 months; and hosts with moderately vascularized corneal beds rejected 65 percent of their grafts in 2 months. Other studies have corroborated this relationship with incidences of rejection being 50 percent [75] and 66 percent [22] in severely vascularized recipient beds. It has also been shown that 95 percent of lamellar grafts and 75 percent of penetrating grafts placed in avascular beds survive a long time, even in hosts sensitized by being permitted to reject large skin grafts from the same donors that provided the corneal buttons. The sensitized lymphocytes of these amply sensitized experimental animals could not reach their avascular corneas [76].

Sensitizing the host with donor tissue increases the rejection rate of corneal grafts placed in vascularized beds. If a skin graft from the same donor as a corneal graft is placed before, after, or simultaneously with the corneal graft, between 80 and 100 percent of these corneal grafts are rejected [77, 78]. If the skin graft is from another donor, however, only 10 percent of the corneal grafts are rejected. Both in vivo and in vitro tests show cross-reactivity between corneal and skin antigens in animals sensitized with either corneal transplants, corneal homogenates in complete Freund's adjuvant, or skin grafts. This expected cross-reactivity can be explained by the common embryologic origin of the two tissues [48]. Sensitization may diminish with time. Recent experimental work seems to indicate that after corneal transplantation the host always becomes aware of the donor antigen despite the absence of clinically recognizable signs of rejection.

The ratio between T4-helper and T8-suppressor lymphocyte sensitization after keratoplasty may reflect the degree of sensitization [79]. Higher ratios indicate enhanced sensitization and low ratios indicate diminished sensitization. Patients who demonstrated elevated levels of T8 suppressor cells after a rejection episode tend to accept their grafts [80].

Desquamated endothelial cells may play a role in this sensitization process [81].

The question arises as to whether sensitization by a graft affects the rejection rate of a second graft placed in the other eye and if the enhanced sensitization induced by the second graft affects the first clear graft.

One group noted a 17 percent chance of rejection within the first year for the first graft after the second was implanted [82]. Others have noted a threefold increase in incidence of rejection in the second eye [83], whereas yet another group reported a statistically insignificant increased rejection incidence in both eyes [84]. The consensus seems to indicate an increased risk of rejection, the precise rate being uncertain.

Repeat grafts should and do have an increased incidence of rejection [75] owing to the previous sensitization and enhanced vascularization or altered vascular permeability secondary to the inflammation and necrosis that follows rejection. Surprisingly, pregnancy and blood transfusions have no effect on the corneal graft rejection rate [85].

The use of eccentric grafts (closer to the limbal lymphatic channels and blood vessels than centered grafts) and of large grafts (closer to the limbus and carrying a larger antigenic load than smaller grafts) can increase the chance of sensitizing the host to the corneal graft and may be associated with increased rejection rates [65, 75].

It has also been observed that the rejection line usually starts at the site of maximum vascularization (Fig. 6-7). Trauma or inflammation that dilates the blood vessels (e.g., associated with combined procedures), and interrupted sutures that are left in place too long or silk sutures that produce neovascularization, can all increase the probability of graft rejection [75].

In patients with severely vascularized corneal beds, and therefore at high risk of rejection, the number of successful grafts was in direct proportion to the number of HLAs shared by the graft donor and recipient. Patients receiving grafts with two matching HLAs had a failure rate of 22 percent after 1 year, whereas grafts with only one matching HLA or with none at all had failure rates of 53 percent and 83 percent respectively [22]. Confirmatory studies have been performed [86, 87]. In dogs,

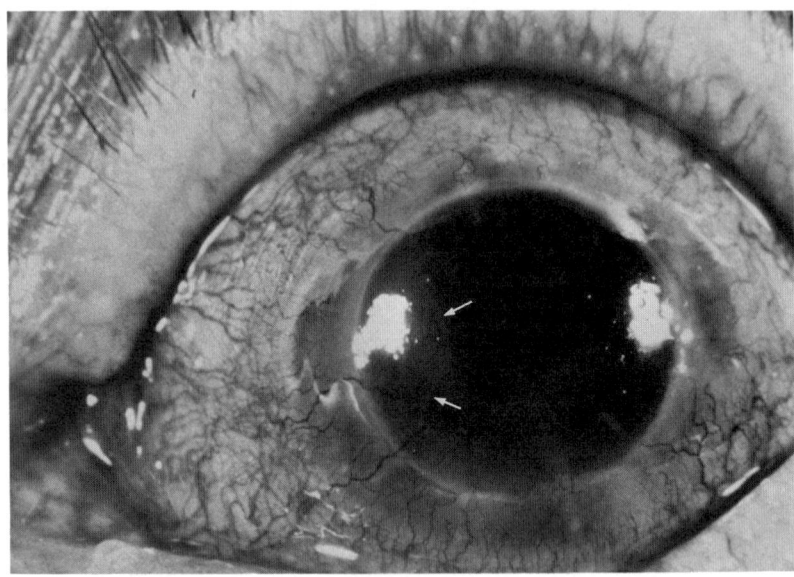

FIG. 6-7   Corneal graft reaction showing endothelial line of rejection (*arrows*) starting at site of maximal vascularization at periphery of graft.

matching the HLA-D locus seems to diminish the incidence of corneal graft reaction notably.

ABH blood-group incompatibility, or an ABH phenotype of the recipient, does not influence graft prognosis [22, 87–89].

In animal experiments, corneas may vary in antigenicity according to species (frog cornea least antigenic, goat cornea most antigenic [90]), and they vary in their ability to reject according to the animal's gender (i.e., male mice reject transplanted tissue less often than female mice. Gender may affect human allograft rejection [85]). Penetrating corneal grafts are rejected slightly more often than lamellar corneal grafts, possibly for the following reasons: (1) the lamellar graft has less antigenic mass; (2) in a lamellar graft the endothelium is in better condition to withstand insult than in a penetrating graft; (3) there is less chance of endothelial damage owing to operation in the lamellar graft; and (4) the endothelium and Descemet's membrane are intact in the lamellar graft, and Descemet's membrane can prevent some sensitized effector lymphoid cells from reaching the endothelium [65].

A retrospective and prospective study has shown that the removal of donor corneal epithelium is associated with a statistically significant lower incidence of allograft reactions and graft loss [91]. The decision to remove epithelium must be tempered by the anticipated postoperative healing problems.

The so-called Lewis antigen was incriminated in the increased rejection rate noted in corneal transplants performed from white donors to black recipients [92].

In chronic herpetic keratitis, antigenic determinants can be incorpo-

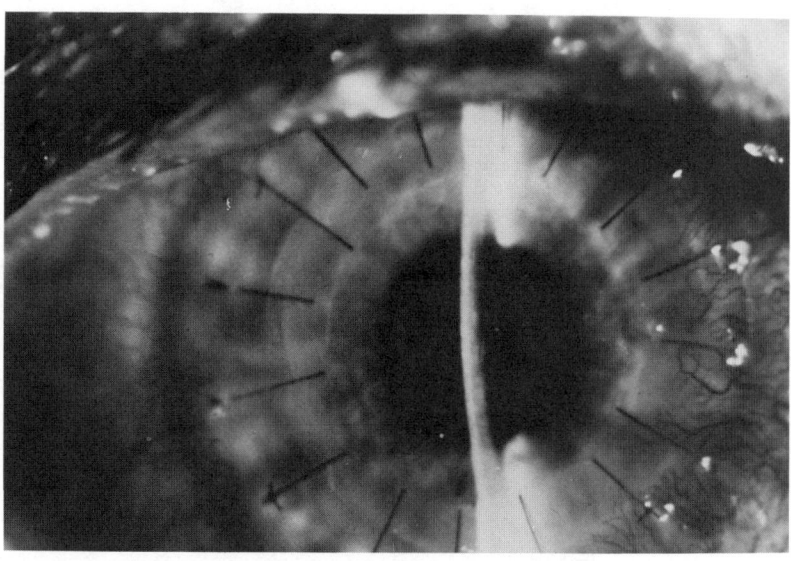

FIG. 6-8   Orthotopically placed human corneal graft with radially placed interrupted 10-0 nylon sutures.

rated into the cell membranes of infected cells, making them permanent sources of antigenicity that may be responsible for an immune reaction in a herpes-sensitized host [93]. In other studies [94, 95], the leukocyte migration technique provided evidence that the chronicity of viral keratitis is caused by corneal antigen and the processes of cellular immunity, and not by the virus. It can be inferred from these studies that when a corneal graft is performed to remove scar tissue from a patient with chronic herpes simplex keratitis, the recipient may be sensitized to corneal tissue and the chances of graft rejection increased.

CLINICAL COURSE AND HISTOLOGIC FEATURES OF REJECTION

Type of Graft

Corneal grafts to remove opaque tissue (lamellar and penetrating) are placed orthotopically (Fig. 6-8). Overlay grafts are used for tectonic purposes and recently for refractive ones (i.e., epikeratophakia). In experimental animals, however, intralamellar placement is sometimes preferred [96, 97] (Figs. 6-9, 6-10). It is simple to perform, less traumatic to the animal, and rarely fails for surgical reasons. Its main use is in the immunologic study of graft reaction. By orthotopic placement in animals, the epithelium, stroma, or endothelium can be transplanted individually, and this capability has greatly helped the researcher to understand the rejection phenomenon in each of these layers.

In epithelium grafted orthotopically in experimental animals, rejection can start in 7 to 10 days, although an interval of 2 to 3 weeks is more usual. A rejection line (best seen when stained with methylene blue) appears at the site of the heaviest vascularization and slowly spreads across the epithelium, sometimes accompanied by stromal edema. It requires

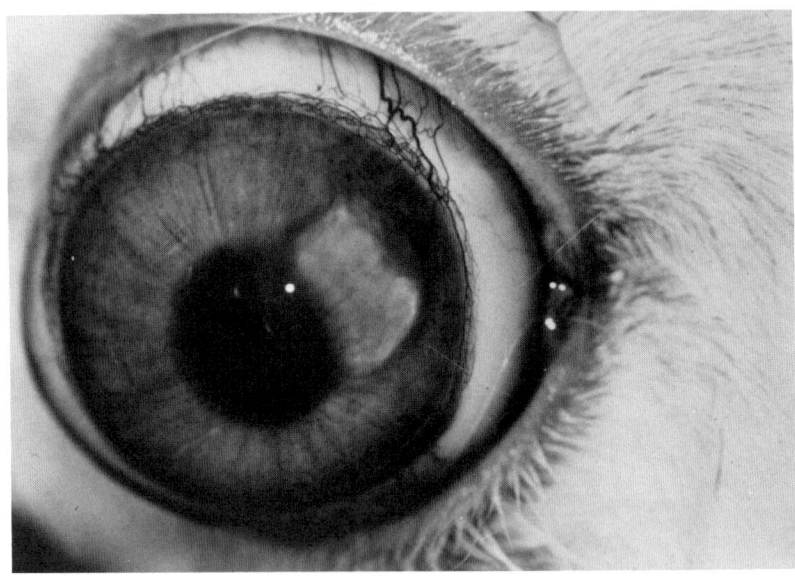

FIG. 6-9   Intralamellar corneal graft in a rabbit. Note absence of sutures.

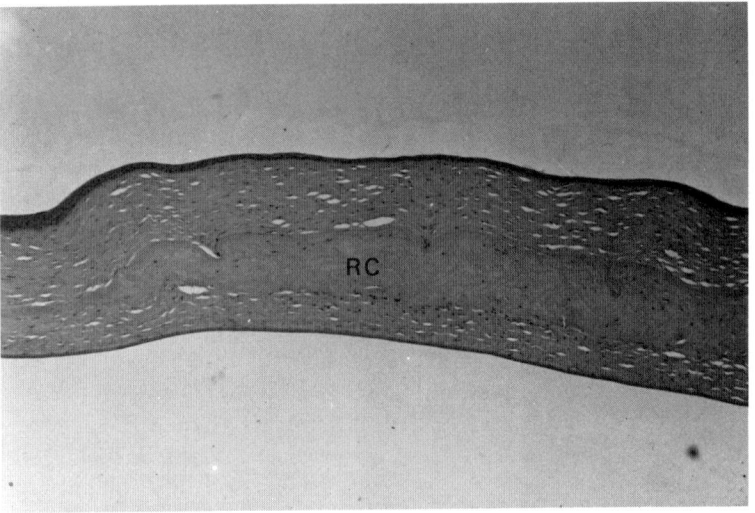

FIG. 6-10   Histologic section of intralamellarly placed rat cornea (RC) in rabbit cornea. Note difference in consistency of rat and rabbit tissues.

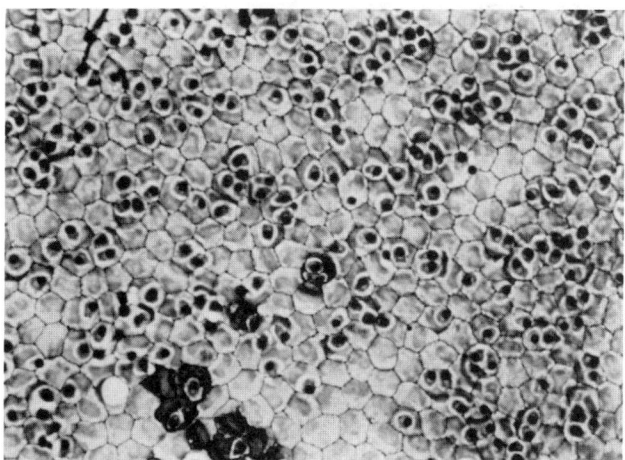

FIG. 6-11 Histologic picture of rabbit endothelium during hyperacute graft reaction. Note numerous plasma cells (heterograft reaction).

only a few days for the entire epithelium to be rejected, but the graft is usually clear thereafter. Only a mild anterior chamber reaction occurs.

In both stromal and endothelial rejection [98], the time of onset is about the same as in epithelial rejection, and again the rejection line begins at the site of the heaviest vascularization. We have seen a line of rejection begin at the site of an iris adhesion to the cornea. Presumably this phenomenon is related to iris vasculature. It requires more time for the stroma and endothelium to be rejected, however, and the graft is usually cloudy after the rejection process is complete. The anterior chamber response is moderate (Fig. 6-11).

In human beings the first corneal allograft rejection may occur as early as 2 to 3 weeks or as late as many years after transplantation. The symptoms of rejection include decreased visual acuity, redness, nonspecific discomfort, and photophobia. Occasionally in instances of mild rejection patients are asymptomatic. Patients must be made aware of these symptoms and the importance of seeing their ophthalmologist within 24 hours after onset.

The diagnosis of rejection can be made or suspected if the following signs are present: graft edema occurring 3 weeks or later in a technically successful clear graft; circumlimbal congestion; flare and cells in the anterior chamber; keratic precipitates (KP) on the graft, especially in excess of that expected from the anterior chamber response; iritis; clouding or an endothelial, stromal, or epithelial line starting near the most proximal and intense vascularization (rejection lines occur in 25–30 percent of patients with graft reaction); elevated intraocular pressure; vascular engorgement around the sutures; and loss of epithelial luster [99]. The first signs are a mild uveal reaction shown by flare and cells, an accumulation of fine KP on the endothelium, and circumlimbal injection.

With the epithelial rejection an elevated line may be present on the

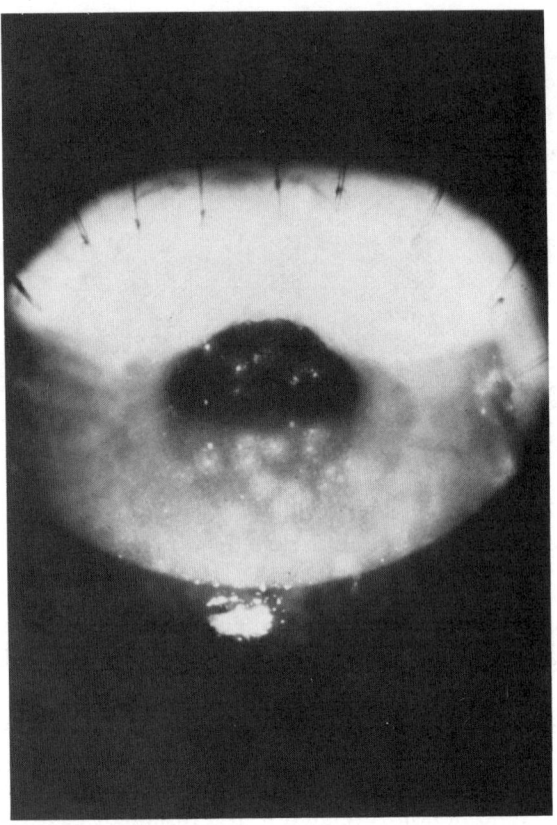

FIG. 6-12   Subepithelial infiltrates in rejecting corneal donor tissue.

epithelium that stains with fluorescein or rose bengal. It first appears at the graft periphery and migrates contripetally within a matter of several days to a few weeks after the process terminates. The graft remains clear. If associated with stromal or endothelial rejection (or both) the epithelial rejection always occurs first. The incidence of epithelial rejection in one large series was 10 percent [100].

Subepithelial infiltrates may be a sign of rejection (Fig. 6-12). These small (0.2–0.5 mm) white infiltrates occur between 6 and 21 months postoperatively. No conjunctivitis is present, and the lesions are present only in the donor tissue (signs that help differentiate this entity from an adenovirus infection). The distribution of the lesions is random in the donor tissue, and the associated anterior chamber inflammatory reaction is minimal. The lesions clear with corticosteroid therapy, sometimes leaving a residual nebular opacity. This type of rejection may accompany epithelial or endothelial rejection. The incidence cited in the literature is 15 percent [101].

In the peripheral type of endothelial graft rejection, the KP are in the lower part of the graft or at its margin. A line of KP (endothelial rejection line) then migrates centripetally, and pigment accumulates on the endothelium. The donor cornea becomes edematous as the endothelium is compromised by an accumulation of lymphoid cells. In the less frequent, diffuse type of rejection, the KP spread diffusely over the donor endothelium, and a few days later the cornea becomes edematous. In both types of response, the development of a membrane on the posterior surface of the corneal button may be a late manifestation [65].

Experimental studies have indicated that donor epithelium, stroma, and endothelium persist for years in the recipient [102–104]. This persistence of foreign antigens may explain the occurrence of late rejection.

Histologic Features of Rejection

Usually one or more areas of linear epithelial breakdown appear at the edge of the graft, and gradually an epithelial rejection line develops. The rejection line stains with methylene blue, and both sides of the line show scattered punctate staining. The rejection line consists of polymorphonuclear leukocytes, and behind them are lymphocytes. Many of the lymphocytes are large and look like blast forms with a light chromatin pattern and abundant endoplasmic reticulum. In the area of the rejection line, epithelial cell alteration and disorganization are noted. Pits or craters form, and debris is deposited on the surface. The rejected (proximal) epithelium is uneven, lumpy, and thicker than the nonrejected epithelium. The superficial layers may even be absent in the nonrejected epithelium next to the rejection line. Massive localized cell destruction affects the whole thickness of the epithelial layer [105].

Repair proceeds from the basal layer and affects both the recipient and the donor tissue [65].

Polymorphonuclear leukocytes and lymphocytes also participate intimately in corneal stromal rejection. Severe cellular alterations—distension of the endoplasmic reticulum, vacuole formation, and the appearance of phagocytized material and high-density crystalline intracytoplasmic material—take place in the keratocytes that are in contact with lymphocytes. Disruption of the normal lamellar structure of collagen of the grafted stroma also occur in areas of leukocytic infiltration [106]. Occasional macrophages and plasma cells are seen as are varying degrees of edema.

The lipid deposition noted in the interface in intralamellar corneal grafts may reflect an allograft reaction.

In endothelial rejections, the rejection line consists primarily of lymphocytes accompanied by fibrin on the endothelial surface. These lymphocytes infiltrate the endothelium, often replacing the endothelial-cell cover of Descemet's membrane in severely damaged areas, and in some areas exposing Descemet's membrane to the anterior chamber. In these circumstances stromal edema overlies the damaged areas. The rejected endothelial cells are often rounded or globular with greatly thickened centers. The endothelial nuclei are irregularly thickened. Junctions between adjacent endothelial cells disappear [107, 108]. The cytoplasmic organelles are fewer in the severely damaged endothelial cells. Precipitates consisting of lymphocytes, monocytes, and fibrin appear on the endothelium. The lymphocytes are said to reach the endothelium through

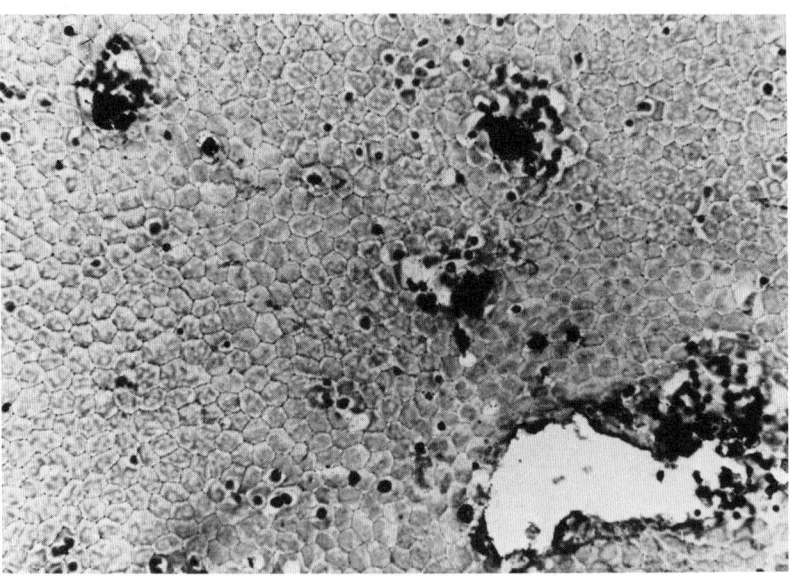

FIG. 6-13 Histologic picture of flat preparation of rabbit corneal endothelium showing pocklike areas of endothelial damage.

the unhealed Descemet's membrane from the blood vessels and wandering cells that have entered the stroma. Descemet's membrane heals in several months, and this route of lymphocyte migration may then close. When grafts are rejected, however, the healing of Descemet's membrane may be delayed [109].

Specular microscopic studies in corneal endothelial rejection have revealed a number of distinct morphologic changes [110]. "Blackout" areas that overlap cell boundaries are present. These may represent wandering inflammatory cells on the endothelium or the pseudoguttata noted secondary to endothelial edema [111]. Intracytoplasmic pinpoint black areas and intracellular bright iridescent oval bodies are present and may represent early cell distress and damage. The endothelial cells may vary in size and shape with the presence of bizarre-shaped, extremely large cells (multinucleated?). In cases in which an endothelial rejection line is present, a sharp demarcation line is noted.

Quantitative studies of conjunctival cytology in relation to corneal grafting revealed an initial neutrophilia in all patients and a late neutrophilia and lymphocytosis in patients with rejection [112].

In rabbit studies in which lymphoid cells sensitized to the histocompatibility antigens of the donor and recipient were introduced into the rabbit's anterior chamber, the formation of local pocklike areas of endothelial damage has been demonstrated (Fig. 6-13). When transferred lymphoid cells are compatible with the tissues of the graft recipient but not with the donor's tissues, the donor graft is severely compromised. If the lymphoid cells are compatible with the graft but not with the tissues of the recipient, the graft remains clear but is surrounded by an area of recipient endothelial destruction [113, 114]. This type of pock lesion differs from the type seen in human beings and suggests to most observers that the sensitized lymphocytes come primarily from the nearest blood vessels and not from the aqueous humor.

The reparative process depends on the surviving endothelial cells of both host and donor spreading. In the rabbit, the host's endothelium can grow to replace the rejected endothelium, and a clear graft results. This regrowth, unfortunately, does not occur to any measurable degree in adult human beings. If the endothelial destruction is severe, a retrocorneal membrane may form. The cells that form the membrane are fibroblasts that come from the edge of the graft through the disrupted Descemet's membrane. A retrocorneal membrane can be produced in the presence of an intact Descemet's membrane by freezing the cornea repeatedly. This experiment led Michels and co-workers [114] to conclude that endothelial-cell metaplasia may be responsible for the retrocorneal membrane even in cases of graft rejection.

TREATMENT AND PREVENTION OF REJECTION

Surgical Maneuvers

Operative techniques can be used to minimize corneal graft rejection. Removing the epithelium decreases the antigenic load and decreases the number of Langerhans' cells presented to the recipient. This procedure should not be performed when an intact epithelium is necessary, however (e.g., in patients with lye burn). The use of a small graft (8.0 mm or less) decreases the antigenic incursion and places the foreign donor tissue further from the recipient's limbal blood vessels. This distancing is also accomplished by centrally placing the graft. The rejection rate increases with grafts larger than 8.5 mm. Smaller grafts also have less Langerhans' cells (Ia-D antigen) because these cells are primarily near the limbus [35].

Removing interrupted sutures as soon as the fibrovascular reparative tissue reaches the graft minimizes neovascularization. (Some workers have induced allograft rejection by leaving interrupted sutures in place as a stimulus to neovascularization [114a].) Running sutures have mitigated the need for early suture removal because they usually evoke a negligible inflammatory response. Nylon sutures rather than silk have reduced the neovascularization caused by the suture material [115].

In vascularized recipient beds, the use of a large lamellar graft followed by a small penetrating graft may help protect the second graft from the surrounding blood vessels. Because repeated grafts may sensitize the recipient, this technique may increase the risk of rejection.

Keratoprostheses have been used in severely vascularized, multiply grafted corneas at certain ophthalmic centers; but although the immunologic rejection phenomenon has been circumvented in this way, a battery of new surgical problems has been introduced [115a, 115b].

Donor Graft Treatment

Several ways of treating the donor cornea have been devised in attempts to alter its antigenicity. The survival of rabbit skin allografts has been prolonged by treating the skin with electrophoresis prior to transplantation [116]. The antigenic substances apparently migrate from the graft in response to the electrical current. This action depletes the antigens and prolongs the life of the graft.

In studies of the antigenic composition of cultured bovine corneas, we found that extracts of cultured corneas did not contain the strong antigen present in extracts of normal corneas or of corneal epithelium [117]. These results are consistent with our observation that little or no epithelium remains on the cultured cornea. Its diminished antigenicity is thus due solely to loss of epithelium. We also found that cultured corneas appear to take up serum proteins from the medium in which they are cultured. At present, culturing corneal tissue may have a technologic function but not an immunologic one.

In contrast, preserving a donor cornea in the recipient's serum prior to a penetrating allograft seems to diminish the incidence of graft rejection [118]. One can assume that the donor's serum proteins are eluted by this method, to be replaced by the recipient's proteins. In addition, passenger leukocytes or macrophages may be removed and donor epithelium lost. This practice may reduce the recipient's sensitization to the donor's antigens.

Prolongation of skin-graft survival by "donor enhancement" can be achieved by pretreating the donor with the recipient's high-titer antidonor serum [119]. The mode of action is obscure, but the two commonly accepted theories are (1) that antidonor serum acts peripherally by blocking antigenic sites and (2) that it acts by inducing central suppression.

We [120] and others [121, 122] have reported that pretreating the donor with antilymphocyte serum (ALS) is a means of prolonging rabbit corneal allografts. Unfortunately, both heterologous ALS and antilymphocyte globulin (ALG) are cytotoxic for corneal cells in the presence of complement. It has been shown, however, that succinylation of ALG produces an antibody that retains its antigen-binding ability but does not combine with complement and is noncytotoxic. Rabbit corneal allografts that are pretreated with succinylated ALG have notably longer survivals than those pretreated with nonsuccinylated ALS or ALG [123, 124].

Cryopreservation of the corneal donor tissue seems to have no measurable effect on its antigenicity [125, 126]. In one earlier contrary claim [127], the freezing technique differed from the technique described in the more recent reports.

Treating corneal donor tissue with hyperbaric oxygen may alter its antigenicity by removing Langerhans' cells (Ia-D antigens) from the donor tissue [128].

Corticosteroids   The mainstay of the treatment of corneal graft rejection is the corticosteroid. Although the lymphocytes of human beings are more steroid-resistant than the lymphocytes of many other species (e.g., rat, rabbit, mouse, hamster), the effect is still dramatic [129]. The mechanism of action of corticosteroids is discussed in Chapter 1.

Some or all of the steroid effects play a role in the suppression or prevention of the corneal graft reaction. For example, it has been shown that phagocytes on the graft endothelium can be completely destroyed in 24 hours by topical dexamethasone [130]. Steroids are not without side effects, however, and these complications are discussed in a later section of this chapter.

POSTOPERATIVE TREATMENT. The postoperative corticosteroid treatment of routine corneal transplants varies markedly among surgeons. In low-risk patients (small first graft in an avascular bed) some surgeons may not even use postoperative corticosteroids whereas others will use high doses. The consensus seems to favor the use of 1% prednisolone four times a day for 1 or 2 weeks and then slowly tapering over the next several weeks. Subconjunctival dexamethasone or betamethasone may be added in the immediate postoperative period. In higher-risk patients topical therapy is mandatory, frequently associated with a subconjunctival or an intravenous bolus of corticosteroids.

In the postoperative period the anti-inflammatory action of corticosteroids is desired and low doses can be employed. The optimal dose for each patient can be determined according to the clinical response (i.e., constriction of blood vessels). If rejection starts, however, immunosuppression and therefore immediate high doses of steroids are mandatory [131].

GRAFT REACTION TREATMENT. In its early stages, the endothelial rejection responds to topical steroid therapy: The endothelial rejection line is still at the periphery, only scattered KP have appeared, and stromal edema is still mild to moderate. If the rejection line has progressed too far, and too much endothelium has been destroyed, steroids can halt the destruction process but cannot maintain a clear graft.

Most ophthalmologists consider topical steroid therapy adequate for the control of the corneal graft reaction.

The type of corticosteroid drop may be important. Prednisone acetate or alcohol penetrates the cornea well if the epithelium is intact, whereas prednisone phosphate does not [132], but if the epithelium has been removed, or if the eye is moderately or severely inflamed, the phosphate preparation penetrates satisfactorily.

Prednisolone 1% or dexamethasone 0.1% (or clobetasone 0.1%) [133] drops are given topically every hour while the patient is awake and as ointment every several hours at night. The dosage can be tapered as the reaction subsides.

If the graft reaction is moderate or severe subconjunctival injections are indicated (some use in mild reactions). When injected subconjunctivally, dexamethasone penetrates the eye much better than triamcinolone. Because dexamethasone is completely soluble, its potency has a short half-life of hours only. In contrast, a subconjunctival depot of Depo-Medrol may remain active for weeks, and triamcinolone may remain active for months. Usually 2 mg of dexamethasone is injected. The injection may be repeated on several successive days [100].

If systemic steroids are necessary (i.e., in patients with moderate to severe graft reactions), 10 to 12 tablets of prednisone per day for 2 weeks, together with the topical medication, is recommended [65]. After 2 weeks, the systemic medication can be decreased and the topical medication increased. Treatment on alternate days, with higher doses given in the morning, may reduce the side effects (caused by adrenal suppression) of long-term therapy [134–136]. Normally, however, long-term systemic therapy (and therefore alternate-day therapy) should not be necessary to counteract corneal graft rejection.

Some authors [99] recommend intravenous corticosteroids immediately.

Other Immunosuppressive Therapy

Other immunosuppressive agents have been used principally in other animal species or in other types of organ transplantation in human beings. They include pyridinolcarbamate [137], diazoacetylglycine amide [138], mercaptopurine [139], cytosine arabinoside [140], adamantoyl cytarabine [141], ε-aminocaproic acid [142], antithymocyte serum [143], asparaginase [144], oxisuran [145], and cyclosporin A (CYA), few of which have been tested in human corneal grafts.

CYA suppresses activation of naive T cells by interleukin 1 and 2 and decreases NK cell activity [146]. Virus (herpes simplex) growth may be enhanced by systemic administration of CYA [147]. Other side effects of systemic administration include nephrotoxicity and hepatotoxicity. When given intramuscularly, CYA can enhance corneal graft survival in rabbits [148, 149]. Surprisingly, topical [150, 151], subconjunctival [152], and retrobulbar [153] application of CYA also enhances corneal graft survival in rabbits. The topical administration of 1% CYA in peanut oil four or five times a day is nontoxic and effective. On rare occasions, azathioprine has been used for this purpose [154]. It is most effective if given 2 or 3 days after grafting [155] and has been reserved for high-risk patients (e.g., sensitized recipients, vascularized recipient beds).

When applied topically, neither azathioprine nor ALS has altered the course of the corneal graft reaction [96, 156].

Systemic ALS has not often been used to treat human corneal graft reactions because of its side effects [157, 158]. In one study [159] ALS was used for 30 days after each of 12 keratoplasties compromised by highly vascularized corneas. The immunologic responses appeared to be inhibitable, even in the highly vascularized, regrafted cases.

Salicylates to modify platelet activity, and of heparin, bishydroxycoumarin, or snake venom to inhibit fibrin deposition and coagulation in the allograft, have been shown to add to the effect of most immunosuppressive agents in preventing kidney damage during rejection [160, 161]. These agents would not be used for corneal graft rejection.

Induction of Immunologic Tolerance

"Tolerance" results when certain antigens fail to evoke response because of their prior administration in a particular form. The induction of transplantation tolerance in adult animals apparently requires the temporary immunosuppression of the recipient animal during the animal's exposure to the antigen [162–164]. Such tolerance has been induced by the transfer of donor spleen cells [165], cell-free tissue extracts [163], and soluble transplantation antigens [164]. The process has been facilitated by also giving the recipients cyclophosphamide, irradiation, or ALS.

Because the immunoglobulin (Ig) molecule is antigenic, antibodies can be made to the variable region of the Ig molecule. These antibodies are called idiotypic antibodies (see Chapter 1). This type of antibody can be developed in in vitro MLC reaction, between the donor's and recipient's lymphocytes. The recipient's sensitized lymphocytes (lymphoblasts) can be given back to the recipient, making him "tolerant" to the specific donor's tissues. Research into this area of graft immunology is still in the early stages.

Induction of Immunologic Enhancement

To increase the survival of foreign cells in a recipient animal, investigators have found that humoral antibodies against foreign antigens, either administered to or produced by the recipient host, can, under the proper conditions, coat the foreign cells and thus protect them from destruction by the lymphocyte-mediated CMI response [166]. "Enhancement" induced in this way has been achieved in renal transplantation [167, 168].

The induction of enhancement and tolerance may lead to the elimination of the use of general immunosuppressive agents and of the risk of the complications associated with their use. These alternatives to immunosuppressive therapy may play an important role in the future treatment of at least some organ transplantations (kidney, liver, heart) in human beings [169].

Anti-inflammatory Agent Treatment

Inflammation caused by factors unrelated to the graft (e.g., trauma, an infectious process) can alter the tissue so that recognition of the antigen and the arrival of effector-sensitized lymphocytes are both enhanced. It is important, therefore, to keep inflammation controlled. The role of cyclic adenosine monophosphate (cAMP) in corneal graft rejection is complex. On the one hand, lowered levels of cAMP are associated with reduced inflammation, and a variety of prostaglandin-E inhibitors (e.g., indomethacin, flurbiprofen, indoxole, meclofenamic acid, naproxen, acetylsalicylic acid, clonixin) are known to reduce both cAMP and inflammation [170]. On the other hand, cAMP also turns off the secretion of immunoglobulins by lymphocytes and inhibits T-cell proliferation and the destructive activities of killer lymphocytes [171]. Systemic PGE_1 treatment in mice has been reported to protect renal grafts from immunologic damage [172]. The role of prostaglandins and their inhibitors in the corneal graft reaction remains uncertain.

Matching Histocompatibility Antigens

This topic is discussed in the section on factors affecting rejection. To reiterate, the use of HLA-matched corneal tissue may be useful in patients at high risk of rejection (i.e., regrafted patients with vascularized recipient beds). It would be especially helpful to avoid any specific HLA antigens of the donor to which the recipient is sensitized.

Stark and colleagues [173] have determined the various serologically defined antigens against which graft-failure patients have already developed antibodies. Prospective donors are then screened to eliminate those who possess major histocompatibility complex antigens to which the recipient is already sensitized.

The use of monoclonal antibodies may be extremely helpful in tissue typing (as well as monitoring and treating allografts) [174]. Many scientists are now using cloning techniques to make antibodies that recognize HLA antigens on the surface of normal leukocytes. By building up a library of antibodies against the HLA antigens, especially at the D locus, tissue-typing procedures should be facilitated.

Regrafting

Rarely, corneal grafts clouded after a rejection process may spontaneously clear months or years later [175]. The pathophysiology of this process is obscure, but recent work has revealed mitoses in the human adult corneal endothelium under certain circumstances [176]. In cases of borderline decompensation the mitosis, along with cell spreading, may be hypothesized to eliminate the corneal cloudiness owing to edema.

If all else fails, the cornea can be regrafted. If the edema, under appropriate maximum therapy (usually corticosteroids), does not disappear within a year, the patient should be prepared for reoperation. In certain circumstances regrafting may be performed sooner. If the edema and the concomitant micronecrosis persist, the graft vascularizes and a less favorable bed for the grafted tissue results. Regrafted patients are at a higher risk of graft rejection than patients grafted for the first time because of the sensitization of the recipient and the increased vasularity of the graft bed.

Side Effects of Treatment

The removal of donor epithelium should be performed only when re-epithelialization is expected to proceed normally. Otherwise, the prolonged exposure of an impaired surface subjects the cornea to a high risk of infection, especially if steroids or other immunosuppressive medications are being used. Partially healed epithelium may release corneal epithelium thymocyte-activating factor, an interleukin-1-like substance, which enhances inflammation by attracting polymorphonuclear leukocytes, lymphocytes, and fibroblasts [177].

Early removal of the sutures may result in a gaping wound, overriding wound edges, leaking from the anterior chamber, and other complications.

When corneas stored in tissue culture medium were transplanted, infection with *Flavobacterium endophthalmitis* followed [178]. Tissue culture medium, if foreign to the recipient, can increase the antigenic load and the rejection rate [179].

Corticosteroids can cause allergic reactions [180, 181] and such other side effects as addiction, skin changes (e.g., ecchymosis, telangiectasis, atrophy, acne, hirsutism) [182], mental changes, peptic ulceration, infection (high incidence) [183–186], certain neoplasms (high incidence) [187, 188], diabetes, osteoporosis, muscle wasting, hypertension, edema,

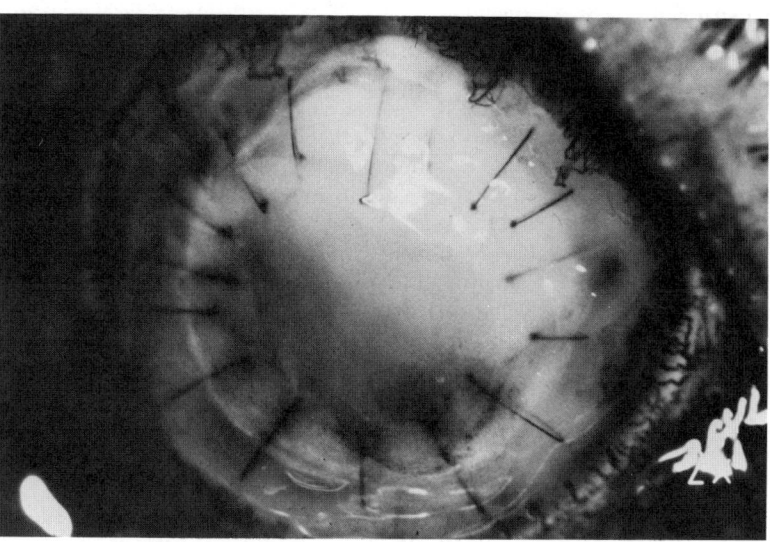

FIG. 6-14 Infected corneal graft.

pseudotumor cerebri, coagulogenic alterations, and a variety of changes in protein and mineral metabolism [189].

One of the ocular side effects from either local or systemic steroid administration is the delay and reduction of quality of corneal wound healing. All the layers of the cornea (epithelium [190], stroma [190], and endothelium [191]) are affected, and the cornea's tensile strength is reduced during the healing process [192, 193]. Fibroblastic activity is inhibited, conversion of procollagen to collagen is diminished, and collagenase activity is enhanced.

The increased risk of infection during local or system corticosteroid therapy has been thoroughly reported [183–186] (Fig. 6-14). If the graft has been performed on a cornea scarred by infection (e.g., infection with herpes simplex virus or *Pseudomonas aeruginosa*), the risk of reinfection is increased by steroid treatment. Cataracts and glaucoma can complicate prolonged corticosteroid therapy [189], a toxic keratopathy may occur, and subconjunctival steroid injections can cause conjunctival scarring, ptosis, and scleral thinning [194]. The injection itself can perforate the globe [195].

The use of other systemic immunosuppressive agents can result in bone marrow suppression [196]. Other troublesome sequelae are hives, rashes, generalized pruritus, serum sickness, and anaphylactic shock.

The increased frequency of infection (bacterial [197], fungal [198, 199], and viral [200, 201]) after immunosuppressive therapy has been extensively reported. The growth of tumors and their transplantation to other animals can be greatly facilitated by immunosuppressive agents [202]. The growth of tumor allografts has been accelerated [203], and there are several reports of more than usually frequent metastases after the immunosuppressive treatment of tumor-bearing animals [204–205].

REFERENCES

1. Roitt, I. *Essential Immunology* (2nd ed.) London: Blackwell, 1974.
2. Kawerau, E., and Ott, H. The soluble proteins of the cornea. *Exp. Eye Res.* 1:134, 1961.
3. Berger, B. Agarose gel electrophoresis of proteins from bovine corneal epithelium. *Acta Ophthalmol.* 47:1026, 1969.
4. Berger, B. Immunoelectrophoresis of extracts from bovine epithelium using antisera specific to individual protein fractions. *Acta Ophthalmol.* 49:685, 1971.
5. Berger, B. A new micromethod for the extraction of tissue protein by ultracentrifugation. *Int. J. Pept. Protein Res.* 2:133, 1970.
6. Nelken, D., and Nelken, E. The serological specificity of the cornea. *Immunology* 5:595, 1962.
7. Nakanishi, S. Studies of corneal antigenicity on the transplantation of a cornea heterograft. *Acta Soc. Ophthalmol. Jpn.* 67:463, 1963.
8. Remky, H. Immunology of keratoplasty. *Int. Ophthalmol. Clin.* 3:559, 1963.
9. Hall, J. M., Smolin, G., and Wilson, F. M., II. Soluble antigens of the bovine cornea. *Invest. Ophthalmol.* 13:304, 1974.
10. Allansmith, M. R., et al. Immunoglobulins in the human eye. *Arch. Ophthalmol.* 89:36, 1973.
11. Allansmith, M. R., and McClellan, B. H. Immunoglobulins in the human cornea. *Am. J. Ophthalmol.* 80:123, 1975.
12. Sapse, A. T., et al. Proteins in human tears. *Arch Ophthalmol.* 81:815, 1969.
13. Holt, W. S., and Kinoshita, J. H. The soluble proteins of the bovine cornea. *Invest. Ophthalmol.* 12:114, 1973.
14. Nelken, E., and Nelken, D. Serological studies in keratoplasty. *Br. J. Ophthalmol.* 49:159, 1965.
15. Stocker, F. W. Soluble Antigens and Isoantibodies. In P. V. Rycroft (Ed.), *Corneoplastic Surgery.* London: Pergamon, 1969, p. 151.
16. Rapaport, F. T. Role of streptococcal and other heterologous antigens in transplantation. *Transplant. Proc.* 2:447, 1970.
17. Nelken, E., et al. Late clouding of experimental corneal grafts. *Arch. Ophthalmol.* 65:584, 1961.
18. Nelken, E., et al. Studies on antigens in the human cornea and their relationship to corneal grafting in man. *J. Lab. Clin. Med.* 49:745, 1957.
19. Foster, C. S., and Allansmith, M. R. Lack of blood group antigen A on human corneal endothelium. *Am. J. Ophthalmol.* 87:165, 1979.
20. Salisbury, J. D., and Gebhardt, B. M. Blood group antigens on human corneal cells demonstrated by immunoperoxidase staining. *Am. J. Ophthalmol.* 91:46, 1981.
21. Allansmith, M. R., Drell, D. W., Kajiyama, G., and Fine, M. ABO blood groups and corneal transplantation. *Am. J. Ophthalmol.* 79:493, 1975.
22. Batchelor, J. R., et al. HLA matching and corneal grafting. *Lancet* 2:551, 1976.
23. Van Rood, J. J., Eernisse, J. G., and Van Leeuwen, A. Leukocyte antibodies in sera from pregnant women. *Nature* 181:1735, 1958.
24. Payne, R., and Rolfs, M. R. Fetomaternal leukocyte incompatibility. *J. Clin. Invest.* 37:1756, 1958.
25. Schaller, J. G., and Omenn, G. S. The histocompatibility system and human disease. *J. Pediatr.* 88:913, 1976.
26. Thorsby, E. The human major histocompatibility system. *Transplant. Rev.* 18:51, 1974.

27. Snell, G. D., Cherry, M., and Demant, P. H-2: Its structure and similarity to HL-A. *Transplant. Rev.* 15:1, 1973.
28. Benacerraf, B., and McDevitt, H. O. Histocompatibility linked immune genes. *Science* 175:273, 1972.
29. Glasser, D. L., and Silvers, W. K. Genetic determinants of immunological responsiveness. *Immunology* 18:1, 1974.
30. Report of Meeting of Sixth International Histocompatibility Testing Workshop, 1975. In F. Kissmeyer-Nielsen (Ed.), *Histocompatibility Testing.* Copenhagen: Ejnar Munksgaard, 1975.
31. Gibofsky, A., et al. The identification of HL-A antigens on fresh and cultured human endothelial cells. *J. Immunol.* 115:730, 1975.
32. Newsome, D. A., et al. Human corneal cells *in vitro:* Morphology and histocompatibility antigens of pure cell populations. *Invest. Ophthalmol.* 13:23, 1974.
33. Whitsett, C. F., and Stulting, R. D. The distribution of HLA antigens on human corneal tissue. *Invest. Ophthalmol. Vis. Sci.* 25:519, 1984.
34. Treseler, P. A., Foulks, G. N., and Sanfilippo, F. The expression of HLA antigens by cells in the human cornea. *Am. J. Ophthalmol.* 98:763, 1984.
35. Mayer, D. J., Daar, A. S., Casey, T. A., Fabre, J. W. Localization of HLA-A, B, C and HLA-DR antigens in the human cornea. *Transplant. Proc.* 15:126, 1983.
36. Young, E., Stark, W. J., Prendergast, R. A. Immunology of corneal rejection. *Invest. Ophthalmol. Vis. Sci.* 26:571–575, 1985.
37. Smolin, G., and Hyndiuk, R. A. Lymphatic drainage from vascularized rabbit cornea. *Am. J. Ophthalmol.* 72:147, 1971.
38. Collin, H. B. Lymphatic drainage of I^{131}-albumin from the vascularized cornea. *Invest. Ophthalmol.* 9:146, 1970.
39. Medawar, P. B. The homograft reaction. *Proc. R. Soc. Lond. (Biol.)* 149:145, 1958.
40. Strober, S., and Gowans, J. L. The role of lymphocytes in the sensitization of rats to renal homografts. *J. Exp. Med.* 122:347, 1965.
41. Elkins, W. L., and Guttman, R. D. Pathogenesis of a local graft versus host reaction: Immunogenicity of circulating host leukocytes. *Science* 159:1250, 1968.
42. Steinmuller, D. Immunization with skin isografts from allogeneic mouse radiation chimeras. *Exp. Hematol.* 15:39, 1968.
43. Lafferty, K. J., and Simeonovic, C. J. Immunology of graft rejection. *Transplant. Proc.* 16:927, 1984.
44. Rubsamen, P. E., McCulley, J., Bergstresser, P. R., and Streilein, J. W. On the Ia immunogenicity of mouse corneal allografts infiltrated with Langerhans' cells. *Invest. Ophthalmol. Vis. Sci.* 25:573, 1984.
45. Chandler, J. W. Pathophysiology of graft failure. *Cornea* 1:281, 1982.
46. Rahi, A. H. S., and Garner, A. *Immunopathology of the Eye.* London: Blackwell, 1976, p. 136.
47. Dyminski, J. W., and Argyris, B. F. *In vitro* sensitization to transplantation antigens. *Cell. Immunol.* 7:198, 1973.
48. Ugrinski, P. S., and Kirkpatrick, C. H. Corneal cellular immunity in the guinea pig. *Am. J. Pathol.* 74:365, 1974.
49. Tagawa, Y., Silverstein, A. M., and Prendergast, R. A. Mechanisms of allograft rejection of corneal endothelium. *Invest. Ophthalmol. Vis. Sci.* 23:32, 1982.

50. Sher, N. A., et al. Macrophage migration inhibition factor activity in the aqueous during experimental corneal xenograft and allograft rejection. *Am. J. Ophthalmol.* 82:858, 1976.
51. Henley, W. L., and Leopold, I. H. Cellular immunity and leukocyte migration inhibition. *Ophthalmol. Digest* 11:812, 1976.
52. Billingham, R. E., Silvers, W. K., and Wilson, D. B. Further studies on adoptive transfer of sensitivity to skin homografts. *J. Exp. Med.* 118:397, 1963.
53. Gowans, J. L., and Uhr, J. W. The carriage of immunological memory by small lymphocytes in the rat. *J. Exp. Med.* 124:1017, 1966.
54. Prendergast, R. A. Cellular changes in the homograft reaction. *J. Exp. Med.* 119:377, 1964.
55. Stastny, P. Bound immunoglobulin and complement in heart allografts undergoing rejection. *Transplantation* 10:248, 1970.
56. Rosenau, W. Interaction of lymphoid cells with target cells in tissue culture. In D. B. Amos and H. Koproski (Eds.), *Cell Bound Antibodies*. Philadelphia: Wistar Institute, 1963, p. 75.
57. Wilson, D. B., and Billingham, R. E. Lymphocytes and transplantation immunity. *Adv. Immunol.* 7:189, 1967.
58. Stark, W. J., et al. Sensitization to human lymphocyte antigens by corneal transplantation. *Invest. Ophthalmol.* 12:639, 1973.
59. Grunnet, N., et al. Occurrence of lymphocytotoxic lymphocytes and antibodies after corneal transplantation. *Acta Ophthalmol.* 54:167, 1976.
60. Mittal, K. K., et al. Lymphocytotoxic antibody response to cardiac allotransplantation in man. *J. Immunol.* 104:1427, 1970.
61. Nelken, E., and Nelken, D. Serological studies in keratoplasty. *Br. J. Ophthalmol.* 49:159, 1965.
62. D'Ermo, F., Lanzieri, M., and Secchi, A. G. Anti-corneal antibodies in rabbits after homologous and heterologous corneal grafts. *Acta Ophthalmol.* 44:233, 1966.
63. Binder, P. S., Chandler, J. W., and Kaufman, H. E. *In vitro* demonstration of cytotoxic antibodies and their possible role in corneal graft rejection. *Invest. Ophthalmol.* 15:481, 1976.
64. Ehlers, N., Olsen, T., Johnsen, H. E. Corneal graft rejection probably mediated by antibodies. *Acta Ophthalmol.* 59:119, 1981.
65. Ciba Foundation Symposium. *Corneal Graft Failure*. Amsterdam: Associated Scientific Publishers, 1973.
66. Perey, D. H. E., and Dupuy, J. M. L. Role of afferent lymphatics and lymph nodes during sensitization and effect on mechanisms of cellular immunity in birds and mammals. *Transplantation* 3:321, 1970.
67. Billingham, R. E., and Silvers, W. B. Studies on the cheek pouch skin homografts in the Syrian hamster. In Ciba Foundation Symposium, *Transplantation*. London: Churchill, 1962, p. 90.
68. Lance, E. M. A functional and morphologic study of intracranial thyroid allografts in the dog. *Surg. Gynecol. Obstet.* 125:529, 1967.
69. Lambert, P. B., et al. The role of lymph trunks in the response to allogeneic skin transplants. *Transplantation* 3:62, 1965.
70. Barker, C. F., and Billingham, R. E. The role of regional lymphatics in the skin homograft response. *Transplantation* 5:962, 1967.
71. Jasani, M. K., and Lewis, G. P. Lymph flow and biochemical composition during homograft rejection. *J. Physiol.* 207:70, 1970.
72. Mitchison, N. A. Passive transfer of transplantation immunity. *Proc. R. Soc. Lond. (Biol.)* 142:72, 1954.

73. Smolin, G., Hall, J. M., and Stein, M. The afferent arc of the corneal immunologic reaction. *Can. J. Ophthalmol.* 7:336, 1972.
74. Smolin, G., and Hall, J. M. Afferent arc of the corneal immunologic reaction. *Arch. Ophthalmol.* 90:231, 1973.
75. Cherry, P. M. H., et al. An analysis of corneal transplantation. *Ann. Ophthalmol.* 11:461, 1979.
76. Khodadoust, A. A., and Silverstein, A. M. Studies on the nature of the privilege enjoyed by corneal allografts. *Invest. Ophthalmol.* 11:137, 1972.
77. Maumenee, A. E. The influence of donor recipient sensitization on corneal grafts. *Am. J. Ophthalmol.* 34:142, 1951.
78. Basu, P. K., and Ormsby, H. L. Studies of immunity with interlamellar corneal homografts in rabbits. *Am. J. Ophthalmol.* 44:598, 1957.
79. Millin, J. A., Boruchoff, S. A., and Kell, P. T-cell subsets following penetrating keratoplasty. *Invest. Ophthalmol. Vis. Sci.* [Suppl.] 24:298, 1983.
80. Young, E., and Stark, W. J. Immunology of corneal allograft rejection. *Ophthalmol.* 92:223, 1985.
81. Silverstein, A. M., Khodadoust, A. A., and Prendergast, R. A. Desquamation of corneal endothelial cells. *Invest. Ophthalmol. Vis. Sci.* 22:351, 1982.
82. Donshik, P. C., Cavanagh, H. D., Boruchoff, S. A., and Dohlman, C. H. Effect of bilateral and unilateral grafts on the incidence of rejections in keratoconus. *Am. J. Ophthalmol.* 87:823, 1979.
83. Malbran, E. S., and Fernandez-Meijide, R. E. Bilateral versus unilateral penetrating graft in keratoconus. *Trans. Am. Acad. Ophthalmol.* 89:38, 1982.
84. Buxton, N., Schurman, M., and Pecego, J. Graft reactions after unilateral and bilateral keratoplasty for keratoconus. *Trans. Am. Acad. Ophthalmol.* 88:771, 1981.
85. Volker-Dieben, H. J., Kok-Van Alphen, C. C., Lansberger, Q., and Persijn, G. G. Different influences on corneal graft survival in 539 transplants. *Acta Ophthalmol.* 60:190, 1982.
86. Volker-Dieben, H. J., Kok-Van Alphen, C. C., Lansberger, Q., and Persijn, G. G. The effect of prospective HLA-A and -B matching on corneal graft survival. *Acta Ophthalmol.* 60:203, 1982.
87. Vannas, S., Karjalainen, P., Ruusuvaara, A., and Tilikainen, A. HLA compatible donor for prevention of allograft reaction. *Albrecht von Graefes Arch. Klin. Ophthalmol.* 198:217, 1976.
88. Billingham, R. E., and Boswell, T. Studies on the problem of corneal homografts. *Proc. R. Soc. Lond. (Biol.)* 141:392, 1953.
89. Stickel, D. L., et al. Immunogenetics of consanguineous allografts in man. *Am. Surg.* 172:160, 1970.
90. Agarwal, L. P., Gupta, A. K., and Mohan, M. Heterogenous keratoplasty. *Orient. Arch. Ophthalmol.* 116:277, 1963.
91. Tuberville, A. W., Foster, C. S., and Wood, T. O. The effect of donor cornea epithelium removal on the incidence of allograft rejection reactions. *Trans. Am. Acad. Ophthalmol.* 90:1351, 1983.
92. Demong, T., Polack, F. M., and Yamaguchi, T. Graft rejection in interracial corneal transplantation. Presented at Eye Bank Association of America, Chicago, Ill., 1980.
93. Polack, F., et al. Immune host response to corneal grafts sensitized to herpes simplex virus. *Invest. Ophthalmol.* 15:188, 1976.
94. Henley, W. L., Shore, B., and Leopold, I. H. Inhibition of leucocyte migration by corneal antigen in chronic viral keratitis. *Natl. New Biol.* 233:115, 1971.

95. Henley, W. L., Okas, S., and Leopold, I. H. Clinical experiments in cellular immunity in eye disease. *Invest. Ophthalmol.* 12:520, 1973.
96. Smolin, G. Corneal homograft reaction following subconjunctival antilymphocyte serum. *Am. J. Ophthalmol.* 67:137, 1969.
97. Smolin, G. Suppression of corneal graft reaction by antilymphocyte serum. *Arch. Ophthalmol.* 79:603, 1968.
98. Khodadoust, A. A., and Silverstein, A. M. The survival and rejection of epithelium in experimental corneal transplants. *Invest. Ophthalmol.* 8:169, 1969.
99. Polack, F. M. Corneal graft rejection. *Ocular Inflammation Ther.* 1:27, 1983.
100. Alldredge, O. C., and Krachmer, J. H. Clinical types of corneal transplant rejection. *Arch. Ophthalmol.* 99:599, 1981.
101. Krachmer, J. H., and Alldredge, O. C. Subepithelial infiltrates. *Arch. Ophthalmol.* 96:2234, 1978.
102. Silverstein, A. M., Rossman, A. M., and DeLeon, A. S. Survival of donor epithelium in experimental corneal xenografts. *Am. J. Ophthalmol.* 69:448, 1970.
103. Polack, R. M., Smelser, G. K., and Rose, J. Long-term survival of isotopically labelled stromal and endothelial cells in corneal homografts. *Am. J. Ophthalmol.* 57:67, 1964.
104. D'Amico, R. A., Chaunico, R., and Castroviejo, R. Suppression of the immune response to corneal xenografts. *Transplant. Proc.* 1:256, 1969.
105. Polack, F. M. Scanning electron microscopy of corneal graft reaction: Epithelial reaction, endothelial rejection, and formation of posterior graft membranes. *Invest. Ophthalmol.* 11:1, 1972.
106. Kanai, A., and Polack, F. M. Ultramicroscopic changes in the corneal graft stroma during early rejection. *Invest. Ophthalmol.* 10:415, 1971.
107. Inomata, H., Smelser, G. K., and Polack, F. M. The fine structural changes in the corneal endothelium during graft rejection. *Invest. Ophthalmol.* 9:263, 1970.
108. Polack, F. M. Scanning electron microscopy of the host-graft endothelial junction in corneal graft reaction. *Am. J. Ophthalmol.* 73:704, 1972.
109. Inomata, H., Smelser, G. K., and Polack, F. M. Fine structure of regenerating endothelium and Descemet's membrane in normal and rejecting corneal grafts. *Am. J. Ophthalmol.* 70:48, 1970.
110. Hirst, L. W., and Stark, W. J. Clinical specular microscopy of corneal endothelial rejection. *Arch. Ophthalmol.* 101:387, 1983.
111. Krachmer, J. H., Schnitzer, J. L., and Fratkin, J. Cornea pseudoguttata. *Arch. Ophthalmol.* 99:1377, 1981.
112. Norm, M. S. Quantitative study of conjunctival cytology in relation to corneal grafting. *Acta Ophthalmol.* 59:810, 1981.
113. Khodadoust, A. A., and Silverstein, A. M. Introduction of corneal graft rejection by passive cell transfer. *Invest. Ophthalmol.* 15:89, 1976.
114. Michels, R. G., Kenyon, K. R., and Maumenee, A. E. Retrocorneal fibrous membrane. *Invest. Ophthalmol.* 11:822, 1972.
114a. Elliott, J. Personal communication, 1975.
115. Moore, T. E., and Aronson, S. B. Suture reaction in the human cornea. *Arch. Ophthalmol.* 82:575, 1969.
115a. Rao, G. N., et al. Results of keratoprosthesis. *Am. J. Ophthalmol.* 88:190, 1979.
115b. Polack, F. M., and Heimke, G. Ceramic keratoprostheses. *Ophthalmology* 87:693, 1980.

116. Kalaue, P., and Jolley, W. B. Prolongation of rabbit skin allograft survival following treatment of the skin with electrophoresis prior to transplantation. *Transplantation* 11:30, 1971.
117. Hall, J. M., et al. Changes in the antigenic composition of cultured bovine corneas. *Invest. Ophthalmol.* 14:295, 1975.
118. Stocker, F. W. Preservation of donor cornea in autologous serum prior to penetrating grafts. *Am. J. Ophthalmol.* 60:21, 1965.
119. Barkin, M., Hambly, E. J., and Dimitriu, D. Prolongation of skin graft survival by donor treatment (donor enhancement). *Transplantation* 13:18, 1972.
120. Smolin, G., and Hyndiuk, R. A. Suppression of corneal graft reaction by antilymphocyte serum. *Arch. Ophthalmol.* 85:451, 1971.
121. Binder, P. S., et al. Immunologic protection of rabbit corneal allografts with heterologous blocking antibody. *Am. J. Ophthalmol.* 79:949, 1975.
122. Chandler, J. W. Immunologic protection of rabbit and allograft. *Invest. Ophthalmol.* 15:213, 1976.
123. Chandler, J. W., et al. Immunologic protection of rabbit corneal allografts. *Transplantation* 17:146, 1974.
124. Binder, P. S., et al. Immunologic protection of rabbit corneal allografts with heterologous blocking antibody. *Am. J. Ophthalmol.* 79:949, 1975.
125. Bourne, W. M. Antigenicity of cryopreserved corneas. *Arch. Ophthalmol.* 93:215, 1975.
126. Brightbill, F. S., and Kaufman, H. E. Paired donor eyes in penetrating keratoplasty. *Ann. Ophthalmol.* 5:161, 1973.
127. Watanabe, S., and Tsutsui, J. Immunochemical alteration of proteins in lyophilized corneal heterografts. *Arch. Ophthalmol.* 67:48, 1962.
128. Strober, S. Strategies promoting allograft acceptance. *Fed. Proc.* 43:261, 1984.
129. Claman, H. N. Corticosteroids and lymphoid cells. *N. Engl. J. Med.* 8:388, 1972.
130. Polack, F. M. Lymphocyte destruction during corneal homograft reactions. *Arch. Ophthalmol.* 89:413, 1973.
131. Meyer, R. F., et al. Effect of local corticosteroids on antibody-forming cells in the eye and draining lymph nodes. *Invest. Ophthalmol.* 14:138, 1975.
132. Kupferman, A., et al. Topically applied steroids in corneal disease. *Arch. Ophthalmol.* 91:373, 1974.
133. Wilhelmus, K. R., Hunter, P. A., and Rice, N. S. C. Equivalence of topical clobetasone and dexamethasone in experimental corneal allograft rejection. *Br. J. Ophthalmol.* 65:699, 1981.
134. Friedman, E. Methylprednisolone therapy and allograft rejection. *Transplantation* 10:552, 1970.
135. Sugar, A., et al. Alternate day versus daily systemic corticosteroids in corneal homograft rejection. *Am. J. Ophthalmol.* 75:486, 1973.
136. Dale, D. C., Fauci, A. S., and Wolff, S. M. Alternate-day prednisone. *N. Engl. J. Med.* 291:1154, 1974.
137. Payrau, P., and Schillinger, G. Action du pyridinolcarbamate sur la réaction de réjét des gréffes de cornée et de peau. *Ann. d'Oculistique* 207:115, 1974.
138. Brambilla, G., et al. The immunosuppressive activity of n-diazoacetylglycine amide in some transplantation systems. *Transplantation* 10:100, 1970.
139. Cleasby, G. W., Webster, R. G., and Vincent, N. J. Modification of the homograft reaction in corneal transplantation. *Arch. Ophthalmol.* 76:282, 1966.
140. Floersheim, G. L. Treatment of hyperacute graft versus host disease in mice with cytosine arabinoside. *Transplantation* 14:325, 1972.

141. Gray, G. D., and Mickelson, M. M. The immunosuppressive effects of adamantoyl cytarabine. *Transplantation* 9:177, 1970.
142. Gillette, R. W., Findley, A., and Conway, H. Prolonged survival of homografts in mice treated with EACA. *Transplantation* 1:116, 1963.
143. Lueker, R. D., Ono, K., and Lueker, D. C. Superiority of antithymus serum to antilymphocyte serum in prolonging cardiac homograft survival. *Proc. Soc. Exp. Biol. Med.* 137:139, 1971.
144. Rapaport, F. T., Shimada, T., and Watanabe, K. Prolongation of canine renal allograft survival by L-asparginase. *Transplantation* 12:217, 1971.
145. Wilson, F. M., II, et al. The effect of oxisuran, a selective inhibitor of cellular immunity, on the rejection of bovine corneal xenografts in rabbits. *Ann. Ophthalmol.* 10:283, 1978.
146. Andrus, L., and Lafferty, K. J. Inhibition of T cell activity by cyclosporin A. *Scand. J. Immunol.* 15:449, 1982.
147. Armerding, D., Scriba, M., Kirchner, H., et al. Modulation by cyclosporin-A of murine natural resistance against herpes simplex virus infection. *Antiviral Res.* 2:13, 1982.
148. Shepherd, W. F., et al. Effect of cyclosporin A on the survival of corneal grafts in rabbits. *Br. J. Ophthalmol.* 64:148, 1982.
149. Bell, T. A. G., Easty, D. L., and McCullogh, K. G. A placebo-controlled blind trial of cyclosporin A in prevention of corneal graft rejection in rabbits. *Br. J. Ophthalmol.* 66:303, 1982.
150. Hunter, P. A., et al. Corneal graft rejection. *Br. J. Ophthalmol.* 66:292, 1982.
151. Coster, D. J. Personal communication, 1984.
152. Kana, J. S., et al. Rabbit corneal allograft survival following topical administration of cyclosporin A. *Invest. Ophthalmol. Vis. Sci.* 22:686, 1982.
153. Salisbury, J. D., and Gebhardt, B. M. Suppression of corneal allograft rejection by cyclosporin A. *Arch. Ophthalmol.* 99:1640, 1981.
154. Hopf, U., et al. Serologische Unteruchungen an Patienten unter Behandlung mit xenogenen Antilymphocytenglobulin. *Klin. Wochenscher.* 48:906, 1970.
155. Leibowitz, H. M., and Elliot, J. H. Corneal grafts. *Arch. Ophthalmol.* 75:826, 1966.
156. Elliot, J. H., and Leibowitz, H. M. Chemotherapeutic immunosuppression of the corneal graft reaction. *Arch. Ophthalmol.* 76:709, 1966.
157. Hall, J. M., Ohno, S., and Pribnow, J. F. The effect of cyclophosphamide on an ocular immune response. *Clin. Exp. Immunol.* 30:309, 1977.
158. Smolin, G., and Wilson, F. M., II. Antilymphocyte serum: A review of general and ophthalmic aspects. *Surv. Ophthalmol.* 18:200, 1973.
159. Alberth, B., and Leovey, A. Immunosuppression with antihuman antilymphocyte globulin in cases of keratoplasty. *Szemszet.* 108:81, 1971.
160. Shehadeh, H., Guttman, R. D., Lindquist, R. R., and Rodriguez-Erdmann, F. Renal transplantation in the inbred rat. *Transplantation* 10:75, 1970.
161. Simpson, K. M., et al. Humoral antibodies and coagulation mechanism in the accelerated or hyperacute rejection of renal homografts in sensitized canine recipients. *Surgery* 68:77, 1970.
162. Rosenberg, E. B., et al. Prolonged skin allograft survival in mice pretreated with soluble transplantation antigens. *Transplantation* 12:492, 1971.
163. Hilgert, P., Vlachov, K., and Viklicky, V. A study of the mechanism of skin allograft tolerance induced by cell-free tissue extracts. *Transplantation* 18:471, 1974.

164. Dietrich, F. M., and Weigle, W. O. Immunologic unresponsiveness to heterologous serum proteins induced in adult mice and transfer of the unresponsive state. *Transplantation* 12:492, 1971.
165. Liacopoulis, P., Bui-Mong-hung, and Dinoeva, S. Transplantation tolerance following transfer of donor spleen cells in adult animals. *Int. Arch. Allergy Appl. Immunol.* 41:101, 1971.
166. Stuart, F. P., et al. Presence of both cell-mediated immunity and serum-blocking factors in rat renal allografts enhanced by passive immunization. *Transplantation* 12:331, 1971.
167. Batchelor, J. R., et al. Immunological enhancement of human kidney graft. *Lancet* 2:1007, 1970.
168. French, M. E., and Batchelor, J. R. Immunological enhancement of rat kidney grafts. *Lancet* 2:1103, 1969.
169. Editorial: Alternatives to immunosuppressive therapy. *J.A.M.A.* 215:1238, 1971.
170. Podos, S., and Becker, B. Comparison of ocular prostaglandin synthesis inhibitors. *Invest. Ophthalmol.* 15:841, 1976.
171. Bourne, H. R., et al. Modulation of inflammation and immunity by cyclic AMP. *Science* 184:19, 1974.
172. Strom, T. B., and Carpenter, C. B. Prostaglandin as an effective anti-rejection therapy in rat renal allograft recipients. *Transplantation* 35:279, 1983.
173. Stark, W. J., Taylor, H. R., Bias, W. B., and Maumenee, A. E. Histocompatibility antigens and keratoplasty. *Am. J. Ophthalmol.* 86:595, 1978.
174. Cosimi, A. B., et al. Use of monoclonal antibodies to T-cell subsets for immunologic monitoring and treatment in recipients of renal allografts. *N. Engl. J. Med.* 305:308, 1981.
175. Baum, J. Late spontaneous clearing of corneal grafts. *Arch. Ophthalmol.* 95:1538, 1977.
176. Laing, R. A., et al. Evidence for mitosis in the adult corneal endothelium. *Trans. Am. Acad. Ophthalmol.* 91:1129, 1984.
177. Grabner, B., Luger, T. A., Smolin, G., and Oppenheim, J. J. Corneal epithelial-cell-derived thymocyte-activating factor. *Invest. Ophthalmol. Vis. Sci.* 23:751, 1982.
178. LeFrancois, M., and Baum, J. Flavobacterium endophthalmitis following keratoplasty. *Arch. Ophthalmol.* 94:1907, 1976.
179. Benezra, D., and Sachs, U. Growth and transplantation of organ-cultured cornea. *Invest. Ophthalmol.* 14:24, 1976.
180. Mendelson, L. M., Meltzer, E. O., and Hamburger, R. M. Anaphylaxis-like reaction to corticosteroid therapy. *J. Allergy Clin. Immunol.* 54:125, 1974.
181. Smolin, G. Medrysone hypersensitivity. *Arch. Ophthalmol.* 85:478, 1971.
182. Koranda, F. C., et al. Cutaneous complications in immunosuppressed renal homograft recipients. *J.A.M.A.* 229:419, 1974.
183. Ley, A. Experimental fungus infections of the cornea. *Am. J. Ophthalmol.* 42:59, 1956.
184. Kimura, S. J., and Okumoto, M. The effect of corticosteroids on experimental herpes simplex keratoconjunctivitis in the rabbit. *Am. J. Ophthalmol.* 43:131, 1957.
185. Smolin, G., and Okumoto, M. Potentiation of *Candida albicans* keratitis by antilymphocyte serum and corticosteroids. *Am. J. Ophthalmol.* 68:675, 1969.
186. Armstrong, D., et al. Cytomegalovirus infections with uremia following renal transplantation. *Arch. Intern. Med.* 127:111, 1971.

187. Penn, I., and Starzl, T. E. Malignant tumors arising de nova in immunosuppressed organ transplant recipient. *Transplantation* 14:407, 1972.
188. Simmons, R. L., et al. Cure of dysgerminoma with widespread metastases appearing after renal transplantation. *N. Engl. J. Med.* 283:190, 1970.
189. Havener, W. H. *Ocular Pharmacology.* St. Louis: Mosby, 1966.
190. Aquavella, J. V., Gasset, A. R., and Dohlman, C. H. Corticosteroids in corneal wound healing. *Am. J. Ophthalmol.* 58:621, 1964.
191. Sanchez, J., and Polack, F. M. Effects of topical steroids on the healing of corneal endothelium. *Invest. Ophthalmol.* 13:17, 1974.
192. Lorenzetti, D. W. C., et al. Subconjunctival corticosteroids. *Can. J. Ophthalmol.* 7:42, 1972.
193. Gasset, A. R., and Dohlman, C. H. The tensile strength of corneal wounds. *Arch. Ophthalmol.* 70:595, 1968.
194. O'Connor, G. R. Periocular corticosteroid injection: Uses and abuses. *Eye Ear Nose Throat Mon.* 55:26, 1976.
195. Schlaegel, T. F., Jr., and Wilson, F. M. Accidental intraocular injection of depot corticosteroids. *Trans. Am. Acad. Ophthalmol. Otolaryngol.* 78:847, 1974.
196. DeMeester, T. R., and Anderson, N. D. The potential bone marrow toxicity of antilymphocyte serum in mice. *J. Surg. Res.* 8:192, 1968.
197. Sell, S. Antilymphocytic antibody: Effects in experimental animals and problems in human use. *Ann. Intern. Med.* 71:177, 1969.
198. Rifkind, D., et al. Systemic fungal infections complicating renal transplantation and immunosuppressive therapy. *Am. J. Med.* 43:28, 1967.
199. Adamson, D. M., and Cozad, G. G. Effect of antilymphocyte serum on animals experimentally infected with *Histoplasma capsulatum* or *Cryptococcus neoformans. J. Bacteriol.* 100:1271, 1969.
200. Edelman, R., and Wheelock, E. F. Enhancement of replication of vesicular stomatitis virus in human lymphocyte cultures. *Lancet* 1:771, 1968.
201. Poste, G. Increased growth of viruses in lymphocytes treated with heterologous antilymphocyte serum. *Transplantation* 10:106, 1970.
202. Rolland, J. M., and Nairn, R. C. Antilymphocyte serum. *Pathology* 4:85, 1972.
203. Lewis, J. L., Jr., Davis, D. C., and Parker, J. T. Modification of immunologic response to human choriocarcinoma in the hamster cheek pouch. *Cancer Res.* 29:1988, 1969.
204. Deodhar, S. D., and Crile, G., Jr. Enhancement of metastases by antilymphocyte serum in allogeneic murine tumor system. *Cancer Res.* 29:776, 1969.
205. Fisher, J. C., and Mannick, J. A. The effect of antilymphocyte serum on the recognition of tumor-specific transplantation antigens. *Proc. Soc. Exp. Biol. Med.* 134:703, 1970.

7 IMMUNOLOGIC DISEASES AFFECTING THE UVEAL TRACT AND RETINA

Many systemic diseases of immunologic origin have been found to affect the uveal tract and retina as opposed to the external structures of the eye.

SERUM SICKNESS

Serum sickness is the prototype of immune complex disease. It stems from the formation of antigen-antibody complexes in the bloodstream of individuals who have received significant doses of heterologous serum proteins such as horse antisera. These complexes circulate as soluble molecular combinations, particularly when antigen is present in excess. They cause pathologic changes when they become localized in blood vessel walls and bind complement. Such antigen-antibody-complement combinations are highly chemotactic to polymorphonuclear leukocytes that enter the sites of immune complex deposition and, in the act of phagocytizing these complexes, release lytic enzymes [1]. The latter may cause necrosis of both the vessel wall and the surrounding tissues. Vessel damage causes leakage of serous fluid into the affected tissues, and deposition of fibrinogen may also occur, leading ultimately to fibrin formation (clotting). If only a single dose of serum protein has been given, the process may resolve spontaneously after the antigen-antibody complexes have been phagocytized and satisfactorily disposed of. If the antigen is administered repeatedly, however, chronic disease may be established in certain target organs (e.g., the kidney).

PATHOGENESIS. It is believed that changes in the permeability of the vascular endothelium are initiated by an IgE-mediated release of vasoactive amines from circulating basophils [2] or choroidal mast cells [3], although vasoactive factors released from platelets may also play a role. In any case, there appears to be an element of the type I reaction even

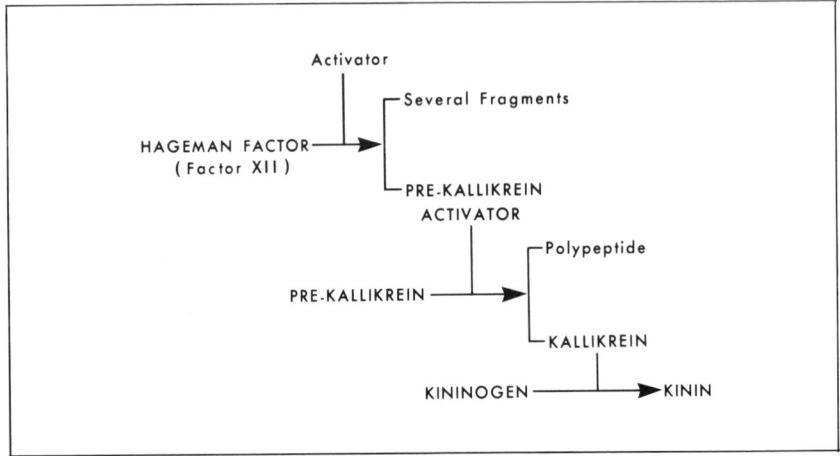

FIG. 7-1 Scheme of kinin formation. (From G. R. O'Connor: Basic mechanisms responsible for the initiation and perpetuation of anterior segment inflammation. *Trans. Am. Acad. Ophthalmol. Otolaryngol.* 79: 56, 1975. Reproduced by permission.)

in classic type III disease. Once small openings have been created in the endothelium of the postcapillary venules by these vasoactive amines, circulating immune complexes can gain access to the subendothelial layer of the vessel wall, and this area is where the major pathologic changes are observed.

Antigen-antibody complexes also activate Hageman factor in the blood, and the result may be clot formation with the appearance of thrombi in certain small vessels of the body. The breakdown products of Hageman factor may precipitate the activation of the kinin system, as indicated in Figure 7-1, and minute quantities of these kinins, the prototype of which is bradykinin, can cause considerable vasodilation and edema. A second source of clot formation is platelet aggregation, the latter being initiated by contact with immune complexes in the circulation.

The signs and symptoms of serum sickness may begin to appear 3 days to 3 weeks after the patient has received an injection of heterologous serum. The complaints generally include malaise, fever, hives, joint pains, and swollen lymph nodes. The signs of iritis may appear as long as 1 month after the original injection of heterologous serum. In the classic case described by Theodore and Lewson [4], photophobia and blurred vision occurred in association with a second bout of serum sickness, 22 days after the initial attack of fever, urticaria, and generalized lymphadenopathy. Their patient, a 40-year-old male, had received 80,000 units of horse antipneumococcal serum intravenously for treatment of a pneumococcal pneumonia. His initial attack of serum sickness occurred 9 days after administration of the serum, his second 22 days later. This cyclic recurrence of disease suggested that sufficient residual antigen was present in the tissues to provoke a second wave of antibody formation.

The patient described by Theodore and Lewson [4] showed marked hyperemia of the conjunctival vessels, perilimbal injection, fine keratic precipitates, and a fibrinous reaction in the anterior chamber. There was no involvement of the posterior segment, and the uveitis cleared spontaneously with no residue. In their description of the case, Theodore and Lewson referred to the early animal experiments of Iga [5], who found that even single intravenous injections of horse serum into rabbits could produce diffuse or nodular infiltrations of the uvea of both eyes, particularly in the region of the choriocapillaris. A transient plastic iritis was also observed in his animals. Iga's work was subsequently confirmed and amplified by Wong et al. [6] who properly identified the uveitis as an immune complex disease and showed a distinct parallelism between the severity of the uveitis observed and the severity of a simultaneously produced glomerulonephritis.

Serum sickness has now become much less of a problem since better alternatives for the prevention and treatment of certain serious infectious diseases have become available. In the modern era some difficulties with this disease have again arisen in connection with the use of antilymphocyte serum to retard the rejection of transplanted organs [7]. Because serious serum sickness inevitably develops when heterologous serum proteins are administered in any form, this therapy has now generally been abandoned.

Elements of serum sickness are still seen in connection with penicillin therapy and in association with certain prolonged bacteremias and bacterial toxemias. Under these circumstances sufficient antigen may be present in the circulation to allow for the intravascular formation of antigen-antibody complexes in antigen excess, and this action is the key to the production of serum sickness.

TREATMENT. The primary treatment of serum sickness is to stop the administration of the offending antigen. In some cases, it can be determined in advance whether patients are hypersensitive to the antigen in question. Minute doses of the substance administered intradermally may produce a wheal-and-flare reaction within an hour, if anaphylactoid responsivity to the substance is present. This test is not a guarantee of freedom from serum sickness, however. In Theodore and Lewson's case [4], the patient failed to manifest dermal hypersensitivity to horse serum. The most that this form of testing can accomplish is to alert the physician to the possibility of sudden anaphylactoid responses in the early phases of treatment.

Treatment with systemic corticosteroids may effectively counter the acute reactions associated with serum sickness. This form of therapy is effective in reducing the joint swelling and urticaria from which these patients suffer. It is likely to be beneficial in the uveitis associated with serum sickness but has not been reliably evaluated.

SYSTEMIC LUPUS ERYTHEMATOSUS (SLE)

A classic collagen-vascular disease, systemic lupus erythematosus (SLE) has now been well characterized. It is without question an immune complex disease, the targeted antigens being the nucleoprotein(s) of the patient's own cells. While lupus patients may show reactivity against other autoantigens as well, there is no consistent pattern [8]. It appears that the disease represents an abnormal response on the part of B cells to signals that come from T lymphocytes. Such abnormal responses result in B-cell proliferation and the production of large amounts of immunoglobulins, mainly IgG. There also appears to be a shift toward autoantibody production to the detriment of more useful antibody formation. Although Gershon [9] indicated that a defect in the control of antibody formation by suppressor T cells might be highly important in the pathogenesis of lupus, such a defect could not have been confirmed in the experimental studies of Theofilopoulos et al. [10]. Moreover, these workers found evidence of excessive T-helper cell activity among lupus-prone mice, such as the MRL/1 strain, as well as an exaggerated response to lipopolysaccharide.

PATHOGENESIS. A fundamental T-cell abnormality is reflected in the fact that lupus patients also have defective delayed hypersensitivity responses [11] and are poorly defended against opportunistic pathogens such as herpes and *Candida*. The origin of the T-cell abnormality is unclear, although Del Giacco [12] has demonstrated the existence of anti-T-cell cytotoxic antibodies in the serum of lupus patients. These antibodies appear to be directed against membrane components of the T cell. In addition to these findings, Kaufman [13] has found a defect in natural killer (NK) cell activity among lupus patients; and this defect appears to be reversible, at least temporarily, when "immune response factor," a soluble mediator produced by concanavalin-A stimulated normal human lymphocytes, is administered. The parallelism between the T-cell deficiency of man and the T-cell deficiency of an excellent animal model of systemic lupus erythematosus, the NZB/NZW hybrid mouse, allows other statements to be made about the disease. First, it appears more than likely that there is a genetic susceptibility to the disease and that it may be influenced by sex hormones. Lupus is about nine times more common in women than in men [14]; the parallel disease that occurs in NZB/NZW mice is much worse in females than in males, but this situation may be altered by gonadectomy [15]. There is an increased prevalence of SLE in the families of patients with the disease [16], indicating a possible genetic predisposition. In this connection, it should be noted that Grumet et al. [17] found that SLE is associated with the HLA type A8 and W15, while this finding could not be confirmed by Statsny [18]. To complete the parallelism, NZB/NZW hybrids probably develop the disease on the basis of peculiarities of their HZ locus (histocompatibility locus). Both mice and man develop hemolytic anemias; both may develop associated Sjögren's syndrome; and both usually die of renal failure, associated with chronic glomerulonephritis.

In addition to Sjögren's syndrome, already discussed in Chapter 5, one

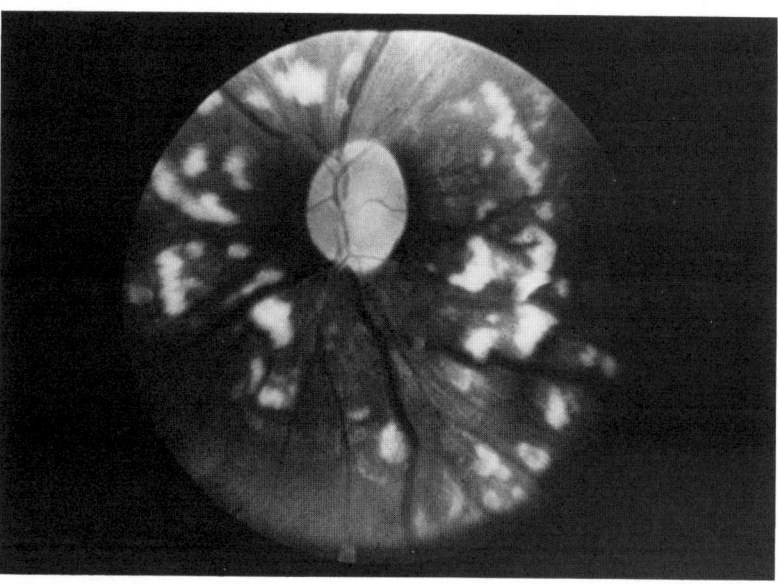

FIG. 7-2　　Fundus photograph showing multiple cotton-wool spots in a patient suffering from lupus erythematosus.

of the principal ocular manifestations of the disease is the development of cotton-wool patches in the retina (Fig. 7-2). This change is presumed to be due to the deposition of antigen-antibody complexes in capillaries supplying the nerve-fiber layer of the retina. Complement is bound in such lesions, and platelet thrombi form in the affected small vessels. It is assumed that the antigen in these complexes is free DNA, for this substance has been identified in lesions elsewhere in the tissues of individuals affected by the so-called fibrinoid necrosis of lupus [19]. Immune complexes have actually been demonstrated by immunofluorescent techniques in basement membranes of human intraocular blood vessels by Aronson et al. [20]. The lesions in the retina are self-limited and generally heal without signs of scarring. Occasionally papilledema and flame-shaped hemorrhages can be seen in SLE [21], and these conditions may also be associated with the thrombotic effects of the disease. However, one must be careful to exclude hypertension as a cause of the papilledema, for it is a common sequela of the chronic renal disease that accompanies lupus. Gold et al. [22] have shown that the classic retinal findings of lupus erythematosus (cotton-wool patches and hemorrhages) are present in only a minority of patients seen with a confirmed diagnosis of SLE. They attribute this discrepancy to the widespread use of corticosteroids in modern treatment.

Uveitis itself is probably only a rare complication of lupus erythematosus. A case of iridocyclitis with calcific band keratopathy was described by Halmay and Ludwig [23] in 1964. Choroiditis is, as a rule, not caused by SLE, although Böke and Baumer [24] demonstrated histologic evidence of fibrinoid necrosis in the choroidal vessels of patients suffering from the disease.

TREATMENT. The use of systemic corticosteroids may produce profound amelioration in cases of SLE, particularly in its acute phases. In chronic SLE, the need for corticosteroid therapy may be constant, and this usage brings on its share of problems, particularly as regards hypertension, psychotic changes, and Cushingism. Various immunosuppressive drugs have been employed, including cyclophosphamide, chlorambucil, and azathioprine. Hayslett et al. [25] obtained good long-term results with a combination of low-dose prednisone (<20 mg/day) and azathioprine (2.5 mg/kg/day). Various forms of therapy for lupus erythematosus, including the use of nonsteroidal anti-inflammatory agents, have recently been reviewed by Stevens et al. [26]. Since circulating substances such as antibody to DNA and other autoantibodies have been directly related to the exacerbations of the disease, plasmapheresis may have some benefit, as demonstrated by Wong et al. [27].

One may ask whether preventive medicine has any role in SLE. The triggers of systemic lupus are certainly multiple. The importance of virus infection has been much debated. Gyorkey et al. [28] have indicated the implication of myxoviruses in acute systemic lupus, but a causative role for them has not been demonstrated, and it would not seem that systemic antiviral therapy could be justified at the moment. Exposure to ultraviolet light may damage cells to the extent that DNA is exposed to the predations of the immunologic defense system. Patients identified as lupus suspects would be well advised to stay out of the sun or to wear protective cremes that filter out the majority of the ultraviolet rays. Systemic lupus is said to have been triggered by the ingestion of drugs such as penicillin, sulfonamides, and iodides [29], but if this is a matter of drug idiosyncrasy, it is difficult to know how it might have been prevented.

BEHÇET'S DISEASE

This syndrome of recurrent aphthous ulcers of the mouth and genitalia, coupled with severe uveitis, was first described by the Turkish dermatologist Behçet in 1937 [30]. Although Behçet believed that this disease was caused by a virus, and although Sezer [31] and others have attempted to substantiate this, there has been no worldwide confirmation of a viral etiology for this disease. Whatever the trigger for the disease, viral or otherwise, it appears that it, too, is a classic immune complex disease with occlusive vasculitis as its principal manifestation.

There are several forms of Behçet's disease, some of which may show signs of overlap with others. One type, producing mainly ocular symptoms, appears to be associated with the HLA type B51, a sub-type of HLA B5. Although Char [32] has stated that Ohno's [33] observations on the association between Behçet's disease and HLA B5 apply only to Orientals, Campinchi [34] and his collaborators have shown otherwise.

Caucasians in France who suffer from Behçet's disease also have a preponderance of HLA B5.

A second form affecting mainly the skin (genitalia) and mucous membranes appears to be associated with the HLA type B12 [35]. A third form, complicated by inflammatory joint disease, seems to be associated with HLA B27 [36]. Although all forms of Behçet's disease may be associated with aphthous stomatitis, this malady is so common by itself that it may not have any special significance. On the other hand, Lehner [37] has shown the existence of antibodies to oral mucosa in the serum of patients with Behçet's disease, and these antibodies have complement-fixing properties.

The ocular form of Behçet's disease is characterized by recurrent hypopyon iritis, choroiditis, and occlusive retinal vasculitis. The disease has an almost uniformly bad prognosis, and left untreated, will produce blindness in a large percentage of patients [38]. Many patients may have incomplete forms of the syndrome, e.g., retinal vasculitis and mouth ulcers but no genital ulcers. Others may have the uveitis and only a vague history of mouth ulcers, but may show erythema nodosum on their legs. The ocular disease has assumed great importance in certain parts of the world, such as Japan and the eastern Mediterranean countries. The reason for this geographic localization is obscure. It may be related to clustering of certain genetic types in these areas, but it seems more likely to be related to exposure to some kind of common environmental factor. Although there is a preponderance of the HLA B51 antigen among patients suffering from this disease, and although Berman et al. [39] have pointed to a genetic role by performing family studies, it is clear that many patients do not have the B51 antigen.

PATHOGENESIS. Shimada and his colleagues [40] have demonstrated chemotactic factors in the aqueous humor of patients suffering from the disease. These factors appear to be a complex of IgG and the C'3 and C'5 components of complement. Together, these chemotactic factors attract great numbers of polymorphonuclear leukocytes into the anterior chamber. Hypopyon sometimes occurs even when the eye does not appear particularly inflamed, indicating that a relatively minor stimulus may trigger the hypopyon. It may then disappear as rapidly as it came.

Williams and Lehner [41] noted circulating immune complexes in the sera of patients with Behçet's syndrome as well as an alteration in the distribution of the third component of complement, suggesting that these factors are important in the pathogenesis of the disease. Shimada et al. [42] have shown a reduction in the levels of serum complement just prior to the onset of an acute attack, indicating that massive amounts of complement may be removed from the circulation (presumably by fixed immune complexes at the tissue sites). The role of immune complexes in the pathogenesis of the occlusive vasculitis so characteristic of Behçet's disease is strongly suggested by the work of Maciejewski and Bandmann et al. [43], Gamble et al. [44], and Graisely et al. [45]. But, Burton-Kee et al. [46] have shown that there are differences in the composition of the immune complexes in different forms of the disease. For example, the composition of the immune complexes in the ocular form of Behçet's disease differs markedly from that of the neurological form. The acute-phase products in the serum of patients with the ocular form are also radically different from those associated with the neurological form [47]. Patients with the ocular form have large amounts of lysozyme and alpha-1-acid glycoprotein in their serum, while patients suffering from neurological complications have large amounts of Factor B in their serum, suggesting activation of the alternate pathway of complement.

If one examines the retina of a patient suffering from Behçet's syndrome, he finds numerous areas of vascular occlusion affecting both the arteries and veins. Eventually the superficial layers of the retina undergo necrosis, which at times may be accompanied by hemorrhage. With progressive loss of its vascular supply, the nerve fiber layer undergoes atrophy, and this change is mirrored by the appearance of the optic nerve, which may ultimately turn chalky white. It is this progressive loss of vascular supply that inevitably produces blindness in these patients, although a certain number will also suffer from vitreous hemorrhages, retinal detachments, and severe glaucoma.

On histologic sections, the affected retinal vessels show a thickened basement membrane, which stains green with Masson's trichrome stain, indicating the deposition of a mucopolysaccharide at this site (Fig. 7-3). The lumen of the vessel shows thrombus formation, and the area around the vessel shows infiltration by polymorphonuclear leukocytes and lymphocytes. This area is eventually subject to necrosis with loss of the normal cellular architecture and eventual infiltration by macrophages that phagocytize the necrotic tissue fragments. A similar sequence of events is said to take place in the brain, which is also subject to focal necrosis.

TREATMENT. If treatment is to be effective, it must be started early. Although corticosteroids appear to be effective early in the course of the disease (particularly in the treatment of the anterior uveitis), they seem to have a minimal effect on the occlusive retinal vasculitis that ultimately blinds the patient. In fact, many investigators in Japan, where Behçet's disease is a significant cause of blindness, feel that systemic corticosteroid therapy is contraindicated in the treatment of the retinal lesions. Treatment with immunosuppressive agents such as chlorambucil seems to be indicated early in the course of the disease before visual function is significantly altered. If patients have already developed extensive electroretinographic signs of impaired visual function, it is generally too late to attempt immunosuppressive therapy.

The regimen described by Godfrey et al. [48] appears to have been effective in the treatment of patients with Behçet's syndrome. Most patients are already on corticosteroid therapy at the time immunosuppressive therapy is initiated. Godfrey's regimen calls for an initial dosage of chlorambucil, 2 mg per day for 1 week, followed by an increase to 4 mg per day in the second week. In each succeeding week the dosage is in-

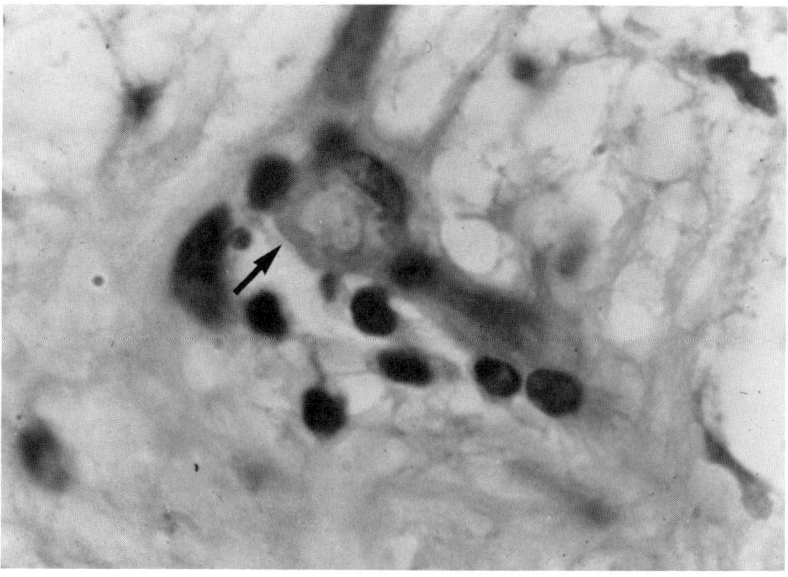

FIG. 7-3 Thickening of the basement membrane and occlusion of a retinal capillary in a patient suffering from Behçet's disease. (H. & E. × 1200.)

creased by 2 mg until either a specific clinical improvement or toxic damage to blood-forming elements is detected. Weekly white blood cell counts and platelet counts are required of all patients on this therapy. Ultimately, the dosage of steroids is reduced by slow increments until the patient is off all corticosteroid medication. Chlorambucil therapy is generally continued for at least 4 or 5 months to assure a sustained remission.

Colchicine, an antimetabolite that inhibits mitotic activity, is currently being investigated as a treatment for acute and chronic Behçet's disease [49]. It would be premature to recommend its general use at this time.

In the area of preventive medicine, patients with an established diagnosis of Behçet's disease should be cautioned against eating English walnuts. Both narrative and scientific evidence [50] suggests that substances contained in walnuts trigger exacerbations of the disease. Possibly certain proteins contained in walnuts bear antigens that coincidentally cross-react with those that trigger the onset of Behçet's syndrome. Although there is still much speculation about this (and very little hard data), it would seem that abstinence from walnuts is a small enough price to pay for reduction of symptoms.

RHEUMATOID ARTHRITIS

Classic rheumatoid polyarthritis of the adult type causes very little disease of the uvea and retina. Various studies give an incidence of 2 to 3% of uveitis among patients with rheumatoid arthritis [51, 52]. The report of Blagojevic et al. [53], in particular, sharply contrasts the difference between the incidence of uveitis in rheumatoid arthritis and the incidence in ankylosing spondylitis. Kimura et al. [54] stated that if cells and flare are seen in the anterior chamber of patients with rheumatoid arthritis, it is because of inflammation of the uvea contiguous to a scleral focus of inflammation; i.e., there is little or no primary uveitis in rheumatoid arthritis. There is no retinal vasculitis, either, except in those patients who have both lupus erythematosus and rheumatoid arthritis.

In contrast to these findings, 2 to 29 percent of subjects with juvenile rheumatoid arthritis manifest uveitis according to Calabro et al. [55], and Spalter [56] gives even higher figures. In the case of the latter report, a good deal of asymptomatic disease was detected by observers who were systematically screening a large group of patients with juvenile rheumatoid arthritis. There are two principal patterns of disease: (1) chronic iridocyclitis in young girls with monoarticular or pauciarticular arthritis, and (2) acute iridocyclitis, mainly in boys, with a tendency to acquire ankylosing spondylitis later in life [57]. The first of these two categories is by far the more serious eye disease, producing highly destructive lesions with progressive synechia formation, complicated cataract, and secondary glaucoma. The eyes of these children are often white and painless, giving rise to the term "white iritis." The second type produces acute attacks of more severe inflammation but tends to clear completely between attacks. The prognosis for vision is definitely better in this type.

PATHOGENESIS. The immunopathology of the uveitis associated with juvenile rheumatoid arthritis (JRA) has not been fully established. At least two authors have described granuloma formation in the uvea with giant cells, epithelioid cells, and lymphocytes [58, 59], suggesting the presence of a particulate foreign antigen as the source of the disease. As yet, no such particulate matter has been identified, but it may be that the cells of the uveal tract themselves are the target of an autoimmune process. Ultimately, the irides of patients suffering from JRA undergo extensive atrophy. This deterioration suggests a necrotizing process that actually destroys stromal components. The granulomatous process that has been seen by both Hinzpater et al. [58] and Sabates et al. [59] may represent a phagocytic reaction to dead or dying cells.

While JRA and ankylosing spondylitis are generally thought of as seronegative forms of arthritis, "rheumatoid factor" may present in up to 20 percent of children with JRA. Moore et al. [60] have shown that rheumatoid factor may be detectable in as many as 40 percent of the patients by a simple separation of the child's serum on a fractionation column (Sephadex G-200). Separation allows for the detection of "hidden rheumatoid factor." This may be nothing more than rheumatoid factor complexed to IgG. This complex would inhibit the binding of rheumatoid factor to IgG on a latex particle. Whatever the status of circulating antibody in JRA, it seems virtually certain that there is a local production of antibody in the diseased uveal tissues. The illustrations of Sabates et al. [59] show the presence of numerous plasma cells in the uveal tissue as well as a few Russell bodies (large crystalline aggregates of immunoglobulins). What the function of these bodies may be in the iris of patients with JRA remains unknown, but the histologic findings suggest that the inflammatory process in the uvea of patients with JRA may be related to locally produced antibody rather than circulating antibody.

Equally baffling is the role of antinuclear antibodies (ANA) in the serum of patients with JRA. Schaller [61] indicates that ANA may be present in 88 percent of patients with chronic iridocyclitis caused by JRA. In eight patients described by her, the ANA test became positive before the onset of the iridocyclitis. Antinuclear antibodies may therefore represent a "marker" for the chronic iridocyclitis associated with JRA, providing predictability as to which patients will develop chronic iridocyclitis. By contrast, patients who are negative for ANA are more likely to have acute attacks of iridocyclitis with periods of complete clinical remission interspersed between these attacks. Such patients are much more likely to develop ankylosing spondylitis later in life, particularly if they are B-27 positive and male. Although the pattern of class I HLA types among patients with juvenile rheumatoid arthritis is generally heterogeneous, Schiavetti et al. [62] found that a majority of patients with JRA of acute onset were positive for HLA BW 35. Glass et al. [63] found a preponderance of HLA DRW5 among JRA patients with iritis and ANA positivity, and Stastny and Fink [64] found that the B-cell allotype TMo was significantly associated with the iridocyclitis of JRA.

TREATMENT. Patients with the chronic iridocyclitis associated with JRA represent a major therapeutic problem. While locally applied corticosteroid drop preparations may reduce the amount of cellular reaction in the anterior chamber, no amount of medication will abolish the inflammatory reaction completely, and with the frequent application of highly concentrated corticosteroids one runs the risk of inducing cataract formation and glaucoma. The latter is a neglected and often disastrous complication of the uveitis associated with JRA in any case. To add steroid-induced glaucoma to an already existent tendency to glaucoma seems manifestly unwise. While orally administered corticosteroids may interrupt the progress of steadily worsening uveitis, the long-term administration of oral steroids cannot be advocated in growing children. Such medication produces premature closure of the epiphyses, cushingoid facial features, and many other side effects that may be damaging not only to the child's body but to his personality as well.

Since it is difficult, if not impossible, to obliterate all the signs of inflammation in the eyes of these children, the aim of therapy should be to reduce the inflammation only to the point that vision-threatening complications can be avoided. Of these, the most important complication is synechia formation. Synechiae often form with frightening rapidity in children affected by JRA. They can be avoided only by scrupulously careful attention to medication schedules. Atropine drops should be given during periods of more serious inflammation, particularly if there is pain or photophobia. Shorter-acting mydriatics such as Mydriacyl may be given during periods of lesser inflammation to keep the pupil moving, and in this instance, it is particularly important to obtain the understanding and cooperation of the parents. Many parents will relax their attention to the giving of drops when the child's eye appears white or when he no longer complains of specific ocular symptoms. Synechia formation can take place even during these periods. Generally, it is wise to instill a drop of a short-acting dilator at bedtime, even if the child's disease appears relatively inactive. This practice causes the pupil to be widely dilated at least once a day and produces no visual disability. Children who must be maintained on long-acting cycloplegics for relief of pain or photophobia should be given bifocals to aid them in their school work.

Nonsteroidal anti-inflammatory agents have been suggested in the treatment of JRA. Benorylate, an ester of aspirin, and Paracetamol have been found effective in controlling the joint symptoms of JRA [65], and ibuprofen, an antagonist of prostaglandin synthesis, may also have some value [66]. A double-blind study on the comparative effectiveness of aspirin and fenoprofen showed that they were of essentially equal benefit, but aspirin in therapeutically effective dosages caused many more side-effects [67]. Within recent years, interest has been reawakened in the therapeutic use of gold salts in the treatment of JRA, and Giannini et al. [68] reported favorable results. As yet, however, none of these agents has been shown to be of definite value in the control of ocular inflammation.

Mention was made earlier of the problem of secondary glaucoma in JRA-associated uveitis. This condition has often been neglected because of the outmoded (but still perpetuated) belief that the secondary glaucomas produce less optic nerve damage than the primary glaucomas. Since the accurate measurement of intraocular pressure in the child requires considerable cooperation on the part of the patient, the physician often "defers" tension measurement or relies upon a tactile tension measurement. This neglect of the secondary glaucoma problem has all too often resulted in irreversible optic nerve damage, insidious in onset but relentless in its progress. When glaucoma is detected in a child with JRA-associated uveitis, it should be treated medically, if at all possible. Agents such as timolol maleate (0.25% or 0.5%) may be used in drop form twice a day. This therapy may be combined with epinephrine 1% twice a day or with the use of oral carbonic anhydrase inhibitors such as acetazolamide 250 mg twice a day. Treatment with miotic agents such as pilocarpine should be avoided because of the irritation that these products cause and because of the strong tendency for synechia formation in this disease. Surgical intervention, a last resort, should be avoided until it is clear that medical therapy will be of no avail. Filtering procedures in the presence of chronic inflammation are notoriously unsuccessful, and cryotherapy may produce a phthisical eye.

Although iridocyclitis associated with ankylosing spondylitis is considered by many authors to be a nonrheumatoid malady, inflammatory involvement of the peripheral joints is occasionally seen in this condition. Its immunopathology is essentially unknown, although the high prevalence of the HLA antigen B-27 among patients suffering from this disease suggests an immunogenetic basis. It may be that antigenic similarity between the B-27 antigen and such bacterial agents as *Klebsiella pneumoniae* allows the bacterial agent to multiply in the tissues of affected individuals ("molecular mimicry"). A report by Ebringer and Cawdell [69] indicates that 76 percent of stool cultures from patients with ankylosing spondylitis and iritis were positive for *Klebsiella pneumoniae*. Whatever the origin of the conditions, prompt treatment with local corticosteroid drop preparations and cycloplegics is required. Prednisolone acetate 1% should be instilled hourly until the pain and photophobia subside. Atropine 1% should be instilled twice a day. Rarely, the inflammation will be so severe as to require a short course of high-dose oral corticosteroid therapy (80 to 100 mg prednisone per day). The pattern of the uveitis associated with ankylosing spondylitis is well known. It produces an acute fibrinous iridocyclitis which usually clears completely in the interval between attacks. Patients whose diagnosis is established should be supplied with cycloplegic drops and local corticosteroid drop preparations at all times. They should begin frequent drop therapy at home at the first sign of a recurrence, as early, intensive therapy will often abort an otherwise disastrous attack. Time otherwise lost in waiting to see the doctor may be the cause of permanent synechia formation.

MULTIPLE MYELOMA

Multiple myeloma may be regarded as a malignant neoplasm of one particular line of B lymphocytes. It is a frequently encountered cause of what is referred to as a monoclonal gammopathy, for such B-cell neoplasms often result in the production of excessively high levels of a single immunoglobulin in the serum. Indeed, studies on patients with IgE-secreting tumors were virtually indispensable to the acquisition of knowledge about the structure of this immunoglobulin. The disease is characterized by the pathologic infiltration of plasma cells into many tissues of the body including the eye. This neoplasm ultimately results in the erosion of bone, inhibition of blood-forming elements, uremia with hypercalcemia, and suppression of normal immunologic competence.

Its direct effects on uveal and retinal tissues include the formation of fluid-filled cysts of the nonpigmented epithelium of the ciliary body [70]. These growths are similar in appearance to cysts that develop in other hyperglobulinemic states such as those associated with hepatic cirrhosis [71]. Congestion of the retinal vessels often occurs as the result of a hyperviscosity syndrome, although this complication may not be so prominent as the retinal vessel change associated with Waldenström's macroglobulinemia [72]. Symptoms related to serum viscosity rarely occur in patients with levels below 4 centipoise, but they occur frequently at levels above 6 centipoise. The characteristic sausage-like dilatation of the retinal vessels is not specific for multiple myeloma, but may be seen in many hyperviscosity syndromes. Glistening crystals of myeloma protein may also be seen in the retina by ophthalmoscopic examination. Here they resemble the appearance of similar crystalline deposits in the conjunctiva and cornea [73].

TREATMENT. The treatment of multiple myeloma is essentially the same as that of the systemic disease. The usual treatment consists of oral melphalan 0.25 mg/kg daily for 4 days combined with oral prednisone 2 mg/kg. This treatment is repeated every 6 weeks. Reduction of blood viscosity may be achieved by frequent phlebotomy with replacement of the plasma by nonviscous balanced electrolyte solutions (plasmapheresis).

MULTIPLE SCLEROSIS

This highly destructive demyelinating disease of the central nervous system is believed to be of autoimmune origin. The evidence that it is an autoimmune disease can be summarized as follows.

1. Circulating antibodies to basic myelin protein can be found in the serum of the majority of patients with this disease [74], and it appears that the levels of these antibodies can be correlated with disease activity.
2. Complement-fixing antibodies have been shown by Berg and Källen [75] to damage the oligodendrocytes that are thought to elaborate myelin.
3. Antimyelin antibody, principally IgG, has been detected, along with complement at the edges of demyelinated plaques in the central nervous system; these studies have been performed by Lumsden [74] using direct immunofluorescence.
4. There is a strong resemblance between experimental allergic encephalitis, produced by repeated injections of autologous brain (with adjuvants), and multiple sclerosis.
5. The peripheral lymphocytes of patients with either pure optic neuritis or the optic neuritis associated with multiple sclerosis undergo lymphocytoblast transformation when stimulated with myelin protein [76]. This change is assumed to be an indication of a cell-mediated reaction (delayed hypersensitivity) to the protein.

PATHOGENESIS. The origin of multiple sclerosis is obscure. It seems likely that a combination of an infectious insult (possibly viral) and an immunogenetic predisposition to react to myelin protein might account for the majority of cases. Considerable interest has been aroused by the finding of antimeasles antibody in the serum and spinal fluid of multiple sclerosis victims [77, 78]. Under those circumstances where IgM antibody has been found, recent infection could be postulated. It is entirely possible that a virus could damage cells of the central nervous system in such a way as to render certain cellular elements antigenic. Once altered or damaged proteins were exposed to the lymphoreticular system of the body, subsequent reactivity to those proteins could be stimulated. Measles and mumps are common infections, and there is reason to believe that a mild encephalitis might accompany virtually every case of these viral exanthems. Why is it that only certain patients develop the disease, and why is it that certain patients develop only mild or self-limited disease while others take a progressive downhill course? These are not easy questions to answer, but it appears that individual variations in immunologic reactivity may account for some of the differences in disease expression. In this regard, the HLA system may play an important role. Paty et al. [79] have implicated HLA DR2 in the pathogenesis of multiple sclerosis, but the association is not entirely convincing. In reviewing this subject, Haile et al. [80] postulate the existence of a "multiple sclerosis susceptibility gene" with reduced penetrance, where full phenotypic expression depends on critical environmental exposures.

Among the ocular signs of multiple sclerosis, optic neuritis and peripheral uveitis figure prominently. Over 50 percent of patients with the isolated sign of optic neuritis will eventually develop other signs of multiple sclerosis. Among the initial signs of optic nerve disease, retrobulbar neuritis is the most common. The occurrence of this sign seems logical in view of the fact that the portion of the optic nerve anterior to the lamina cribrosa represents only a small portion of the total myelinated structure. Occasionally, however, an acute papillitis will be observed in the optic neuritis associated with multiple sclerosis. Under these circumstances, edema of the nerve head, minor hemorrhages, and exudation into the overlying vitreous may be seen.

Uveitis develops in a significant number of patients with multiple sclerosis. Indeed, Breger and Leopold [81] found evidence of uveitis in 14 out of 52 patients with otherwise classic signs of multiple sclerosis. The majority showed evidence of pars plana exudates, snowball opacities in the vitreous, and sheathing of the peripheral retinal vessels. While most showed only mild anterior chamber reactions (1^+ cells and flare), one patient showed a moderate number of fine keratic precipitates and another showed large numbers of KPs along with posterior synechiae. Three of the nine patients described by Porter [82] also showed posterior synechiae, indicating that these patients must have had a moderately severe iritis at one time or another.

The relationship between the uveal inflammation and the central nervous system disease is not easy to understand at the outset. While the optic nerve and retina may be thought of as embryologic extensions of the brain, the uvea is for the most part of mesodermal origin. Rahi and Garner [83] suggest that the uveitis is simply a response to an antigenic stimulus originating in the retina. They point to the observation of Wickremesinghe and Yates [84] that astrocytes, oligodendrocytes, and myelin may possess at least one common antigen and that this antigen may be present in the retina as well as in the central nervous system. Along this line, it is interesting to note that Snyder et al. [85] found evidence of antiganglioside antibodies in 44 percent of pars planitis patients and in 71 percent of patients with the Vogt-Koyanagi-Harada syndrome. We have already seen that the Vogt-Koyanagi-Harada syndrome is essentially a uveameningitis involving the central nervous system, the cochlea, and a number of ocular structures including the choroid, the optic nerve, and the retina. Pars planitis (peripheral uveitis, "intermediate uveitis") appears to be the principal uveal manifestation of multiple sclerosis. Indeed, Curless and Bray [86] and Smith et al. [87] have shown that pars planitis can precede the onset of classic multiple sclerosis by several years. Although the majority of patients with the pars planitis syndrome never go on to develop central nervous system disease, it is nevertheless possible that the two diseases are etiologically linked, and the antiganglioside antibodies described by Snyder et al. [85] provide additional evidence of that link.

TREATMENT. Multiple sclerosis has a highly variable and unpredictable course. Its ultimate course depends upon a number of variables including age at onset and the targeted areas of attack. From the point of view of visual health, the optic neuritis that so often precedes or accompanies the main central nervous system afflictions is of paramount importance. There is no uniform opinion about the usefulness of corticosteroids in modifying the course of multiple sclerosis. Many authors feel that corticosteroids, administered by either the oral or retrobulbar route, alter the course of the optic neuritis. At the same time, it should be noted that a certain amount of spontaneous recovery often takes place after the acute edema and infiltration of the optic nerve have subsided. Bowden et al. [88] have published the results of double-masked control studies showing that corticosteroids have no net effect on visual impairment in the patient suffering from multiple sclerosis.

Since the disease is almost certainly of autoimmune origin and since its acute attacks are accompanied by lymphocytic infiltration and edema of the affected tissues, it would seem logical to treat patients in the acute phase of the attacks with corticosteroids. On the other hand, since structures that have been subjected to demyelinization will not regenerate, and since the acute inflammatory phase of the disease generally does not last more than a few weeks, treatment beyond one month's time seems pointless.

Other treatments have recently been proposed in the management of multiple sclerosis. These include the use of hyperbaric oxygen, particularly in acute exacerbations of the disease [89]. The perivascular infiltrates that accompany this disease may preclude the normal transmission of oxygen to the tissues, and hyperoxygenation of the blood may overcome this problem, at least temporarily. Hauser et al. [90] found intensive intravenous cyclophosphamide therapy, coupled with intramuscular ACTH administration, to be highly effective in controlling the disease, but it seems clear that the ideal regimen has not yet been established.

CRANIAL ARTERITIS

Cranial arteritis, more popularly called temporal arteritis, is a thrombotic disease affecting middle-sized branches of the aortic arch as well as other major vessels of the body such as the renal arteries. The affected arteries are subject to segmental damage of the internal elastic lamina and smooth muscle layer with infiltration by lymphocytes, giant macrophages, and eosinophils. Ultimately, the intima of the vessel is disrupted, providing a site for platelet aggregation and eventually for thrombus formation. The most commonly observed effect on the eye is an ischemic optic atrophy due to involvement of the short posterior ciliary arteries and of the branches which they supply to the juxtapapillary choroid. In some cases, the optic nerve head itself is spared, but damage to the retrobulbar portion of the nerve occurs as a result of occlusion of the pial branches of the ophthalmic artery. Rarely, central retinal artery occlusion may be produced.

PATHOGENESIS. The disease is presumed to be of immunologic origin, but there is as yet no very good evidence of this, and undue emphasis has probably been placed on the eosinophils that may be present in the inflammatory infiltrate of the vessel wall. Cranial arteritis affects a group of patients older in age than most individuals subject to autoimmune diseases. Commonly, victims of the disease are in their sixth or seventh decade of life and have been in good general health prior to the attack. Since the disease affects only certain segments of the arteries and not others, it might be appropriate to postulate that degenerative changes have occurred in certain areas of the smooth muscle, followed by inflammatory reaction to the necrotic muscle cells. However, as Rahi and Garner [91] point out, such inflammatory reactions do not occur in the presence of hypertension-associated medial necrosis. It seems more likely that initial damage to the smooth muscle or to the internal elastic layer might occur as the result of an attack on these structures by an infectious agent, which, like herpes zoster, preferentially affects patients in an older age group. Such individuals are known to have compromised T-cell immunity and are, in general, more susceptible to the ravages of viral diseases. Once altered by viral attack, smooth muscle cells might act as autoantigens. Again, the presence of giant cells in the arterial lesions suggests the presence of particulate antigenic matter, which must be removed by phagocytosis. The nature of the antigens remains a mystery.

Hazleman and associates [92] have found evidence of lymphocytoblast transformation in the lymphocytes of patients with polymyalgia rheumatica, a related disease, when such lymphocytes were exposed to soluble extracts of arterial tissue. This finding may have some relevance, since polymyalgia rheumatica may precede or accompany cranial arteritis, and like it, is greatly benefited by corticosteroid therapy.

The histologic picture of cranial arteritis appears to be quite different from that of polyarteritis nodosa, which may also cause coagulative necrosis of retinal vessels. In polyarteritis nodosa there is severe fibrinoid necrosis with marked polymorphonuclear leukocyte infiltration. Moreover, this affection appears to be more typical of an immune complex disease. IgG and complement have been identified in the arterial lesion [93], and in addition, a specific role for Australia antigen, the agent of hepatitis-B, has been described. Gocke et al. [94] found evidence of Australia antigen-antibody complexes in the circulating blood of patients with polyarteritis nodosa and have been able to demonstrate these complexes, together with complement, in the vascular lesions. It must also be stated that patients with polyarteritis give evidence of more generalized illness. They are subject to hypertension, hematuria, eosinophilia, and periodic fever, whereas patients with cranial arteritis are generally well except for headaches and signs of visual impairment.

Laboratory studies on patients with cranial arteritis show elevated levels of α-2 globulin, fibrinogen, and occasionally of IgM. The presence of these proteins may account for rouleaux formation among the circulating erythrocytes of the patient and hence for the elevated sedimentation rate that characterizes the disease. No other laboratory tests are diagnostic, and a temporal artery biopsy, even when selected from a site of maximum tenderness, will occasionally be negative.

TREATMENT. Systemic corticosteroid administration is mandatory once the diagnosis of cranial arteritis has been made. This therapy has been proven to be sight saving and has brought about the recovery of tissues temporarily compromised by inflammatory disease of the nutrient arteries. If macular fibers within the optic nerve or the central retina itself have been affected by arterial occlusive disease, a return of good visual function cannot be expected. All too often the disease has not been suspected until the optic nerve of one eye has been found to be atrophic and the optic nerve of the second eye has begun to be affected. The aged patient with ischemic optic atrophy and an elevated erythrocyte sedimentation rate should be considered a cranial arteritis victim until proven otherwise.

SARCOIDOSIS

Ocular sarcoidosis is best described as a diffuse uveitis affecting both the anterior and posterior uvea as well as the retina and, occasionally, the optic nerve. The basic lesion is noncaseating granuloma containing lymphocytes, epithelioid cells, and giant cells, often arranged in a well-circumscribed or tuberculoid granuloma. Although ocular sarcoidosis is generally assumed to be part and parcel of a generalized granulomatous disease, it is often difficult to prove the existence of characteristic lesions elsewhere in the body. However, the classic cases are said to show evidence of hilar adenopathy or intralobar infiltration of the lungs, erythema nodosum, peripheral lymphadenopathy, and occasionally infiltrative lesions of the parotid and lacrimal glands. Erosive lesions of the bones of the hands and feet may occasionally be detected by roentgenograms, particularly in areas where there are overlying lesions of the skin. Occasionally, the arthritic lesions of sarcoid may mimic those of JRA.

In the United States sarcoidosis is seen with the greatest frequency among black patients, but the disease is assumed to have a worldwide distribution and there are important foci of this disorder among the Caucasian populations of central and northern Europe, particularly in Scandinavia.

PATHOGENESIS. The etiology of sarcoidosis is unknown, but the persistence of epithelioid cells and giant cells in the lesions suggests a "frustrated macrophage" function, i.e., a function in which macrophages are present in the lesion but are unable to complete their task of phagocytosis. Numerous organisms, including mycoplasma [95], various viruses [96], and *Mycobacteria* spp. [97], have been thought to play a role in the causation of sarcoidosis, but Koch's postulates have not been fulfilled for any of these organisms, nor has any one organism been found with regularity in the tissue lesions. The lesions of sarcoid also have superficial resemblances to foreign body granulomas such as those caused by beryllium or inhaled pollen granules, but here again, no causative foreign body has been observed with any regularity. Sarcoidosis has a higher prevalence in certain southeastern states where particular species of pine trees cast allergenic pollens into the air, but this may merely reflect higher numbers of blacks in these areas or other factors causally related to the disease but as yet unidentified.

Patients with sarcoidosis appear to have adequate B-cell functions; in fact, they may show higher than usual amounts of immunoglobulins (principally IgG) in their serum. Circulating immune complexes have been described in patients with sarcoidosis [98], but the antigenic component of these complexes has not been characterized, nor has it been established that immune complexes play any role in the development of the tissue lesions. Indeed, the classic lesions of sarcoidosis bear no resemblance to other lesions known to be associated with immune complex deposition (e.g., glomerulonephritis, lupus, the Arthus phenomenon).

A special type of T-cell deficiency appears to be characteristic of sarcoidosis. Patients suffering from this disease manifest cutaneous anergy to tuberculin as well as to other skin-test antigens representing common infectious agents to which the patient should normally have been exposed earlier in life (e.g., *Trichophyton, Candida,* mumps). The defect is said to be related to a deficiency in the production or recognition of "transfer factor," a lymphokine secreted by antigen-stimulated T lymphocytes. Failure to utilize this substance appears to be responsible for a failure to recruit noncommitted lymphocytes to a cutaneous antigen depot. This defect may be responsible for the fact that sarcoid patients are immunologically compromised hosts. They are unable to defend themselves adequately against the human tubercle bacillus, to which many such patients eventually succumb. They also manifest less than optimal responses to such common facultative pathogens as *Candida albicans*. Another immunologic factor possibly connected with decreased resistance to opportunistic pathogens is the decrease in natural killer (NK) cell activity encountered among patients suffering from sarcoidosis. Antonaci et al. [99] found natural killer cell activity reduced to about 50 percent of normal in a significant number of patients with active sarcoidosis.

Anergy is not universal among sarcoidosis patients (some 11 to 15 percent of patients manifesting normal skin-test responses), nor do they show a complete failure to attract lymphocytes to certain sites. The Kveim test, in which a cutaneous granuloma develops in response to a subcutaneous inoculation of an extract of human sarcoid-laden spleen, probably represents just such a reaction. Lenzini et al. [100] have described an in vitro correlate of this reaction: 9 to 12 patients with established sarcoidosis showed positive leukocyte migration inhibition (LMI) tests when their leukocytes were stimulated with Kveim antigen. In a similar vein, Jones-Williams et al. [101] have described a Kveim macrophage inhibiting factor (KMID), which gives a much more rapid result than the standard Kveim test, avoids biopsy, and avoids the possible transmission of hepatitis virus.

The clinical appearance of ocular sarcoid is highly variable, depending upon the structures affected and the duration of the lesions. In its earliest stages, the ocular inflammation may be asymptomatic, and the anterior chamber may show only a few cells and slight flare. In this stage, it might not be easy to distinguish the clinical appearance of the disease from a nongranulomatous uveitis. Later, more acute forms of iridocyclitis may be seen, some with mutton-fat keratic precipitates, synechia formation, and secondary glaucoma. Hyperfluorescent dots may be seen in the ciliary body band, as noted by Kimura [102] in 1982. In the more chronic forms of iridocyclitis, vascularized nodules of the iris stroma may be seen, particularly in the chamber angle. Here they may ultimately be a source of peripheral anterior synechia formation. At the pupillary margin, Koeppe nodules may form; these, however, are by no means diagnostic of sarcoidosis. Behind the lens, snowball opacities may be seen, and some of these may settle down to the inferior pars plana area, giving rise to the characteristic pars plana "snowbank" usually associated with peripheral ("intermediate") uveitis. Examination of the peripheral retinal vessels located near such snowbanks may show extensive perivascular inflammation. While this condition may appear as regular sheathing of the vessels in this location, elsewhere particularly in the posterior pole of the retina, heavy irregular coating of the retinal vessels ("candle wax drippings") (Fig. 7-4) may be observed. Lastly patchy chorioretinitis, usually associated with actual granuloma formation in the retina and choroid, may be seen, as described by Gass and Olson [103].

Direct involvement of the optic nerve is relatively rare and, as pointed out by Gould and Kaufman [104], is usually associated with simultaneous involvement of the central nervous system. While the latter may produce localizing neurological signs, infiltrates of the brain may be visualized in "silent areas" by CT scanning.

Biopsy remains the most reliable way of making a diagnosis of sarcoid. While the classic biopsy sites include the scalene or supraclavicular nodes, biopsy of a skin nodule or a conjunctival nodule yields equivalent information. In our hands, blind biopsy of the conjunctiva has not yielded worthwhile information. One should find a yellowish-pink nodule of the conjunctiva, usually a little larger and a little more irregular than a conjunctival follicle, before proceeding with biopsy. The palpebral portion of the lacrimal gland is another easily accessible site for biopsy and has yielded useful results.

Ancillary blood tests that might support the diagnosis of sarcoidosis (serum lysozyme and serum angiotensin converting factor) have been described in Chapter 2, Testing Procedures. The uptake of gallium 67

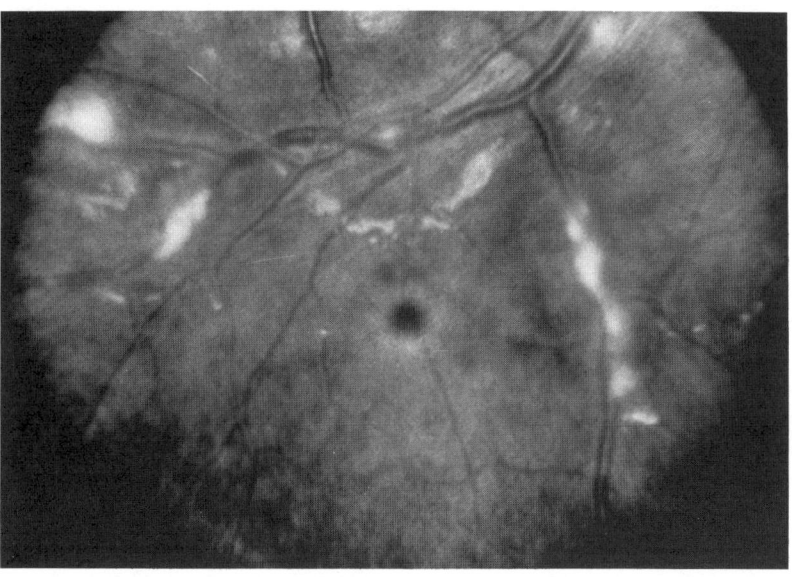

FIG. 7-4   Perivascular exudates of the "candle-wax dripping" type in the fundus of a patient suffering from ocular sarcoidosis. (From G. R. O'Connor: Ocular sarcoidosis. In E. A. Klein (Ed.), *Symposium on Medical and Surgical Diseases of the Retina and Vitreous*. St. Louis, Mosby, 1982, p. 215. Reproduced with permission.)

by the mediastinal nodes, lacrimal gland, and parotid gland also provides a helpful clue as to the existence of sarcoid infiltrates in these structures. This technique, described by Lauver and Gooneratne [105], is useful, particularly when roentgenograms of the mediastinal area prove inconclusive.

TREATMENT. The use of corticosteroids is beneficial in ocular sarcoidosis and is mandatory in those cases that show vision-threatening lesions. Patients who manifest iridocyclitis alone should be treated with prednisolone acetate 1% drops (or an equivalent preparation) as well as a corticosteroid ointment at bedtime. Careful attention should be given to the pupil, particularly in the more darkly pigmented patients, where synechia formation of an intractable nature may take place insidiously. Atropine drops (1%) should be instilled at least twice a day during acute, painful episodes, and shorter acting mydriatics should be employed frequently to keep the pupil moving during the chronic phases of inflammation. Sub-Tenon's injection of depot steroids may be useful in patients whose compliance is not optimal for the instillation of drops. Such medication is also useful to relieve cystoid macular edema in those cases where the intraocular inflammation has become chronic.

Posterior involvement, particularly that involving the central retina or optic nerve, generally requires the use of systemically administered corticosteroids. Daily doses of 80 to 100 mg of prednisone may be required initially. This glucocorticoid may be given in divided doses at first. Later, after a good anti-inflammatory effect has been achieved, one might shift to an alternate-day form of therapy, administering twice the usual daily dose at 8:00 every other morning. This schedule has obvious advantages in that it helps avoid adrenal suppression [106], but as Fauci points out [107], the regimen may not be so effective for the treatment of the uveitis. Symptoms on the day between the treatment days may be considerably worse. Cytotoxic immunosuppressive therapy is generally not considered in sarcoidosis, because patients with this disease are already considered to be immunologically depressed.

ACQUIRED IMMUNE DEFICIENCY SYNDROME (AIDS)

The bizarre, tragic malady of acquired immune deficiency syndrome (AIDS) was first reported among homosexual men by Gottlieb et al. [108] in 1981. AIDS is marked by the occurrence of Kaposi's sarcoma or opportunistic infections, or both, in previously healthy persons less than 60 years of age whose immunosuppression has no known cause. In addition to homosexuals, the disease is known to affect users of intravenous drugs, hemophiliacs, recent Haitian immigrants, female sexual partners of men suffering from the syndrome, and infants of women in the known risk groups. The immune deficiency is manifested as a defect in cellular immunity that permits the overgrowth of one or more opportunistic infections, some of which may be fatal. These include *Pneumocystis carinii*, oral and esophageal candidiasis, disseminated cytomegalovirus, persistent invasive herpes (particularly in the perianal regions), atypical mycobacterial infections, and disseminated toxoplasmosis. Death is often associated with fatal *Pneumocystis* pneumonia or with cerebral necrosis due to invasive lesions caused by *Toxoplasma* or cytomegalovirus.

The ocular disorders associated with AIDS were described by Holland et al. in 1982 [109]. This report was complemented by a prospective study of 26 patients with AIDS, examined on multiple occasions by Freeman et al. [110] at the Lenox Hill Hospital in New York City. Nineteen of the patients examined had ophthalmic lesions at some point in the course of their disease, and 16 of these had lesions confined to the retina. Seven patients had isolated cotton-wool patches as the only ophthalmic manifestation of their disease, and two patients showed only isolated retinal hemorrhages. The cotton-wool patches appeared to be identical to those seen in diabetes and hypertension. It was unusual to see them in patients with Kaposi's sarcoma; on the other hand, they were commonly observed in patients with *Pneumocystis* pneumonia with or without other opportunistic infections. Cotton-wool spots could not be correlated with deterioration or improvement in the general condition of the patient; their distribution was seemingly random. On the other hand, the development of cytomegalovirus retinitis (Fig. 7-5), which was observed in 3 of the 26 patients, was an indication of grave prognosis, and death generally followed in 2 or 3 months.

The cotton-wool spots, which represent such a common ophthalmic sign in AIDS, have been subjected to intensive study by Kwok et al. [111]

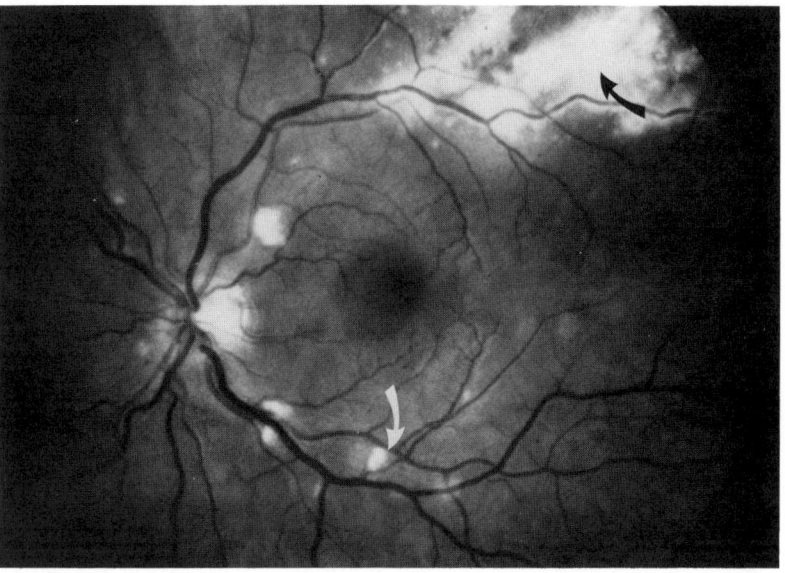

FIG. 7-5 Fundus photograph of a patient suffering from acquired immune deficiency syndrome (AIDS). Black arrow denotes retinal lesion of cytomegalovirus infection. White arrow denotes cotton-wool spot. (Courtesy of Dr. Gary N. Holland, University of California, Los Angeles.)

and by Pepose et al. [112]. The former found electron-microscopic evidence of *Pneumocystis* infection at the site of a cotton-wool patch that had been observed in the fundus of an AIDS patient just before death. Pepose et al. [112] were not able to confirm this observation in pathologic specimens taken from the eyes of several other AIDS patients post mortem, nor were they able to document immune complex deposition in the lesions. Direct immunofluorescence staining for IgG, IgM, and C3b showed no differences between the cotton-wool spots examined and sections of normal retina.

Another interesting feature of their study was the finding of an abnormal ratio of helper to suppressor/cytotoxic T-lymphocytes in the choroid of a patient with cytomegalovirus retinitis. The analysis of T-cell subsets in the ocular tissue was performed by an indirect immunoperoxidase technique designed to detect specific T-cell antigens on the surfaces of the sectioned lymphocytes. The average ratio of helper (OKT4$^+$) to suppressor/cytotoxic (OKT8$^+$) lymphocytes in the circulation of normal individuals is approximately 1.85. Among AIDS patients this ratio may be 0.5 or lower, while in patients with an AIDS-related complex (generalized persistent adenopathy, fever, weight loss, and malaise) the ratio may be in the range of 0.85. The abnormal ratio of OKT4$^+$ cells to OKT8$^+$ cells is reflected in the ocular tissue lesions of patients with AIDS and may be connected with the failure of ocular tissues to withstand attack by common opportunistic pathogens such as the cytomegalovirus. The latter is only one of a number of opportunistic agents that have been positively identified in postmortem specimens of eyes from AIDS patients. Others include *Cryptococcus* [113], *Mycobacterium avium intracellulare* [114], and *Toxoplasma gondii* [115].

PATHOGENESIS. The etiology and pathogenesis of AIDS have not been established with certainty. When it was discovered that hemophiliacs and abusers of intravenously administered drugs developed the same disease as homosexuals indulging in potentially traumatic sexual practices (e.g., anal intercourse), an intense search was made for a blood-borne agent that might cause the disease. Isolation of a T-lymphotrophic retrovirus from a patient at risk for acquired immune deficiency was reported by Barré-Sinoussi et al. [116] in 1983. Subsequent reports such as that of Gallo et al. [117] showed that a human T-cell leukemia virus (HTLV-III) could be isolated with some regularity from patients with AIDS or from patients at risk for the development of AIDS. The latter also were found to produce antibody against HTLV-III, but the usefulness of testing for antibody to HTLV-III has not been determined. Large numbers of asymptomatic homosexuals appear to be antibody-positive but fail to develop the disease. As a precautionary measure blood banks are now screening donors for anti-HTLV-III antibodies, but the risk/benefit ratio of such procedures has not been determined.

If HTLV-III has a predilection for attacking OKT4$^+$ cells in some individuals, the reduced numbers of such cells might contribute to the deficiency of immunologic responsiveness that characterizes the disease. Patients suffering from AIDS typically show deficiencies in delayed hypersensitivity, as manifested by poor skin-test responses to commonly employed injectable antigens (*Candida,* mumps, streptokinase-streptodornase, etc.) In vitro tests on their cultured lymphocytes show poor lymphoblastogenic responses to many antigens. Thus the mechanisms for both stimulation and recruitment of lymphoid responses seem to be disturbed. It is not known why some HTLV-positive individuals develop the disease while others do not; in this connection, it is particularly mysterious that elderly individuals are usually spared, while young, otherwise healthy individuals appear to be more regularly attacked. The apparent attack rate may be influenced by the fact that the disease seems to have a very long incubation period (possibly in excess of two years), so nothing of a definitive nature can be said at present about who will be attacked and who will be spared. A large number of factors other than viral infection (immunogenetic, hormonal, or even climatic) may eventually be shown to be of significance in the causation of this disease. One or more cofactors may be necessary to develop the disease. A certain level of cellular activation, found only among young, otherwise healthy individuals, may be necessary for the propagation of HTLV in vivo, and this has been suggested by Sonnabend et al. [118] as a requisite cofactor.

TREATMENT. Despite the therapeutic use of lymphokines such as interferon and interleukin-2, as well as other manipulations including thymic epithelial cell transplantation and lymphocyte transfusions, little success has been achieved in restoring immunologic competence to the affected individuals. Over 80% of those afflicted for more than two years have now died. Attempts to produce an antiviral vaccine, possibly one with specific antireverse transcriptase activity, are underway; and these efforts have been greatly aided by the fact that HTLV-III can now be mass-produced.

The major thrust of therapy has been to quell those opportunistic infections that might be lethal. *Pneumocystis* infections have been treated with pentamidine, cryptococcal infections with amphotericin B and 5-fluorocytosine, and *Toxoplasma* infections with pyrimethamine and sulfonamides, all with some success, at least on a temporary basis. Little headway has been made against invasive forms of cytomegalovirus infection, which may ultimately be lethal.

SYMPATHETIC OPHTHALMIA

The term *sympathetic ophthalmia* was coined by MacKenzie in 1840 to describe a mysterious and sometimes devastating inflammation of both eyes that followed in the wake of penetrating injury to one eye. MacKenzie, however, was not the first to observe the disease. Kraus-Mackiw [119] recently cited an obscure reference to the subject in the early work of Bartisch, who published his treatise in Dresden in 1583. This form of uveitis has long been assumed to represent an autoimmune disease, but in fact, its etiology is still unknown.

The inflammation has an insidious onset and a progressive course. It appears in the second ("sympathizing") eye as early as 10 days after injury to the first ("exciting") eye. Kraus-Mackiw [119] states that 50% of her cases developed inflammation in the sympathizing eye within 3 months of the injury, and 70% had developed the disease by the end of two years. In a minority of cases, the onset of sympathetic ophthalmia may be delayed as much as 40 or 50 years.

Sympathetic ophthalmia begins as a choroiditis affecting the most posterior portions of the eye first. Spitznas [120] has documented this pattern of inflammation beautifully in a series of fluorescein angiograms performed on a patient who sought medical attention very early in the course of his disease. Somewhat later, cells may appear in the vitreous and vision may decline because of vitreous opacities or because of macular edema. A serous detachment of the retina may be produced, although the retina itself will show no damage except for focal areas of perivasculitis. Ultimately, the anterior uvea may become involved. Edema and infiltration of the ciliary body may cause loss of accomodation. Cells and flare will be seen in the anterior chamber; keratic precipitates will form on the endothelial surface of the cornea; and posterior synechiae may form between the iris and the lens. Complicated cataract and secondary glaucoma may ensue in the later course of the disease.

PATHOGENESIS. The histologic picture of sympathetic ophthalmia is highly characteristic, if not pathognomonic. The cellular infiltrates are primarily mononuclear and are restricted, at least in the early phases of

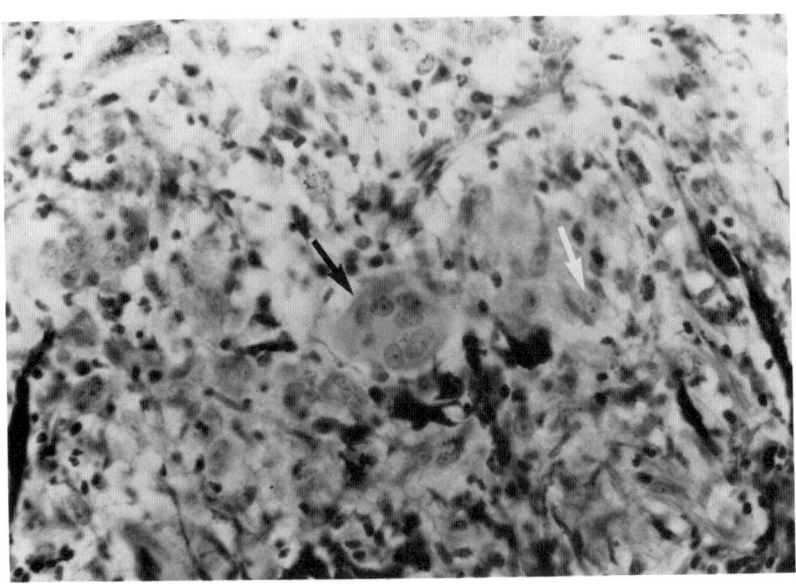

FIG. 7-6 Histologic picture of sympathetic ophthalmia. *Black arrow* denotes giant cell in the choroid. *White arrow* denotes epithelioid cell. Note scattered melanin. (H. & E. × 800.)

the disease, to the posterior pole. Active migration of mononuclear cells through the endothelium of the post-capillary venules can be seen in the choroid. Initially, eccentric crescents of these cells can be seen surrounding the venules. Later the mononuclear cells form a more or less uniform thickening of the uveal tract, punctuated here and there by focal infiltrates. Later, clusters of epithelioid cells, now known to be activated macrophages, form clusters of cells within the otherwise exclusively lymphocytic infiltrates (Fig. 7-6). These epithelioid cells fuse, in some cases, to become multinucleated giant cells. Eosinophils may be seen in great numbers beneath the choriocapillaris, although the latter layer remains uninvolved in most cases. Anterior to Bruch's membrane, however, other highly characteristic cellular infiltrates may be observed in the form of Dalén-Fuchs nodules. These consist of accumulations of monocytes and epithelioid cells beneath a detached "hillock" of the pigmented epithelium of the retina. In some cases the integrity of the pigmented epithelium may be destroyed, allowing the round infiltrate of the Dalén-Fuchs nodule to be seen ophthalmoscopically as a small, yellow-grey spot in the periphery of the fundus.

Considerable effort has been expended to identify the origin and function of the various types of cells that participate in sympathetic ophthalmia. Jakobiec et al. [121] have shown that the majority of lymphocytes in the choroidal infiltrate are T cells of the suppressor/cytotoxic subset (OKT8$^+$), only 5 percent of the cells being immunoglobulin-producing B cells. The epithelioid cells were found to be Ia$^+$ and OKM1$^+$, antigenic determinants that are characteristic of bone-marrow-derived cells.

Although some of the epithelioid cells contained single melanin granules in the cytoplasm, these granules were membrane-bound and frequently associated with lysosomal material. The authors felt that these characteristics, together with the histochemical reactivity of the cells' cytoplasm for alpha-1-antichymotrypsin and lysozyme, marked them as monocytes of bone-marrow origin rather than tranformed choroidal melanocytes, as suggested earlier by Ishikawa and Ikui [122]. In like manner, Jakobiec et al. [121] identified the majority of the monocytes within Dalén-Fuchs nodules as $OKT8^+$. However, these cells also reacted with the monoclonal antibody OKT20, suggesting that the cells represented activated cytotoxic/effector cell populations rather than resting suppressor-cytotoxic cells. The cells of the Dalén-Fuchs nodules were also in large part, Ia^+ and OKM1 positive, suggesting a bone-marrow origin. This is in contrast to the earlier studies of Font and Fine [123], which concluded that the majority of the cells were pigmented epithelial cells that had undergone epithelioid transformation.

The histopathology of sympathizing eyes is essentially the same as that of the exciting eyes except that Müller-Hermelink [124] has found a greater tendency to anterior uveitis in sympathizing eyes, particularly when there was an associated lens-induced uveitis. Inflammatory infiltrates in the ciliary body may show clusters of epithelioid cells characteristic of the disease.

It is of interest that the inflammatory infiltrates of sympathetic ophthalmia bear a strong resemblance to those seen in the Vogt-Koyanagi-Harada syndrome (VKH). The syndrome is a chronic bilateral granulomatous uveitis affecting mainly Orientals and other dark-skinned peoples. It is characterized by a cyclical or sometimes unremitting course that may eventually produce blindness. Depigmentation of the skin, eyelashes, and scalp hair may occur in the later stages of the disease, while acoustic nerve dysfunction, headache, and other signs of meningeal irritation may occur in the early stages. These same signs and symptoms may occur in sympathetic ophthalmia. The principal differences between the two diseases appear to be as follows: (1) Sympathetic ophthalmia is always associated with penetrating trauma to the eye. (2) Pronounced alteration of the retina with scarring, perhaps associated with prolonged serous detachment of the retina is regularly seen in VKH but not in sympathetic ophthalmia. (3) Pigment migration into the inner layers of the retina is frequently seen in VKH but not in sympathetic ophthalmia. (4) Plasma cell infiltration is frequently seen in VKH but not in sympathetic ophthalmia.

The etiology of both diseases remains obscure, although they have been intensely studied in recent years. Char and associates [125] recently found evidence of increased cellular reactivity to crude ocular antigens in both diseases, while Uthoff [126] el al. showed that only VKH patients showed evidence of hyperreactivity to both uveoretinal antigens and brain tissue antigens. Multiple studies [127, 128, 129] have implicated S-antigen, a soluble antigen derived from the outer segments of the photoreceptors in the causation of sympathetic ophthalmia. It appears that patients with sympathetic ophthalmia show exaggerated cell-mediated responses to this antigen when their lymphocytes are maintained in tissue culture in the presence of minute quantities of it. If this is the case, it is not clear how the antigen, which is mainly found in the posterior structures of the eye, could be released by perforating injuries of the globe, the majority of which are anterior in location.

Nevertheless, animal studies performed by Wacker [127] and others indicate that when purified S-antigen is administered to experimental animals in specific small doses, along with complete Freund's adjuvants, a disease very similar to sympathetic ophthalmia in both its clinical and histologic aspects is produced. It should be emphasized that the experimentally produced disease is *low-dose specific*, other forms of uveitis being produced by higher doses of S-antigen.

It is also of interest that the experimental disease can be produced much more readily in certain strains of rats (such as the Lewis strain) than in others, suggesting a genetic predisposition. If experimental studies on animals can be extended by analogy to humans, we might also gain additional understanding of the fact that so few patients develop sympathetic ophthalmia after penetrating trauma. Perhaps the disease only develops in individuals of a certain immunogenetic background. In this connection, Azen et al. [130] have found that a high percentage of patients suffering from sympathetic ophthalmia possess the HLA type A-11.

Rao et al. [131] have shown that S-antigen injected into the vitreous body of rabbit's eye will not cause chronic uveitis, whereas a subconjunctival injection of the same antigen will do so. They suggest that the route of antigen administration is important, for the internal eye has no lymphatics, while the subconjunctival space is drained by local lymph nodes capable of processing an injected antigen. By analogy, penetrating trauma to the human eye would cause a spillage of uveal antigens into the subconjunctival space and thus provide for the initial sensitization to the exposed antigens.

To explain the fact that S-antigens, though absent from the anterior ocular structures, may nevertheless play a role in sympathetic ophthalmia, Jakobiec [121] proposes that sympathetic ophthalmia represents a cell-mediated response to surface antigens shared by the membranes of photoreceptors, retinal pigmented epithelial cells, and choroidal melanocytes, all of which, incidentally, are derived from common neuroectodermal origins. Similarly the common appearance of phakoanaphylaxis in sympathetic ophthalmia "may also have an embryologic underpinning with shared antigens, in view of the induction of the lens by the neuroectodermal optic cup."

Another theory for the origin of sympathetic ophthalmia proposes that is infectious in origin. Ikui et al. [132] reported the presence of a presumptive virus in ultra-thin sections of such eyes. This theory remains unconfirmed, although the possibility of an infectious origin cannot be ruled out.

TREATMENT. Every penetrating injury is recognized as a possible source of sympathetic ophthalmia. If an injured eye is both blind (no light perception) and persistently painful, it is generally agreed that it should be removed, preferably before two weeks have elapsed. The question of whether the exciting eye should be removed once sympathetic ophthalmia has developed has been much debated. Winter [133] had stated that at an arbitrary point 90 days after the onset of symptoms in the sympathizing eye, enucleation of the exciting eye made no difference as to the final visual outcome in the sympathizing eye. Lubin et al. [134], however, showed that if the exciting eye were removed within two weeks of the onset of symptoms in the sympathizing eye, the visual prognosis for the sympathizing eye was far better, particularly with the adjunctive use of corticosteroid therapy. This is a view shared by Kraus-Mackiw [135] but disputed by Marak [136].

Although many cases of sympathetic ophthalmia are symptomatically improved by the use of systemically administered corticosteroids, the disease is difficult, if not impossible, to eradicate by this means. The long-term use of corticosteroids, even in the best of hands, is fraught, moreover, with multiple undesirable side-effects, particularly in children. Recent advances in the use of cytotoxic immunosuppressive drugs [137] and in the use of selective anti-T-cell agents such as cyclosporine [138] indicate that improved therapeutic results with fewer undesirable side effects can be achieved.

LENS-INDUCED UVEITIS

Although the crystalline lens, under normal conditions is neither toxic nor autoantigenic, a number of intraocular inflammations may arise from circumstances that result in an abnormal exposure of the central lymphoreticular organs to lens materials. These inflammations are referred to collectively as lens-induced uveitis. They include a number of special variants such as phakolytic glaucoma, granulomatous lens-induced uveitis, and phakoanaphylactic uveitis, which may be distinguished from one another by the peculiar histological picture that characterizes each of them. The term *phakoanaphylaxis* has generally been abandoned because there is nothing in the reaction that is anaphylactoid. That is to say, the condition is not abrupt in onset; it is not IgE-mediated; and it appears to have nothing to do with classical type I immunological reactions such as hay fever conjunctivitis.

PATHOGENESIS. Although the lens is surrounded by a capsule of very limited permeability, it is now known that small amounts of lens proteins may leak through the lens capsule throughout life. Lens proteins are therefore no longer thought of as completely "sequestered" antigens; and in fact, as the permeability of the lens capsule increases in later life, considerable amounts of lens proteins may leak into the internal milieu of the eye. Such proteins may then gain access to venous channels such as the episcleral venous plexus, and ultimately they might be processed

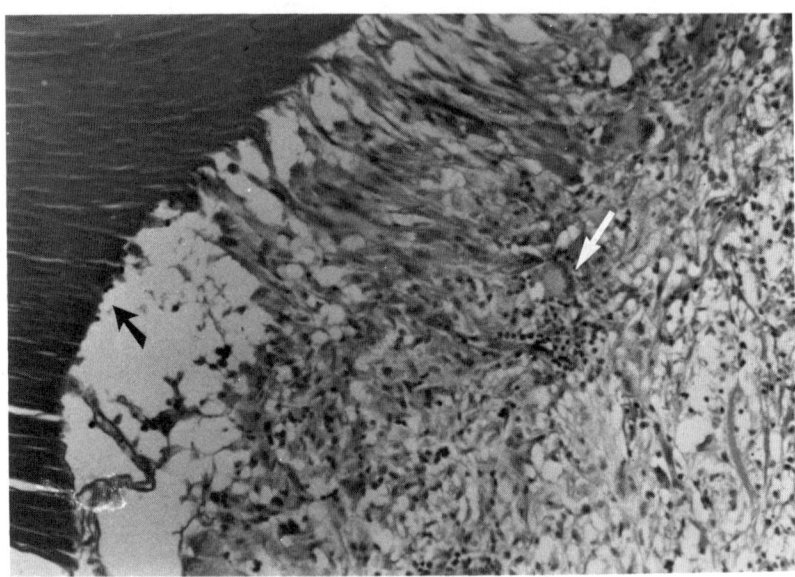

FIG. 7-7 Granulomatous reaction in lens-induced uveitis. *Black arrow* denotes edge of degenerated mass of lens fibers. *White arrow* denotes giant cell. (H. & E. × 44.)

as any other intravenously injected antigen. The finding that lens proteins normally initiate very little immunologic reaction is attributed to two factors: (1) Such substances are not normally very antigenic, and (2) the body builds up a "low zone tolerance" [139] to them, provided that they are continuously fed into the system in low doses. When, however, large amounts of lens proteins are released into the eye or gain access to the subconjunctival spaces, as from traumatic rupture of the lens capsule or from extra-capsular cataract extraction with retention of large amounts of cortical material, lens-induced uveitis may result.

The clinical picture may take one of a number of different forms, as described by Müller-Hermelink [140]. According to him, type I inflammations consist of simple foreign body reactions with macrophages in abundance at the site of rupture of the lens capsule. Foreign body giant cells may also appear. This type of reaction may or may not be accompanied by a nongranulomatous anterior uveitis. The acute inflammatory reaction subsides within several weeks and a fibrous scar forms in the defect of the lens capsule. Type II reactions, formerly referred to as phakoanaphylactic endophthalmitis had been described by Verhoeff and Lemoine [141] in 1922. Subcortically, in the lens nucleus, polymorphonuclear leukocytes and debris are seen. Peripheral to these cells palisading macrophages and multinucleated giant cells can be identified (Fig. 7-7). The outer most layer consists of lymphocytes, plasma cells, and macrophages. The iris and ciliary body are infiltrated with lymphocytes and plasma cells, but only rarely does the process involve the pars plana or the choroid.

The immunologic reaction appears to be of the Arthus type. It is antibody-mediated and complement-dependent, according to Marak [142]. The disease has a sympathizing tendency; i.e., certain individuals are prone to develop inflammatory disease of the other eye. This happens most often in aging individuals whose lens capsule (in the healthy eye) begins to leak large amounts of lens proteins in the later decades of life. In this way, the lens appears to be both inductor and target of an immunologically induced inflammation. Marak [143] has been able to show that serum factors, presumably antibodies or soluble immune complexes are of great importance in the induction of the inflammation, since the disease can be produced in healthy rats by passive transfer of serum. The presence of polymorphonuclear leukocytes in the lesion, which is the sine qua non of this lesion also speaks for the presence of immune complexes in the lesion. Marak [144] has recently been able to show the importance of oxidative metabolites, namely peroxides and superoxides in the destructive phases of these lesions, and these products are liberated principally by polymorphonuclear leukocytes.

Participation of delayed hypersensitivity in type II reactions has not been so conclusively demonstrated, although Verhoeff and Lemoine reported positive skin-tests to lens antigens and Hammer and Olah [145] reported positive lymphocytoblast transformation tests in individuals with this type of inflammation.

Type III lesions are classed by Müller-Hermelink as granulomatous lens-induced uveitis. The main features of such lesions are tumor-like thickenings of the iris and ciliary body, which, on microscopic examination, show multiple clusters of epithelioid cells, most prominent in the immediate area of the lens remnants. Plasma cells and lymphocytes are seen in areas remote from the damaged lens. The plasma cells appear to be producing a mixture of IgG and IgA, according to Müller-Hermelink [140].

Phakolytic glaucoma is designated as a type IV reaction by Müller-Hermelink, although he freely admits that some features of this disease may be encountered in other types of lens-induced inflammation. Clusters of macrophages loaded with phagocytized lens material are characteristic of this form of the inflammation. These clusters form cohesive precipitates on the corneal endothelium and may also clog the trabecular meshwork giving rise to severe glaucoma. Phakolytic glaucoma may occur as a result of lens damage from penetrating injury or as a result of spontaneous capsule rupture in various types of complicated cataracts. Occasionally the features of phakolytic glaucoma overlap those of the type II reactions. In both conditions keratic precipitates may be seen on the corneal endothelium and macrophages laden with lens material may block the trabecular spaces.

Type V and type VI reactions will be described only briefly. The former consists of scars in the injured eye, giving indications of a previous acute or chronic inflammation but providing no clue as to the responsible mechanisms. Type VI inflammations consist of lens injuries complicated by infection. Such lesions may occur as a result of direct spread of infection from the vitreous in cases of bacterial endophthalmitis, or the lens lesions may be caused by the penetration of an infected foreign body. Occasionally, lesions of this type, which are virtually abscesses of the lens, may be confused with type II reactions. In both cases, enormous numbers of polymorphonuclear leukocytes are present in the lens. Examination of a MacCallum-stained section for bacteria, however, will generally allow the careful observer to make the distinction. Endogenous septicemic involvement of the lens may be seen in immunologically compromised patients; Müller-Hermelink [140] records one interesting case of Aspergillus infection of the lens in a patient who developed Aspergillus fungemia following the treatment of acute leukemia by cytostatic agents.

It is of interest that Müller-Hermelink [146] and Kraus-Mackiw have reproduced in rats all of the six forms of lens-induced uveitis observed by them in human autopsy specimens or enucleated eyes. For example, type III lesions (granulomatous lens-induced uveitis) have been produced in rats by performing lens discission and an iridotomy. It is of further interest that these lesions could be produced in only four of the 50 rats on which they operated. Furthermore, different strains of rats appeared to be prone to develop different kinds of lens-induced inflammation, indicating that immunogenetic factors might play a role in the type of inflammation that developed after a given stimulus. This may have some bearing on the fact that many individuals following lens trauma develop no inflammation at all, whereas others develop severe bilateral disease. Discission and needling of congenital cataracts was an accepted form of surgical therapy for many years, and relatively few cases of lens-induced uveitis developed from this procedure. Thus the age of the individual, the type of cataract he has developed, and his genetic background may all represent significant factors in his disease.

TREATMENT. Although the use of topically applied or systemically administered corticosteroids may mitigate lens-induced uveitis, surgical removal of damaged lenses or of lens remnants is essential for the cure of such conditions. Several cases of lens-induced uveitis have recently been seen in patients who have undergone extracapsular cataract extraction and pseudophakos implantation in the second of two eyes. Operation on the first eye may have sensitized the patient, but no inflammation was seen in this eye. Severe, intractable inflammation developed in the second eye several weeks after a seemingly identical operation was performed on it. The inflammation produced large granulomatous keratic precipitates composed of macrophages laden with lens material. Cure was produced only by performing vitrectomy on the second eye with removal of the residual cortical lens remnants.

Another patient of interest developed a sympathizing uveitis in his left eye 50 years after blunt, nonpenetrating injury to his right eye. The right eye, blind and intermittently painful, showed evidence of acute and chronic inflammation with a completely opaque cataract and seclusion of the pupil. The patient agreed to enucleation of his right eye, which showed a type II reaction on histologic examination (Fig. 7-7). Following operation, the inflammation in his left eye, which had consisted mainly of a mild nongranulomatous iridocyclitis, promptly remitted and has not recurred.

REFERENCES

1. Movat, H. Z. Tissue injury and inflammation induced by immune complexes: the critical role of the neutrophilic leukocyte. *Exp. Mol. Pathol.* 31:201, 1979.
2. Egido, J., et al. Evidence of an immediate hypersensitivity mechanism in systemic lupus erythematosus. *Ann. Rheum. Dis.* 39:312, 1980.
3. De Kozak, Y., et al. Evidence for immediate hypersensitivity phenomena in experimental autoimmune uveoretinitis. *Eur. J. Immunol.* 11:612, 1981.
4. Theodore, R. H., and Lewson, A. C. Bilateral iritis complicating serum sickness. *Arch. Ophthalmol.* 21:828, 1939.
5. Iga, R. Ueber Herdreaktionen an den unberührten Augen nach parenteraler Zufuhr von artfremden *Serum. Klin. Monatsbl. Augenheilkd.* 84:449, 1930.
6. Wong, V. G., Anderson, R. R., and McMaster, P. R. B. Endogenous immune uveitis. *Arch. Ophthalmol.* 85:93, 1971.
7. Niblack, G. D., et al. Antilymphocyte serum for preventing graft rejection. *Proc. Clin. Dial. Transplant. Forum* 10:160, 1980.
8. Hughes, G. R. V., and Lachman, P. J. Systemic lupus erythematosus. In P. G. H. Gell, R. R. A. Coombs, and P. J. Lachmann (Eds.), *Clinical Aspects of Immunology* (3rd ed.). Oxford: Blackwell, 1975. P. 1132.
9. Gershon, R. K. Suppressor T cell dysfunction as a possible cause for autoimmunity. In N. Talal (Ed.), *Autoimmunity.* New York, Academic, 1977. P. 171.
10. Theofilopoulos, A. N., et al. Splenic immunoglobulin-secreting cells and their regulation in autoimmune mice. *J. Exp. Med.* 151:446, 1980.
11. Ziff, M. Viruses and the connective tissue diseases. *Ann. Intern. Med.* 75:951, 1971.
12. Del Giacco, G. S. Antilymphocyte antibodies and diseases. In M. Ricci, A. S. Fauci, et al. (Eds.), *Developments in Clinical Immunology.* London: Academic, 1978. P. 136.
13. Kaufman, D. B. Natural killer augmentation in systemic lupus erythematosus via a soluble mediator derived from human lymphocytes. *Arthritis Rheum.* 25:562, 1982.
14. Estes, D., and Christian, C. L. The natural history of systemic lupus erythematosus by prospective analysis. *Medicine* 50:85, 1971.
15. Howie, J. B., and Helier, B. J. The immunology and pathology of NZB mice. *Adv. Immunol.* 9:215, 1968.
16. Leonhart, T. Family studies in systemic lupus erythematosus. *Clin. Exp. Immunol.* 2:743, 1967.
17. Grumet, R. C., et al. Histocompatibility (HL-A) antigens associated with systemic lupus erythematosus. A possible genetic predisposition to the disease. *N. Engl. J. Med.* 285:193, 1971.
18. Statsny, P. The distribution of HL-A antigens in black patients with SLE. *Arthritis Rheum.* 15:455, 1972.
19. Gueft, B., and Laufer, A. Further cytochemical studies on systemic lupus erythematosus. *Arch. Pathol.* 57:201, 1954.

20. Aronson, A. J., et al. Immune complex deposition in the eye in systemic lupus erythematosus. *Arch. Int. Med.* 139:1312, 1979.
21. Lessell, S. J. Some ophthalmological and neurological aspects of systemic lupus erythematosus. *J. Rheumatol.* 7:398, 1980.
22. Gold, D. H., Morris, D. A., and Henkind, P. Ocular findings in systemic lupus erythematosus. *Br. J. Ophthalmol.* 56:800, 1972.
23. Halmay, O., and Ludwig, K. Bilateral band-shaped deep keratitis and iridocyclitis in systemic lupus erythematosus. *Br. J. Ophthalmol.* 48:558, 1964.
24. Böke, W., and Baumer, A. Klinische und histopathologische Augenbefunde beim akuten Lupus erythematodes disseminatus. *Klin. Monatsbl. Augenheilkd.* 146:175, 1965.
25. Hayslett, J. P., et al. The effect of azathioprine on lupus glomerulonephritis. *Medicine* 51:393, 1972.
26. Stevens, M. B., et al. Management of systemic lupus erythematosus. *Bull. Rheum. Dis.* 32:35, 1982.
27. Wong, K., et al. Visual loss as the initial symptom of systemic lupus erythematosus. *Am. J. Ophthalmol.* 92:238, 1981.
28. Gyorkey, F., et al. Systemic lupus erythematosus and myxovirus. *N. Engl. J. Med.* 280:333, 1969.
29. Grayson, M. *Diseases of the Cornea.* St. Louis: Mosby, 1979. P. 314.
30. Behçet, H. Ueber rezivierrende Aphthose, durch ein Virus verursachte Geschwüre am Mund, am Auge, und an den Genitalien. *Dermatol. Wochenschr.* 105:1152, 1937.
31. Sezer, N. The isolation of a virus as a cause of Behçet's disease. *Am. J. Ophthalmol.* 35:301, 1953.
32. Char, D. H. *Immunology of Uveitis and Ocular Tumors.* New York: Grune & Stratton, 1978. P. 30.
33. Ohno, S., et al. Specific histocompatibility antigens associated with Behçet's disease. *Am. J. Ophthalmol.* 80:636, 1975.
34. Campinchi, R., Bloch-Michel, E., and Faure, J. P. L'uvéite-aspects cliniques. *Trans. XIII Intl. Congr. Ophthalmol.* 1:95, 1979.
35. Lehner, T., et al. An immunogenetic basis for the tissue involvement in Behçet's syndrome. *Immunology* 37:895, 1979.
36. Ibid.
37. Lehner, T. Characterization of mucosal antibodies in recurrent aphthous ulceration and Behçet's syndrome. *Arch. Oral Biol.* 14:843, 1969.
38. O'Connor, G. R. Behçet's disease. In E. A. Klein (Ed.), *Symposium on Medical and Surgical Diseases of the Retina and Vitreous.* St. Louis: Mosby, 1983. P. 199.
39. Berman, L., and Trappler, B. Behçet's syndrome: family study and elucidation of a genetic role. *Ann. Rheum. Dis.* 38:118, 1979.
40. Shimada, K., Yaoita, H., and Shikano, S. Chemotactic activity in aqueous humor of patients with Behçet's disease. *Jpn. J. Ophthalmol.* 16:84, 1972.
41. Williams, B. D., and Lehner, T. Immune complexes in Behçet's syndrome and recurrent oral ulcerations. *Br. Med. J.* 1:1387, 1977.
42. Shimada, K., et al. Reduction of complement in Behçet's disease and drug allergy. *Med. Biol.* 52:234, 1974.
43. Maciejewski, W., and Bandmann, H. J. Immune complex vasculitis in a patient with Behçet's syndrome. *Arch. Dermatol. Res.* 264:253, 1979.
44. Gamble, C. N., et al. Immune complex pathogenesis of glomerulonephritis and pulmonary vasculitis in Behçet's disease. *Am. J. Med.* 66:1031, 1979.
45. Graisely, B., et al. Maladie de Behçet. Immuns complexes circulants et

anomalies du chemotactism des polynucleaires chemotaxis. *Nouv. Presse Med.* 8:867, 1979.
46. Burton-Kee, J. E., et al. Different cross-reacting circulating immune complexes in Behçet's syndrome and recurrent oral ulcers. *J. Lab. Clin. Med.* 97:559, 1981.
47. Lehner, T., and Adinolfi, M. Acute phase proteins, C9, factor B, and Lysozyme in recurrent oral ulceration and Behçet's syndrome. *J. Clin. Pathol.* 33:269, 1980.
48. Godfrey, W. A., et al. The use of chlorambucil in intractable idiopathic uveitis. *Am. J. Ophthalmol.* 78:415, 1974.
49. Yamana, S., et al. Long term observation of patients with Behçet's disease treated with colchicine. In G. Inaba (Ed.), *International Conference on Behçet's Disease. Pathogenetic Mechanisms and Clinical Future.* Tokyo: Univ. of Tokyo, 1981. P. 585.
50. Marquardt, J. L., et al. Depression of lymphocyte transformation and exacerbation of Behçet's syndrome by ingestion of English walnuts. *Cell. Immunol.* 9:263, 1973.
51. Woods, A. C. *Endogenous Inflammations of the Uveal Tract.* Baltimore: Williams & Wilkins, 1961.
52. Sorsby, A., and Gormaz, A. Iritis in the rheumatic affections. *Br. Med. J.* 1:597, 1946.
53. Blagojevic, M., et al. Aspects clinique et immunitaire des uveites rheumatismales. *Bull. Soc. Ophthalmol. Fr.* 83:71, 1970.
54. Kimura, S. J., et al. Uveitis and joint diseases: clinical findings in 191 cases. *Arch. Ophthalmol.* 77:309, 1967.
55. Calabro, J. J., et al. Chronic iridocyclitis in juvenile rheumatoid arthritis. *Arthritis Rheum.* 13:554, 1975.
56. Spalter, H. F. The visual prognosis in juvenile rheumatoid arthritis. *Trans. Am. Ophthalmol. Soc.* 73:554, 1975.
57. Smiley, W. K. The eye in juvenile rheumatoid arthritis. *Trans. Ophthalmol. Soc. U. K.* 94:817, 1974.
58. Hinzpater, E. N., Naumann, G., and Bartelhaimer, H. K. Ocular histopathology in Still's disease. *Ophthal. Res.* 2:16, 1971.
59. Sabates, R., Smith, T., and Apple, D. Ocular histopathology in juvenile rheumatoid arthritis. *Ann. Ophthalmol.* 11:733, 1979.
60. Moore, T., et al. Hidden rheumatoid factor in seronegative juvenile rheumatoid arthritis. *Ann. Rheum. Dis.* 33:255, 1974.
61. Schaller, J. G., et al. The association of anti-nuclear antibodies with the chronic iridocyclitis of juvenile rheumatoid arthritis. *Arthritis Rheum.* 17:409, 1974.
62. Schiavetti, L., et al. On the heterogeneity of HLA association in juvenile rheumatoid arthritis. *Arthritis Rheum.* 24:1216, 1981.
63. Glass, D., et al. Early onset pauciarticular juvenile rheumatoid arthritis associated with HLA DRW5, iritis, and antinuclear antibody. *J. Clin. Invest.* 66:426, 1980.
64. Stastny, P., and Fink, C. W. Different HLA-D associations in adult and juvenile rheumatoid arthritis. *J. Clin. Invest.* 63:124, 1979.
65. Powell, R. H., and Ansell, B. M. Benorylate in the management of Still's disease. *Br. Med. J.* 1:145, 1974.
66. Ansell, B. M. Ibuprofen in the management of Still's disease. *Practitioner* 211:659, 1974.

67. Brewer, E. J., et al. Aspirin and fenoprofen (Nalfon) in the treatment of juvenile rheumatoid arthritis. Results of the double-blind trial. A segment I study. *J. Rheumatol.* 9:123, 1982.
68. Giannini, E. H., et al. Auranofin in the treatment of juvenile rheumatoid arthritis. *J. Pediatr.* 102:138, 1983.
69. Ebringer, R., and Cawdell, D. *Klebsiella pneumoniae* and acute anterior uveitis in ankylosing spondylitis. *Br. Med. J.* 1:383, 1979.
70. Slansky, H., Bronstein, M., and Gartner, S. Ciliary body cysts in multiple myeloma. *Arch. Ophthalmol.* 76:686, 1966.
71. Johnson, B. Proteinaceous cysts of the ciliary epithelium. II. Their occurrence in nonmyelomatous hypergammaglobulinemic conditions. *Arch. Ophthalmol.* 84:171, 1970.
72. Fahey, J. L., Barth, W. F., and Solomon, A. Serum hyperviscosity syndrome. *J.A.M.A.* 192:464, 1965.
73. Grayson, M. *Diseases of the Cornea.* St. Louis: Mosby, 1979. P. 367.
74. Lumsden, C. E. The immunogenesis of the multiple sclerosis plaque. *Brain Res.* 28:365, 1971.
75. Berg, O., and Källen, B. Gliotoxic effect of serum from patients with neurological diseases. *Lancet* 1:1051, 1962.
76. Lessel, S., et al. Sensitivity to encephalitogenic protein in optic neuritis. *Br. J. Ophthalmol.* 54:731, 1970.
77. Millar, J. H., et al. Immunoglobulin M specific for measles and mumps in multiple sclerosis. *Br. Med. J.* 2:378, 1971.
78. Haire, M., Millar, J. H., and Merritt, J. D. Measles virus specific IgG in cerebrospinal fluid of multiple sclerosis. *Br. Med. J.* 4:192, 1974.
79. Paty, D. W., et al. HLA in multiple sclerosis—relationship to measles antibody, mitogen responsiveness, and clinical course. *J. Neurol. Sci.* 32:371, 1977.
80. Haile, R. W., et al. Genetic susceptibility to multiple sclerosis: a review. *Int. J. Epidemiol.* 12:8, 1983.
81. Breger, B. C., and Leopold, I. H. The incidence of uveitis in multiple sclerosis. *Am. J. Ophthalmol.* 62:540, 1966.
82. Porter, R. Uveitis in association with multiple sclerosis. *Br. J. Ophthalmol.* 56:478, 1972.
83. Rahi, A. H. S., and Garner, A. Immunopathology of the Eye. Oxford: Blackwell, 1976. P. 234.
84. Wickremesinghe, H. R., and Yates, P. O. Immunological properties of normal tissues. *J. Neurol. Sci.* 15:225, 1972.
85. Snyder, D. A., Tessler, H. H., and Yokoyama, M. M. Immunologic studies on Vogt-Koyanagi-Harada syndrome and pars plantitis. In A. M. Silverstein and G. R. O'Connor (Eds.), *Immunology and Immunopathology of the Eye.* New York: Masson, 1979. P. 71.
86. Curless, R. G., and Bray, P. F. Uveitis and multiple sclerosis in an adolescent. *Am. J. Dis. Child.* 123:149, 1972.
87. Smith, R., Godfrey, W., and Kimura, S. Chronic cyclitis. I. Course and visual prognosis. *Trans. Am. Acad. Ophthalmol. Otolaryngol.* 77:760, 1973.
88. Bowden, A. N., et al. A trial of corticotropin gelatin injection in acute optic neuritis. *J. Neurol. Neurosurg. Psychiatry* 37:869, 1974.
89. Fischer, B. H., et al. Hyperbaric oxygen treatment of multiple sclerosis. A randomized, placebo-controlled, double-blind study. *N. Engl. J. Med.* 308:18, 1983.
90. Hauser, S. L., et al. Intensive immuno-suppression in multiple sclerosis. A

randomized, three-arm study of high-dose intravenous cyclophosphamide, plasma exchange, and ACTH. *N. Engl. J. Med.* 308:173, 1983.
91. Rahi, A. H. S., and Garner, A. *Immunopathology of the Eye.* Oxford: Blackwell, 1976. P. 304.
92. Hazleman, B. L., MacLennan, I. C. M., and Esiri, M. M. Lymphocyte proliferation to artery antigen as a possible diagnostic test in polymyalgia rheumatica. *Ann. Rheum. Dis.* 34:122, 1975.
93. Paronetto, F., and Strauss, L. Immunocytochemical observations in periarteritis nodosa. *Ann. Intern. Med.* 56:289, 1962.
94. Gocke, D. J., Hsu, K., Morgan, C., et al. Vasculitis in association with Australia antigen. *J. Exp. Med.* 134:330, 1971.
95. Jansson, E., et al. Isolation of mycoplasma from sarcoid tissue. *J. Clin. Pathol.* 25:837, 1972.
96. Byrne, E. B., et al. Serological hyperreactivity to Epstein-Barr virus and other viral antigens in sarcoidosis. In K. Iwai and Y. Hosada (Eds.), *Proceedings of the Sixth International Conference on Sarcoidosis.* Baltimore: University Park, 1974. P. 218.
97. Barth, C. L., et al. Isolation of an acid-fast organism from the aqueous humor in a case of sarcoidosis. *Henry Ford Hospital Med. J.* 27:127, 1979.
98. Hedfors, E., and Norberg, R. Evidence for circulating immune complexes in sarcoidosis. *Clin. Exp. Immunol.* 16:493, 1974.
99. Antonaci, S., et al. Natural and antibody-dependent cellular cytotoxicity in patients with active sarcoidosis. *Allergol Immunopathol.* 11:40, 1983.
100. Lenzini, L., et al. Test d'inhibition de migration leukocytaire en sarcoidose. *Nouv. Presse Med.* 2:2751, 1973.
101. Jones-Williams, et al. The Kmif (Kveim induced macrophage migration inhibition factor) test in sarcoidosis. *J. Clin. Pathol.* 25:951, 1972.
102. Kimura, R. Hyperfluorescent dots in the ciliary body band in patients with granulomatous uveitis. *Br. J. Ophthalmol.* 66:322, 1982.
103. Gass, J. D. M., and Olson, C. L. Sarcoidosis with optic nerve and retinal involvement: a clinicopathologic case report. *Trans. Am. Acad. Ophthalmol. Otolaryngol.* 77:739, 1973.
104. Gould, H., and Kaufman, H. E. Sarcoid of the fundus. *Arch. Ophthalmol.* 65:454, 1961.
105. Lauver, J. W., and Gooneratne, N. S. Lacrimal, parotid, and mediastinal uptake of gallium 67 in sarcoidosis. *Br. J. Radiol.* 52:582, 1978.
106. Harter, J. G., Reddy, W. J., and Thorn, G. W. Studies on an intermittent corticosteroid dosage regimen. *N. Engl. J. Med.* 269:591, 1963.
107. Fauci, A. S. Alternate-day corticosteroid therapy. *Am. J. Med.* 64:729, 1978.
108. Gottlieb, M. S. *Pneumocystis carinii* pneumonia and mucosal candidiasis in previously healthy homosexual men. Evidence of a new acquired cellular immunodeficiency. *N. Engl. J. Med.* 305:1424, 1981.
109. Holland, G. N., et al. Ocular disorders associated with a new severe acquired cellular immunodeficiency syndrome. *Am. J. Ophthalmol.* 93:393, 1982.
110. Freeman, W. R., et al. A prospective study of the ophthalmological findings in the acquired immune deficiency syndrome. *Am. J. Ophthalmol.* 97:133, 1984.
111. Kwok, S., et al. Retinal cotton-wool spots in a patient with *Pneumocystis carinii* infection. *N. Engl. J. Med.* 307:104, 1982.
112. Pepose, J. S., et al. An analysis of retinal cotton-wool spots and cytomegalovirus retinitis in the acquired immunodeficiency syndrome. *Am. J. Ophthalmol.* 95:118, 1983.

113. Newman, N. M., et al. Clinical and histologic findings in opportunistic ocular infections. Part of a new syndrome of acquired immunodeficiency. *Arch. Ophthalmol.* 101:396, 1983.
114. Holland, G. N., et al. Acquired immune deficiency syndrome. Ocular manifestations. *Ophthalmology* 90:859, 1983.
115. Schuman, J. S. Ocular effects in the acquired immune deficiency syndrome. *Mt. Sinai J. Med.* 50:443, 1983.
116. Barré-Sinoussi, F., et al. Isolation of a T-lymphotropic retrovirus from a patient at risk for acquired immune deficiency syndrome. *Science* 220:868, 1983.
117. Gallo, R. C., et al. Isolation of human T-cell leukemia virus in acquired immune deficiency syndrome (AIDS). *Science* 220:865, 1983.
118. Sonnabend, J. A., et al. Acquired immunodeficiency syndrome, opportunistic infections, and malignancies in male homosexuals. A hypothesis of etiologic factors in pathogenesis. *J.A.M.A.* 249:2370, 1983.
119. Kraus-Mackiw, E. Exogenous uveitis: Sympathetic uveitis. In E. Kraus-Mackiw and G. R. O'Connor (Eds.), *Uveitis: Pathophysiology and Therapy*. New York: Thieme-Stratton, 1983.
120. Spitznas, M. Fluoreszenzangiographie der sympatischen Ophthalmie. *Klin. Mbl. Augenheilk.* 169:195, 1976.
121. Jakobiec, F. A., et al. Human sympathetic ophthalmia. An analysis of the inflammatory infiltrates by hybridomamonoclonal antibodies, immunochemistry, and correlative electron microscopy. *Ophthalmology* 90:76, 1983.
122. Ishikawa, T., and Ikui, H. The fine structure of the Dalén-Fuchs nodule in sympathetic ophthalmia. Report 1. Changes of the pigment epithelial cells within the Dalén-Fuchs nodule. *Jap. J. Ophthalmol.* 16:254, 1972.
123. Font, R. L., and Fine, B. S. Light and electron microscopic study of Dalén-Fuchs nodules in sympathetic ophthalmia. *Invest. Ophthalmol.* 14:(Suppl. ARVO Abstracts) 24, 1975.
124. Müller-Hermelink, H. K. Recent topics in the pathology of uveitis. In E. Kraus-Mackiw and G. R. O'Connor (Eds.), *Uveitis: Pathophysiology and Therapy*. New York: Thieme-Stratton, 1983. P. 177.
125. Char, D. H. Vogt-Koyanagi-Harada syndrome and sympathetic ophthalmia: clinical and immunologic characteristics. In R. J. Helmsen, A. Suran, I. Gery, and R. B. Nussenblatt (Eds.), *Immunology of the Eye, Workshop II*. Washington: Information Retrieval, 1981. P. 67.
126. Uthoff, D., et al. Vogt-Koyanagi-Harada Syndrome. Ein Beitrag zur Frage der Immunopathogenese. *Albrecht v. Graefes Arch. Klin. Exp. Ophthalmol.* 210:251, 1979.
127. Wacker, W. B., et al. Experimental Sympathetic Ophthalmia. In A. M. Silverstein and G. R. O'Connor (Eds.), *Immunology and Immunopathology of the Eye*. New York: Masson, 1979. P. 121.
128. Nussenblatt, R. B., et al. Cellular immune responsiveness of uveitis patients to retinal S-antigen. *Am. J. Ophthalmol.* 89:173, 1980.
129. Marak, G. E. Recent advances in sympathetic ophthalmia. *Surv. Ophthalmol.* 24:141, 1979.
130. Azen, S. P., et al. Histocompatibility antigens in sympathetic ophthalmia. *Am. J. Ophthalmol.* 98:117, 1984.
131. Rao, N. A., et al. Role of penetrating wound in development of sympathetic ophthalmia. 101:102, 1983.
132. Ikui, H., et al. Electron microscopic study of ultrathin sections of sympathetic ophthalmia (preliminary report) *Jpn. J. Ophthalmol.* 2:13, 1958.

133. Winter, F. C. Sympathetic uveitis. A clinical and pathological study of the visual result. *Am. J. Ophthalmol.* 39:340, 1955.
134. Lubin, J. R., et al. Sixty-five years of sympathetic ophthalmia. A clinicopathologic review of 105 cases (1913–1978). *Ophthalmology* 89:109, 1980.
135. Kraus-Mackiw, E. Exogenous uveitis. In E. Kraus-Mackiw and G. R. O'Connor (Eds.), *Uveitis: Pathophysiology and Therapy.* New York: Thieme-Stratton, 1983. P. 145.
136. Marak, G. E. Letter to the Editor. *Ophthalmology* 89:1291, 1982.
137. Martenet, A. C. Therapie der endogenen uveitis: immunosuppression. *Ber. Zusammenkunft Dtsch. Ophthalmol. Ges.* 78:223, 1981.
138. Nussenblatt, R. B., et al. Cyclosporin A therapy in the treatment of intraocular inflammatory disease resistant to corticosteroids and cytotoxic agents. *Am. J. Ophthalmol.* 96:275, 1983.
139. Sandberg, H. O., and Closs, O. Lens crystallins and low-zone tolerance. In A. M. Silverstein and G. R. O'Connor (Eds.), *Immunology and Immunopathology of the Eye.* New York: Masson, 1979. P. 325.
140. Müller-Hermelink, H. K. Recent topics in the pathology of uveitis. In E. Kraus-Mackiw and G. R. O'Connor (Eds.), *Uveitis: Pathophysiology and Treatment.* New York: Thieme-Stratton, 1983. P. 157.
141. Verhoeff, F. H., and Lemoine, A. N. Endophthalmitis phacoanaphylactica. *Am. J. Ophthalmol.* 5:737, 1922.
142. Marak, G. E., et al. Pathogenesis of lens-induced endophthalmitis. In A. M. Silverstein and G. R. O'Connor (Eds.), *Immunology and Immunopathology of the Eye.* New York: Masson, 1979. P. 135.
143. Marak, G. E., et al. Experimental lens-induced granulomatous endophthalmitis: Passive transfer with serum. *Ophthalmic Res.* 8:117, 1976.
144. Marak, G. E., et al. Free Radicals and Phacoanaphylaxis. In G. R. O'Connor and J. W. Chandler (Eds.), *Advances in Immunology and Immunopathology of the Eye.* New York: Masson, 1985. P. 144.
145. Hammer, H., and Olah, M. Cellular hypersensitivity to lenticular protein in lens-induced uveitis. *Albrecht v. Graefes Arch. Klin. Exp. Ophthalmol.* 192:339, 1974.
146. Müller-Hermelink, H. K., et al. Lens as Inducer and Target in Uveitis. In G. R. O'Connor and J. W. Chandler (Eds.), *Advances in Immunology and Immunopathology of the Eye.* New York: Masson, 1985. P. 155.

INDEX

Acquired immune deficiency syndrome (AIDS), 110, 125, 328–331
  pathogenesis, 330
  treatment, 330–331
Addison's disease, 72, 236
Adenovirus infection, 215
Adherent cells, 33–36
Adjuvants, 3
Adult celiac disease, 5
Agar diffusion test, 110
Aging, amyloidosis associated with, 225–226
Adrenergic receptors
  alpha, 52
  beta, 52, 141
AIDS. *See* Acquired immune deficiency syndrome (AIDS)
Allergy. *See* Anaphylactic response; Atopy
ALS (Antilymphocyte serum), 73, 292
Allogeneic antigens, 4
Allografts, 273–297
  reactions, 83
Amyloid deposits
  in palpebral conjunctiva, 226
  in the vitreous, 224
Amyloid neuropathy, 223
Amyloidosis, 221–229
  associated with aging, 225–226
  complement, 222
  Crohn's disease, 222
  heredofamilial, 223–224
    Mediterranean fever, 224
    signs, 223–224

  ocular lesions, 223
  primary localized, 226–227
    conjunctival, 226
    gelatinous droplike dystrophy, 227
    lattice dystrophy, 227
    ptosis, 227
  primary systemic, 222–223
    clinical lesions, 223
    chronic sensomotor polyneuropathy, 223
    heart failure, 223
    macroglossia, 223
  secondary localized, 228–229
    corneal opacification, 228
    corneal scarring, 228
  secondary systemic, 224–225
Anaphylactic response, 48–56, 80–81
  basophils, 49–52
  cyclic adenosine monophosphate, 52–53
  feedback inhibition, 54–55
  helper and suppressor T cells, 55–56
  HLA antigen associations, 48
  immunoglobulin A and allergy, 55
  insect bites or stings, 182
  mast cells, 49–52
  mechanisms, 48–52
  pharmacologic mediators, 53–54
  treatment, 56
Anaphylactoid response, 263–264
  treatment, 264
Anaphylatoxins, 39, 43
Anaphylaxis, 193

Anemia, pernicious, 72
Angioedema, 154
Ankylosing spondylitis, 5
Anterior chamber, 75–76
  flare and cells in, 287
Anterior uveitis, 150
Antibiotics, 73
  ointment, 206
  staphylococcal infections, 206
Antibodies
  combining with antigen, 9
  excess, 60–61
  humoral, 281, 295
  idiotypic, 295
  to nucleic acid constituents, 115–116
  production, 3
  response, 14
  structure, 7
Antibody tests, 104–129
  allergen-specific IgG, 114
  autoantibodies, 114–115
  chlamydia, 109
  chromium release test, 122
  complement components and levels, 116
  cytomegalovirus serology, 110–111
  electrophoresis, 112–113
  FTA-absorption tests, 107–109
  histoplasma serology, 110
  IgE determinations, 114
  immune complexes, 116–117
  immunoelectrophoresis, 112–113
  infectious diseases, 104–111
  indirect fluorescent, 105
  monoclonal antibodies, 124–125
  noninfectious diseases, 111–129
  nucleic acid constituents, 115–116
  products of activated lymphocytes, 122
  radial diffusion, 113–114
  rheumatoid factor, 115
  skin tests, 117–120
  tears and aqueous humor, tests on, 126–129
  toxocara, 111
  toxoplasma dye-test, 104–105
  VDRL, 107–109
Antibody-dependent cytotoxicity, 121–122
Anti-donor serum, 292
Antigens, 3–6, 274–279
  adjuvants, 3
  allogeneic, 4
  antibody complexes, 14–16
  antibody production, 3
  cell-mediated immunity, 3
  excess, 59–60
  haptens, 4
  heterologous, 4
  histocompatibility, 4, 276
  homologous, 4
  human leukocyte (HLA), 4, 276–277
  immune associated (Ia), 4, 277
  immune cytotoxic reactions, 277
  immunologic tolerance, 3
  individual specific, 4
  major histocompatibility complex (MHC), 4–6
  matching histocompatibility, 295–296
  ocular tissue, 80
  organ specific, 4
  S-antigen, 334
  T-cell activation by, 21
  T-cell recognition of, 20–21
  T-independent, 30
  xenogenic, 4
Antihistamines, 142
Anti-inflammatory agents. See Nonsteroidal anti-inflammatory agents (NSAIAs)
Antilymphocyte serum (ALS), 73, 292
Aqueous humor
  aqueous/serum ratio in diagnosis, 128
  immune complexes, 128–129
  immunoglobulins, 127
Arachidonic acid metabolites, physiologic effects, 54
Arthritis, rheumatoid, 60, 72. See also Rheumatoid arthritis
Arthus reaction, 60–61, 337
Aspergillus fungemia, 338
Aspergillus sp., 218
Aspirin, 170
Asthma, 136
Ataxia telangiectasia, 172
Atopic dermatitis, 37
  cause, 171–172
  clinical features, 173–174
    skin, 173–174
  diagnostic criteria, 176
  history, 171
  interferon, 172
  ocular manifestations, 171–174
Atopic diseases, 112, 135–184
  allergens, 136–137
  diagnosis, 139
  giant papillary hypertrophy, 179–181
  hay fever, 147–157
  heredity, 135–136

immunoglobulins, 112
incidence, 135–136
keratoconjunctivitis, 174–179
ocular considerations, 145–184
  allergen exposure, 145–146
  sensitization, 146–147
onset, 135–136
radioallergosorbent test, 138
specific ocular diseases, 147–184
treatment, 139–145
vernal keratoconjunctivitis, 157–171
Atopic keratoconjunctivitis (AKC), 153, 174–179
atopic uveitis, 179
retinal detachment, 178
signs, 175
Atopic reactions to insect bites or stings, 181–184
treatment, 184
Atopic uveitis, 179
Atopy, 6
definition, 135
pathogenesis of sensitization, 136–137
treatment, 139–145
  antihistamines, 142
  avoidance of exposure, 140–141
  corticosteroids, 143–144
  immunotherapy, 144–145
  interferon, 144
  levamisole, 144
  psychotherapy, 141
  specific drug therapy, 141–145
Auer reaction, 59
Autoantibodies, 114–115, 268
Autoimmune diseases, multiple sclerosis, 320–322
Autoimmune reactions, 57
Autoinoculation, 216

Bacterial infections, 202–209
  ligneous conjunctivitis, 207, 208
  membranous conjunctivitis, 207, 209
  pseudomonas, 209
  staphylococcal infections, 202–207
Basophils, 49–52, 62
B-cell differentiation factor (BCDF), 31
B-cell dysfunction, 28
  Bruton's disease, 28
B-cell growth factor (BCGF), 31
B-cell lymphoma, 68
B-cells triggered without help, 30
BCDF (B-cell differentiation factor), 31

BCGF (B-cell growth factor), 31
Behçet's disease, 312–315
  English walnuts, 315
  pathogenesis, 313–314
  treatment, 314
Benign mucous membrane pemphigoid, 257–259
Biological activity of complement, 43
Blastomycosis, 209
Blood vessels, 74–76
B-lymphocytes, 6–13
  antibody structure, 7
  homogenous myeloma proteins, 6–7
  immunoglobulin, 6
Breast cancer, 68
Bronchiectasis, 225
Bruton's disease, 28
Burkitt's lymphoma, 29
Burns, chronically infected, 225

Candida, 119
  acquired immune deficiency syndrome (AIDS), 328
  agar diffusion test, 110
  albicans, 218, 235
    phlyctenulosis, 235
  endophthalmitis, 109
  serology, 109–110
Candidiasis, 37
  esophageal, 328
Cataract, atopic, 165
Cat-scratch disease, 209
Celiac disease, adult, 5
Cell-division TSTA, 67
Cell-mediated immune response, 61–70, 83, 235–242
  impaired, 62
  infection and CMI depression, 66
  infections, 63–66
  Jones-Mote reaction, 61
  non-organ-specific diseases, 72
  nonspecific immune defenses, 64
  phlyctenulosis, 235–238
  specific immune defenses, 64
  treatment, 72–74
  tumors, 66–70
    therapy, 69–70
Cell-mediated immunity, 3
Cellular factors in inflammation, 44–45
Cervical carcinoma, 69
Chalazion, 209
Chancroid, 209
Chédiak-Higashi syndrome, 37, 38
Chemical TSTA, 66–67
Chemotaxis, 37, 40

Chlamydia, 109, 211
Chorioretinitis, 111
Choroiditis, 313
Chromium release test, 122
Chymotrypsin, 207
Cicatricial pemphigoid, 257–259
   treatment, 259
Cimetidine, 142
Circumlimbal congestion, 287
Clotting factor XII, 39
Clotting systems, 38–40
Clq binding test, 116
CMI response. See Cell-mediated immune response
Coccidioides immitis, 119, 235
Coccidioidin, 119
Coccidioidomycosis, 209
Colitis, ulcerative, 225
Collagenase inhibitor, 201
Complement, 222
   components and levels, 116
   defects, 43–44
   fixation test, 105
Complement system, 40–44
   anaphylatoxins, 43
   biologic activity of, 43
   C1 through C9, 40–44
   cytolsis, 43
   immunoconglutinins, 42
   pathway of complement activation, 40–42
   regulation, 42
Conjunctiva, 78
Conjunctival excision, 201
Conjunctival flaps, 201
Conjunctivitis, 109
   giant papillary, 180
   granulomatous, 207–208
   inclusion, 109
      chlamydia, 109
   ligneous, 207, 208
   membranous, 207, 209
Connective tissue disorders, 83
Contact dermatitis, 62–63, 83, 152, 179, 193, 238–242
   clinical features, 241
   histopathologic features, 241–242
   patch test, 239
   pathogenesis, 240–241
      prostaglandins, 241
   poison oak, 179
   treatment, 242
Contact lenses, 146
   hydrophilic, 201
   peripheral catarrhal infiltrations, 204
   scleral, 266
   staphylococcal infections, 204

Coomb's test, 58
Cornea
   acute corneal epithelial HSV keratitis, 216
   burns, 46, 219
   chronic corneal herpetic disease, 75
   ectatic, 198
   Mooren's ulcer, 196–202
   Neovascularization of, 46
   perforation in peripheral, 198
   peripheral infiltrates, 220–221
   Salzmann's nodular degeneration, 236
   Wessely ring, 219–220
Corneal allograft reaction, 193
Corneal edema, 150
Corneal epithelium, 78
Corneal graft
   clinical course of rejection, 285–291
   epithelium removal, 284, 296
   histologic features of rejection, 289–291
   immunologic mechanisms of rejection, 274–285
      antigens, 274–279
      hypersensitivity responses, 279–282
   induction of immunologic enhancement, 295
   induction of immunologic tolerance, 294–295
   intralamellar, 286
   lamellar, 284, 285
   matching histocompatibility antigens, 295–296
   penetrating, 284
   reaction, 273–297
   regrafting, 296
   rejection
      line, 283, 284
      rate, 283
      symptoms, 287
      treatment and prevention, 291–297
         anti-inflammatory agents, 295
         corticosteroids, 292–294
         donor graft, 291–292
         immunosuppressive therapy, 294
         side-effects, 296–297
         surgical maneuvers, 291
   type of graft, 285–289
Corneal immune response, 280
Corneal immune ring, 220
Corneal stromal herpes simplex, 65
Corticosteroids, 46–48, 65, 72, 143–144
   adenoviral infections, 215

chronic iridocyclitis, 317
complications of therapy, 48
contact dermatitis, 242
corneal graft rejection, 292–294
  postoperative treatment, 293
cranial arteritis, 324
disciform keratitis, 214
graft reaction treatment, 293–294
herpes simplex, 216
Mooren's ulcer, 201
multiple sclerosis, 322
sarcoidosis, 327
scleritis, 235
serum sickness, 309
side effects, 296–297
Sjögren's syndrome, 269–270
staphylococcal infections, 206
Stevens-Johnson syndrome, 265–266
sympathetic ophthalmia, 335
systemic lupus erythematosus, 312
treatment of atopy, 143
vernal keratoconjunctivitis, 170
Cotton-wool spots, 328
Counterimmunoelectrophoresis, 110
Cranial arteritis, 322–324
  pathogenesis, 323
  treatment, 324
Crohn's disease, 83, 222
Cryopreservation, 292
Cutaneous eruptions, 193
Cyclic adenosine monophosphate, 52–53
Cyclitis, 83
Cyclophosphamide, 201
Cycloplegics, iridocyclitis, 318
Cyclosporine, 74, 216
  herpes simplex, 216
Cystoid macular edema, 46, 327
Cysts, fluid-filled, 319
Cytokines, 21
Cytolysis, 43
Cytomegalovirus
  acquired immune deficiency syndrome (AIDS), 328
  ELISA test, 110–111
  retinitis, 328
  serology, 110–111
    AIDS, 110
Cytotoxic antibodies, 67
Cytotoxic reactions, 193–202
  corneal allograft reaction, 193
  Mooren's ulcer, 196–202
Cytotoxic response, 56–58, 81
  acute endocarditis, 57
  acute nephritis, 57
  Coombs' test, 58
  drug reactions, 57–58, 193–196
  quinidine, 58
  methyldopa, 58
  organ transplantation, 57
  rhesus incompatibility, 57
  systemic lupus erythematosus, 57
  transfusion reactions, 57
Cytotoxicity, antibody-dependent, 121–122
Cytotoxins, 23
  lymphotoxin, 23

Debridement, in treatment of eye infections, 216
Delimiting keratectomy, 201
Dendritic herpetic lesion, 214
Dermatitis, 43. *See also* Atopic dermatitis; Contact dermatitis
  hay fever, 136
  herpetiformis, 5
Dermatomyositis, 72, 267
Desensitization, 184
Diabetes, 37, 38, 225
Diathermy, 207
Di George's disease, 28, 55
Direct agglutination test, 105
Disciform edema, 215
Disciform keratitis, 214
Discoid lupus, 72
Down's syndrome, 37
Drug fever, 193
Drug-related reactions, 193–196
Dysfunction of T- and B-lymphocytes, 28–29
  immune deficiency disorders, 28
Dysproteinemia, 225

Echothiophate iodide, 194
Ectatic cornea, 198
Edema, 38, 40, 148
  disciform, 215
Electrophoresis, 112–113, 291
ELISA. *See* Enzyme-linked immunosorbent assay
Embryonic TSTA, 67
Endocarditis, acute, 57
Endophthalmitis
  Candida, 109
  lens induced, 83
  phakoanaphylactic, 336
Endothelial-cell metaplasia, 291
Enhanced phagocytosis, 37
Enhancement, immunologic, 295
Enucleation, 335
Enzyme-linked immunosorbent assay, 105, 106–107, 110
  cytomegalovirus, 110–111
  toxocara, 111
Eosinophils, 53–55

Epidemic keratoconjunctivitis, 152
Epinephrine, 184
Episcleritis, 229–231
  diffuse, 230
  nodular, 230, 237
Erythema multiforme, 264–265
External eye, immunologic reactions in, 193–242. *See also* Cytotoxic reactions; Immune complex-mediated reactions; Cell-mediated immune response
Extracapsular cataract extraction, 338
Eye patching, 201

Familial chemotactic defect, 37
Farmer's lung, 61
Feedback inhibition, 54–55
Fibrinolytic systems, 38
Flocculation test, 105
Focal necrotizing retinochoroiditis, 118
Folic acid, 73
Foreign body under upper lid, 154
FTA-absorption test, 108–109

Gelatinous droplike dystrophy, 227
Gentamicin, 194
Giant papillary conjunctivitis, 180
Giant papillary hypertrophy, 179–181
  treatment, 181
Glanders, 209
Glaucoma
  iridocyclitis, 318
  secondary, 318
Glomerulonephritis, 310
  acute poststreptococcal, 60
Goodpasture's syndrome, 72
Graft, corneal. *See* Corneal graft
Graft edema, 287
Granuloma formation, 316
Granulomatous conjunctivitis, 207–208
Granulomatous disease, chronic, 37, 38

Hageman factor (clotting factor XII), 39
Hansen's disease (leprosy), 28, 209, 225
Haptens, 4
Hashimoto's thyroiditis, 72, 267
Hay fever, 147–157
  atopic dermatitis, 136
  clinical features, 148–154
  diagnosis, 151–154
  history and cause, 148

radioallergosorbent test, 152
  treatment, 154–157
Heart failure, 223
Heart transplants, 281
Helper and suppressor T-cells, 55–56
Hemagglutination test, 105
Hemolytic anemias, 193, 310
Hepatitis, chronic, 5
Hepatocellular carcinoma, 69
Hereditary angioedema, 154
Herpes simplex, 65, 75, 121, 211–218, 265
  chronic corneal herpetic disease, 75
  clinical features, 213–216
  corneal stromal, 65
  dendritic lesion, 214
  interferon, 212
  keratitis, 215
    acute corneal epithelial, 216
    chronic, 284
    disciform edema, 215
  lid vesicles and ulcers, 213
  treatment, 216–218
    debridement, 216
    topical chemotherapy, 216
  uveitis, 46, 216
Herpes zoster, 125
  monoclonal antibodies, 125
Heterologous antigens, 4
Heterophil antigens, 4
Histocompatibility antigens, 4
Histoplasmin, 119
  capsulatum, 110, 119
  skin tests, 110, 119
HLA (Human leukocyte antigen), 4, 5, 6
Hodgkin's disease, 5, 28, 35, 68, 225
Homologous antigens, 4
Hordeolum, 205
Horner's points, 160
HSV. See Herpes simplex
Human leukocyte antigen (HLA), 4
  major histocompatibility complex (MHC), 4–6
Humoral antibodies, 281, 295
Hyaluronidase, 207
Hydrophilic contact lens, 201
Hyperbaric oxygen, 292
  multiple sclerosis, 322
Hyperimmunoglobulin E syndrome of Buckley, 172
Hypersensitivity responses, 48–74, 80–83, 193–202, 279–282
  anaphylactic response, 48–56, 81–82
  atopic diseases affecting the eye, 137–139

cell-mediated immune (CMI)
  response, 61–70, 83, 279
cyclic adenosine monophosphate,
  52–53
cytotoxic response, 56–58, 81, 193–
  202
delayed, 119–120
  in vitro tests for, 120–124
feedback inhibition, 54–55
helper and suppressor T cells, 55–
  56
humoral antibodies, 281
immune-complex response, 58–61,
  81–83
immunoglobulin A and allergy, 55
leukocyte migration inhibition
  (LMI), 280
migration inhibition factor (MIF),
  280
nephrotoxic nephritis, 60
pharmacologic mediators of
  anaphylaxis, 53–54
sensitization, 279
stimulatory response, 70–72
treatment, 56, 72–74
  alkylating agents, 73
  alkaloids, 74
  antibiotics, 73
  cyclosporine, 74
  folic acid, 73
  purine antagonist, 73
  pyrimidine antagonist, 73
Hypogammaglobulinemia, 225
Hypoparathyroidism, 236
Hypopyon iritis, 313
Hyposensitization, 184
Hypothyroidism, 154

Idiotypic regulation, 26–27
Ig. *See* Immunoglobulins (Ig)
Immune associated antigen (Ia), 4
Immune complexes
  in aqueous humor, 128–129
  tests for, 116–117
    Clq binding test, 116
    polyethylene glycol technique,
      117
    Raji cell technique, 117
Immune-complex mediated-reactions
  bacterial infections, 202–209
  chlamydial infections, 211
  related to infection, 202–235
  viral infections, 211–218
Immune-complex response, 58–61,
  81–83
  antibody excess, 60–61

antigen excess, 59–60
Arthus reaction, 60–61
Auer reaction, 59
Immune cytotoxic reactions, 277
Immune defenses, 64
Immune deficiency disorders, 28
  severe combined
    immunodeficiency, 28
Immune globulin. *See*
    Immunoglobulins (Ig)
Immune reaction, 3–27
  antibody response, 14
  antigens, 3–6
  B-lymphocytes, 6–11
  idiotypic regulation, 26–27
  immunoglobulins (Ig), 8–13
  monoclonal antibodies, 13–14
  T-lymphocytes, 16–26
Immune response to tumors, 67–69
  cytotoxic antibodies, 67
  interferon, 67–68
  lymphokines, 67
Immunoconglutinins, 42
Immunoelectrophoresis, 112–113
Immunoglobulin A and allergy, 55
Immunoglobulin E determinations,
  114
Immunoglobulins (Ig), 6, 8–13, 216
  allergen-specific, 114
  in aqueous humor, 127
  characteristics, 10
  evaluation of, 111–112
  syphilis, 13
Immunologic considerations, 1–74.
    See also under specific
    considerations, e.g., Phylogenic
    considerations
  immune reaction, 3–27
  antigens, 3–6
Immunologic deficiency, 120
Immunologic diseases affecting the
  eye, 255–272
Immunologic enhancement, 30
Immunologic mechanisms of
  rejection, 274–285
  factors affecting rejection, 282
Immunologic principles, 1–74
  phylogenic considerations, 1–3
Immunologic reactions in the external
  eye, 193–242
Immunologic testing
  antibody tests, 104–129
  procedures, 103–129
    general considerations, 103–104
    relationship to bodily disease, 104
    usefulness, 103–104
Immunologic tolerance, 3, 29

Immunology, ocular considerations, 74–83
Immunosuppression, 72–74, 236
  antilymphocyte serum (ALS), 73
Immunosuppressive therapy, 294
  Behçet's disease, 314
  Mooren's ulcer, 201
  side-effects, 197
  systemic lupus erythematosus, 312
Impaired cellular immunity, 55
In vitro lymphocyte transformation, 120
In vitro tests for delayed hypersensitivity, 120–124
Indirect fluorescent antibody test, 105
Individual specific antigens, 4
Infections, 63–66
  bacterial. *See* Bacterial infections
  CMI depression and, 66
  mycotic, 218
  natural killer cells, 65–66
Infectious diseases
  antibody tests, 104–111
Infectious mononucleosis, 209
Inflammation, 38–48
  acute, 152
  anti-inflammatory agents, 45–48
  cellular factors, 44–45
  complement system, 40–44
  confused with hay fever, 152–154
  Kinin, fibrinolytic and clotting systems, 38–40
  toxic or irritating substances, 152
Inflammatory bowel disease, 220
Ingested allergens, 137
Inhaled allergens, 136–137
Insect bites or stings, 181–184
  atopic reactions to, 181–184
  cornea, 182
  treatment, 184
Interaction of suppressor and helper T-cells, 32
Interferon, 24, 67–68
  atopic dermatitis, 172
  herpes simplex, 212
  treatment of atopy, 144
Interleukin, 3, 24–26, 146
Interstitial nephritis, 193
Intralamellar corneal graft, 285. *See also* Corneal graft
Intraocular pressure (IOP), 46, 287
IOP (Intraocular pressure), 46, 287
Iridocyclitis, 316–318
  acute, 316
  chronic, 316, 317
    treatment, 317

rheumatoid arthritis, 316, 317
  secondary glaucoma, 318
Iris, 78
Iritis, 287
Isoproterenol, 184

J chain, 9
Job-Buckley syndrome, 37
Jones-Mote reaction, 61

Kaposi's sarcoma, 68
Keratectomy
  delimiting, 201
  lamellar, 201
Keratic precipitates (KP), 287
Keratitis, 82
  acute corneal epithelial HSV, 216
  chronic herpetic, 216, 284
  disciform, 214
  fascicular, 237
  recurrent immunogenic interstitial, 82
  sclerokeratitis, 232
Keratoconjunctivitis
  herpetic, 238
  rosacea, 238
  sicca, 267
Keratoconus, 165
Keratopathy, 261, 266
Keratoprostheses, 291
Kidney grafting, 281
Killer cells, 8, 18, 20, 33
Kinin fibrinolytic and clotting systems, 38
Kveim test, in sarcoidosis, 262

Lacrimal apparatus, 76–77
Lactoferrin, 76
Lamellar corneal grafts, 284. *See also* Corneal graft
Lamellar keratectomy, 201
Langerhans' cells, 277–278, 292
Lazy leukocyte syndrome, 37
Leiner's disease, 44
Leishmania sp., 235
Lens-induced uveitis, 115, 335–339
  granulomatous, 337
  pathogenesis, 335–338
  treatment, 338–339
    surgical removal, 338
Leprosy (Hansen's disease), 28, 209, 225
Leukemia, 28, 68, 220
  chronic lymphatic, 29
  chronicytic, 28
  lymphoblastic, 29

Leukocyte migration inhibition (LMI), 280
Leukocyte migration inhibition factor (LIF), 124
Levamisole, 144, 216–217
LIF (Leukocyte migration inhibition factor), 24
Ligneous conjunctivitis, 207, 208
Linear catarrhal infiltrate, 204
Listeriosis, 209
LMI (Leukocyte migration inhibitor), 280
Lupus erythematosus, systemic, 6, 37, 43, 57, 60, 72, 116, 220, 265, 267, 310–312
 pathogenesis, 310–312
 treatment, 312
Lymphadenopathy, 209
Lymphatics, 74–76
Lymphocytes
 products of activated, 122
 transformation in vitro, 120
Lymphogranuloma venereum, 209
Lymphoid reactions, 67
Lymphokines, 21–24, 61
 cytokines, 21
 interferon, 24
 lymphotoxin, 23
 monokines, 21
 tumor cells and, 67
Lymphoreticular neoplasm, 267
Lymphosarcomas, 29
Lymphotoxin, 23
Lysozyme, 76

Macroglossia, 223
Macrophage migration inhibition factor (MIF), 122–124
Macrophages (adherent cells), 33–36
 Hodgkin's disease, 35
Major histocompatibility complex (MHC), 4
Malignancies, 29, 83
 chronic lymphatic leukemia, 29
Malignant melanoma, 37, 125
 monoclonal antibodies, 125
Malnutrition, 37, 38
Mantoux skin test, 118
Mast cells, 49–52
Measles, 265
Mechanisms of anaphylactic response, 49–52
Mediterranean fever, 209, 224
Medullary carcinoma of the thyroid gland, 225
Meibomian gland infection, 205

Melanoma, 68, 70
Membranous conjunctivitis, 207, 209
Methotrexate, 73
Methyldopa, 58
MHC (Major histocompatibility complex), 4
Microimmunofluorescence test, 109
MIF (Macrophage migration inhibition factor), 122–124, 280
Moisture chamber spectacles, 269
Monoclonal antibodies, 13–14, 70, 124–125, 296
 herpes zoster, 125
 malignant myeloma, 125
Monoclonal gammopathy, 267, 319
Monokines, 21
Mooren's ulcer, 196–202, 221
 clinical features, 196–199
 diagnosis, 199–200
 histopathologic findings, 200–201
 immune disease, 196
 pathogenesis, 196–197
 treatment, 201–202
Mucosal tissue, 77–80
Multiple myeloma, 68, 104, 225, 266–267, 319–320
 treatment, 266, 320
Multiple sclerosis, 6, 320–322
 pathogenesis, 320–322
 treatment, 322
Myasthenia gravis, 5, 220
Mycosis fungoides, 29
Mycotic corneal infiltrate, 219
Mycotic infections, 218
 Aspergillus sp., 218
 Candida albicans, 218
Myotonic dystrophy, 37

Natural killer cells (NK), 18, 33, 34, 47, 65–66, 68, 211, 325
 sarcoidosis, 325
Necrotizing vasculitis, 43
Neoplasms
 lymphoreticular, 267
 multiple myeloma, 319–320
Neovascularization of the cornea, 46
Nephritis
 acute, 57
  poststreptococcal glomerulonephritis, 60
 interstitial, 193
 nephrotoxic, 60
Neuritis, optic, multiple sclerosis, 321
Neuroretinal edema, 150
Nezelof's syndrome, 28

NK. *See* Natural killer cells (NK)
Nodular episcleritis, 237
Non-Hodgkin's lymphoma, 68
Noninfectious diseases, 111–129
Nonspecific immune defenses, 64
Nonsteroidal anti-inflammatory
 agents (NSAIAs), 45–46, 142–
 143
 iridocyclitis, 318
NSAIAs. *See* Nonsteroidal anti-
 inflammatory agents (NSAIAs)
Null cells, 20

Occlusive vasculitis, 82, 313
Ocular anatomy and physiology, 74–
 80
 anterior chamber, 75–76
 blood vessels, 74–76
 lacrimal apparatus, 76–77
 lymphatics, 74–76
 mucosal tissue, 77–80
 tear film and lacrimal apparatus,
 76–77
Ocular considerations in immunology,
 74–83
Ocular pemphigoid, 257–259
Ocular sarcoidosis, 125
Ocular tissue antigens, 80
Ocular toxocariasis, 111
Ocular toxoplasmosis, 118, 120
Ocular tumors, 83
Ophthalmia, sympathetic, 72, 83
Opportunistic infections, 109–111
 Candida, 109–110
 cytomegalovirus, 110–111
Optic neuritis, 72, 321
Organ specific antigens, 4
Organ transplantation, 57
Osteogenic sarcoma, 68
Osteomyelitis, 225

Pannus trachomatosus, 238
Parinaud's oculoglandular syndrome,
 208–209
Pars planitis, 321
Patch test, 238
Patching the eye, 201
Pemphigoid, 72, 81, 255–259
 cicatricial, 257–259
 treatment, 256
Pemphigus, 257–259
 treatment, 255–256
 vulgaris, 255–256
Penetrating corneal grafts, 284. *See
 also* Corneal graft
Penicillin, 150
 urticaria, 150

Periarteritis nodosa, 220
Peripheral corneal infiltrates, 220–
 221
Peripheral uveitis, 321
Pernicious anemia, 72
Phacogenic uveitis, 72
Phagocytes
 activation, 37
 destruction of foreign material, 37
 function, 37–38
 attachment to material, 37
 chemotaxis, 37
 ingestion, 37
 random movement, 37
Phakolytic glaucoma, 337
Pharmacologic mediators of
 anaphylaxis, 53–54
Phlyctenulosis, 83, 235–238
 cause, 235–236
 clinical features, 236–237
 fascicular keratitis, 237
 herpetic keratoconjunctivitis, 237–
 238
 histopathologic features, 237–238
 limbal vernal keratoconjunctivitis,
 238
 pannus trachomatosus, 238
 pingueculitis, 238
 rosacea keratoconjunctivitis, 238
 staphylococcal, 236
 treatment, 238
Phylogenic considerations, 1–3
Physiologic effects of arachidonic acid
 metabolities, 54
Pigeon-fancier's disease, 61
Pingueculitis, 238
Plasmapheresis
 multiple myeloma, 320
 systemic lupus erythematosus, 312
Plasmin system, 39
Plate hemolysin test, 105
Platelet-activating factor, 53
Pneumocystis carinii, 328
POHS (Presumptive ocular
 histoplasmosis syndrome), 110
Poison oak, 179
Polyarteritis nodosa, 81, 200
Polyethylene glycol technique, 117
Polymyalgia rheumatica, 323
Polyneuropathy, choriosensomotor,
 223
Preciptin test, 105
Prednisone, 46
Presumed ocular histoplasmosis
 syndrome, 119
Presumptive ocular histoplasmosis
 syndrome (POHS), 110

Primary myxedema, 72
Progressive systemic sclerosis, 267
Proparacaine hydrochloride, 150
 urticaria, 150
Prostaglandins, 45, 68, 241
 contact dermatitis, 241
Pseudomonas, 202, 209
Pseudophakos implantation, 338
Psoriasis, 6, 220
Psoriatic arthritis, 267
Psychotherapy, 141
Ptosis, 223
Punctal occlusion, 269
Purine antagonists, 73
Pyelonephritis, 225
Pyogenic infections, 43, 44
Pyrimidine antagonists, 73

Quinidine, 58

Radial diffusion, 113–114
Radiation, 170, 229
 amyloidosis, 229
 vernal keratoconjunctivitis, 170
Radioallergosorbent test, 138, 152
 hay fever, 152
Radiopaque dyes, 150
 urticaria, 150
Raji cell technique, 117
Reactions not related to infection, 219–235
Regional enteritis, 225
Reiter's syndrome, 109, 225
Rejection
 factors affecting, 282
 line, 283, 285, 287, 289
 rate, 283
 skin allograft immunity, 282
 T4-T8 ratio, 283
Renal cell carcinoma, 225
Renal disease, 43
Retina, 78
 detachment, 178
 diseases of, 307–339
 hemorrhages, 328
Retrobulbar neuritis, 321
Retrocorneal membrane, 291
Rhesus incompatibility, 57
Rheumatoid arthritis, 37, 60, 72, 112, 200, 220, 225, 265, 267, 315–319
 ankylosing spondylitis, 316
 juvenile, 115
Rheumatoid factor, 13, 115, 268
 immunoglobulin M (IgM), 13
Rhinitis, vasomotor, 136
Rosacea keratoconjunctivitis, 238

Sabin-Feldman dye-test, 105
Salicylates, 150
 urticaria, 150
Salzmann's nodular corneal dystrophy, 236
S-antigen, 334
Sarcoidosis, 83, 119, 209, 259–263, 324–328
 clinical appearance, 326
 diagnosis, 326
 pathogenesis, 324–327
 treatment, 262, 327–328
S. aureus, 202–203
Scleritis, 230–235
 anterior, 231–232
 brawny, 232
 necrotizing, 232
 sclerokeratitis, 232
 scleromalacia perforans, 232
Scleroderma, 72, 267
Sclerosis, progressive systemic, 267
Sensitization, 146–147
Sensomotor polyneuropathy, chronic, 223
Sepsis, 37, 38
Serum angiotensin converting enzyme (ACE), 125–126
Serum lysozyme, 125
Serum sickness, 59–60, 193, 307–309
 pathogenesis, 307–309
 signs and symptoms, 308
 treatment, 309
Severe combined immunodeficiency, 28
Sezary's disease, 29
Sykes-Moore chamber, 123
Sjögren's disease, 115, 267–269
Sjögren's syndrome, 6, 29, 72, 115, 262, 267–270, 310
 treatment, 269
Skin tests, 117–120
 coccidioidin, 119
 delayed hypersensitivity, 119–120
 histoplasmin, 119
 Mantoux, 118
 toxoplasmin, 118
 tuberculin, 118
SLE. *See* Systemic lupus erythematosus
Smallpox vaccination, 216, 265
Sporotrichosis, 209
Squamous cell carcinoma, 68
Staphylococcal abscesses, 37
Staphylococcal infections, 202–207
 acute poststreptococcal glomerulonephritis, 60
 antibiotic ointment, 206

Staphylococcal infections—*Continued*
  pseudomonas, 202
  S. aureus, 202–203
Staphylococcal phlyctenulosis, 236
Steroids, 47
Stevens-Johnson syndrome, 216, 264–266
  treatment, 265–266
Stimulatory response, 70–72
Sulfonamides, 150
  urticaria, 150
Suppressor T cells, 55–56
Sutures, 291, 296
Symblepharon, 265
Sympathetic ophthalmia, 72, 83, 331–335
  histologic picture, 332
  pathogenesis, 331–334
  S-antigen, 334
  treatment, 335
Synechia formation, 317
Syphilis, 13, 209, 225
  FTA-absorption test, 108–109
  VDRL test, 107–109
Systemic lupus erythematosus (SLE), 6, 37, 43, 57, 60, 72, 116, 220, 265, 267, 310–312
  pathogenesis, 310–312
  treatment, 312

T- and B-lymphocyte interaction, 30–32
  T-independent antigens, 30
T-cells, 55–56
  activation by mitogens, 25–26
  dysfunction, 28
    B-cells vs, 19–20
    Di George's syndrome, 28
    Hansen's disease (leprosy), 28
    Hodgkin's disease, 28
  recognition of antigen, 20–21
Tear film and lacrimal apparatus, 76–77
Tear IgA and IgG, 126–127
Tear substitutes, 269
Temporal arteritis, 220
Terrien's degeneration, 199–200
Tests
  agar diffusion, 110
  antibody. *See* Antibody tests
  aqueous humor, 127–129
  chlamydial, 109
  chromium release, 122
  Clq binding, 116
  coccidiodin, 119
  complement fixation, 105, 110
  Coombs', 58
  direct agglutination, 105
  enzyme-linked immunosorbent assay (ELISA), 105, 106–107, 110, 111, 128
  FTA-absorption, 108–109
  flocculation, 105
  hemagglutination, 105
  histoplasmin, 110
  histoplasmosis, 110
  in vitro, 120–124
  indirect fluorescent, 105
  immune complexes. *See* Immune complexes, tests for
  immunologic. *See* Immunologic testing
  mantoux, 118
  microimmunofluorescence, 109
  patch, 239
  plate hemolysin, 105
  precipitin, 105
  radioallergosorbent, 138
  Sabin-Feldman, 105
  serum angiotensin converting enzyme (ACE), 125
  serum lysozyme, 125
  skin. *See* Skin tests
  toxoplasma, 104–105
  toxoplasmin, 118
  toxoplasmosis. *See* Toxoplasmosis
  tuberculin, 118
  Venereal Disease Research Laboratory (VDRL), 107–109
Thrombocytopenia, 193
Thymidylate, 73
Thymopoietin pentapeptide, 144
Thyrotoxicosis, 72
T-lymphocytes, 16–26
  distribution of T-cells, 17
  interleukins, 24–25
  lymphokines, 21–24
  macrophage-aggregation factor (MAF), 22
  migration-inhibition factor (MIF), 22
  surface markers on human peripheral blood T-cells, 18
  surface markers on non-T-cells, 20
Tolerance, immunologic, 294–295
Topical chemotherapy, 216
Toxocara serology, 111
Toxoplasma
  acquired immune deficiency syndrome (AIDS), 328
  dye-test, 104–105

T. gondii, 118
Toxoplasmin, 118
Toxoplasmosis
  complement fixation test, 105
  direct agglutination test, 105
  enzyme-linked immunosorbent assay, 105, 106–107
  flocculation test, 105
  hemagglutination test, 105
  indirect fluorescent antibody test, 105
  plate hemolysin test, 105
  preciptin test, 105
  Sabin-Feldman dye-test, 105
Trachoma, 109, 168, 225, 238
  chlamydia, 109
  hyperendemic, 109
  vernal keratoconjunctivitis, 168
Transfer factor, 217, 325
  sarcoidosis, 325
Transfusion reactions, 57
Transfusions, multiple, 225
Transplantation, organ, 57
Trantas' dots, 157, 160
Trichophyton, 119
Trifluorothymidine, 216
T-suppressor lymphocytes, 196
  Mooren's ulcer, 196
TSTA (Tumor-specific transplantation antigens), 66–67
Tuberculin skin test, 118
Tuberculosis, 209, 225
Tularemia, 209
Tumors, 66–70
  antigenicity, 68
  blocking factors, 69
  cell-division TSTA, 67
  chemical TSTA, 67
  embryonic TSTA, 67
  host immune responsiveness, 68
    effect on, 69
  immune response to, 67–69
  macrophages, 68
  medical treatment, 69
  natural killer cells, 68
  ocular, 83
  prostaglandin, 68
  therapy, 69–70
    prophylaxis, 69
    surgical treatment, 69
  tolerance, 69
  tumor-specific transplantation antigens, 66–67
  viral TSTA, 66–67
Tumor-specific transplantation antigens (TSTA), 66–67

Ulcerative colitis, 225
Urticaria, 149–150, 193
  drug induced, 149–150, 193
  foods, 150
  infections, 150
  inhalants, 150
  systemic diseases, 150
Uveal tract diseases, 307–339
Uveitis, 83, 309
  anterior, 150
  atopic, 179
  Behçet's disease, 312
  chronic bilateral granulomatous uveitis, 333
  herpes simplex, 216
  herpetic, 46
  lens-induced, 115, 335
  multiple sclerosis, 321
  phacogenic, 72
  rheumatoid arthritis, 315–316
  sarcoid, 261
  scleritis, 232
  serum sickness, 309
  systemic lupus erythematosus, 311
Uveitis. See also Lens-induced uveitis

Vaccines, 150, 216
  smallpox, 216, 265
  urticaria, 150
Vascularization, 287
Vasoconstrictors, 170
Vasodilation, 40
Vasomotor rhinitis, 136
VDRL (Venereal disease research laboratory tests), 107–109
Venereal disease research laboratory tests (VDRL), 107–109
Vernal keratoconjunctivitis (VKC), 152–153, 157–171
  cause, 157–158
  clinical features, 159–167
    signs, 159–165
    symptoms, 159
  diagnosis, 167–168
  epidemiologic findings, 158
  histopathologic findings, 167
  history, 157
  limbal, 157, 238
  mixed, 157
  palpebral, 157
  prognosis, 165–167
  trachoma, 168
  Trantas' dots, 157
  treatment, 168–171
    drug therapy, 169–171
    general measures, 168–169

Viral infections, 211–218
  adenovirus infection, 215
  herpes simplex, 211–218
  treatment, 216–218
Viral TSTA, 66–67
Vitamin A, 218
VKC. *See* Vernal keratoconjunctivitis (VKC)
Vogt-Koyanagi-Harada syndrome (VKH), 83, 321, 333

Waldenström's macroglobulinemia, 29, 266, 319
Wegener's granulomatosis, 81, 200, 220

Wessely ring, 214, 219–220
Whipple's disease, 225
Wiskott-Aldrich syndrome, 37, 55, 172

Xenogenic antigens, 4
  antibody combining with, 9
  heterophil, 4
  T-cells vs, 19–20
X-linked agammaglobulinemia, 172

Yersinia, 209